Forensic mental health nursing

Ethics, debates and dilemmas

CW01656467

Note

Healthcare practice and knowledge are constantly changing and developing as new research and treatments, changes in procedures, drugs and equipment become available.

The author and publishers have, as far as is possible, taken care to confirm that the information complies with the latest standards of practice and legislation.

Forensic mental health nursing

Ethics, debates and dilemmas

edited by

Michael Coffey and Richard Byrt
on behalf of the National Forensic Nurses' Research and Development Group

QUAY BOOKS
A division of MA Healthcare Ltd

Quay Books Division, MA Healthcare Ltd, St Jude's Church, Dulwich Road, London
SE24 0PB

British Library Cataloguing-in-Publication Data
A catalogue record is available for this book

© MA Healthcare Limited 2010

ISBN-10: 1-85642-407-3
ISBN-13: 978-1-85642-407-3

All rights reserved. No part of this publication may be reproduced, stored in a retrieval system or transmitted in any form or by any means, electronic, mechanical, photocopying, recording or otherwise, without prior permission from the publishers

Edited by Jessica Anderson

Printed by CLE, Huntingdon, Cambridgeshire

Contents

About the editors

Richard Byrt is Lecturer-Practitioner, Nursing, at Arnold Lodge Medium Secure Unit, Nottinghamshire Healthcare NHS Trust and the School of Nursing and Midwifery, De Montfort University, Leicester.

Michael Coffey is a Senior Lecturer at Swansea University. He previously worked as a community mental health nurse in both generic and forensic mental health services. His research focuses upon health policy and aspects of service delivery and organisation with reference to community mental health nursing and particularly people's experiences of receipt of these services.

The National Forensic Nurses' Research and Development Group is an organisation that seeks to develop forensic nursing practice and research and to contribute to relevant Government policy.

List of contributors

Mary Addo is a Lecturer in Mental Health Nursing at the School of Nursing and Midwifery and a Member of the Institute for Health and Welfare Research (IHWR) Neurological and Mental Health Theme, Robert Gordon University. Her interest lies in promoting positive acceptance of people living with mental illness and supporting pre-registration nursing students to develop values that underpin mental health practice. She is involved in research and has published on forensic nursing and related issues. Her specific research interests are mental health/psychiatric/forensic nursing, mentoring and clinical supervision, values-based practice and observation of acutely ill patients.

"Billy B" is an expert by experience, with many ideas about forensic nursing and services. Among other roles, he is currently a patient in a medium secure unit.

Frances Barrone is a Certified Lifeskills Consultant, speaker and coach living in the South West of England with her husband and two children. She runs lifeskills courses, workshops and is involved in community work.

Giotto Bonomaully is Senior Lecturer, at the School of Nursing and Midwifery, De Montfort University, Leicester.

Trevor Broughton is a Specialist Registrar in Forensic Psychiatry, currently working at Rampton Hospital, Nottinghamshire Healthcare NHS Trust.

Jacqueline Davies teaches social science at City University School of Community and Health Sciences and is convenor of the British Sociological Association Risk Study Group. Her research interests include health, youth work, forensic mental healthcare and service user involvement.

Tony Earp is Care Programme Approach Manager and Workforce Development Coordinator at Arnold Lodge Medium Secure Unit, Nottinghamshire Healthcare NHS Trust.

Paul Godin is a Reader in Risk Studies at City University School of Community and Health Sciences and is editor of *Risk and Nursing Practice* in the Palgrave Sociology and Nursing Practice series. His research interests include community mental healthcare, the history of madness, forensic mental healthcare and service user involvement in research.

Keith Halsall has experience in journalism, public speaking and working with other people with service user experience. He has taken a lead role in research on forensic patients' views.

Tim Hardie is Consultant Forensic Psychiatrist in Leicester. He has published papers in the areas of needs assessment for prisoners, consent to treatment, diminished responsibility, fitness to plead, inpatient violence, cultural awareness and language development in Deaf people.

Jeanette Hewitt is Lecturer in the Philosophy of Healthcare and Mental Health Nursing. Her research interests include the ethics of suicide, schizophrenia and the therapeutic relationship.

Andrew Higgins, Mandy Laird, Monica Elaine Mantey, Phineas Mapfumo, Tapiwa Mugabe and Folorunso Olubukola were formerly student nurses.

Wendy Ifill is an author who, amongst other work, has used her expertise and experience as a service user in several publications.

Satnam Kaur, at the time of writing, is a student nurse, mental health branch in the School of Nursing and Midwifery, De Montfort University. Her dissertation is on seclusion.

Alyson M Kettles is Research and Development Officer (Mental Health) for NHS Grampian and is based at the Royal Cornhill Hospital in Aberdeen, Scotland. She is also Honorary Senior Lecturer for the Centre for Advanced Studies in Nursing at the University of Aberdeen where she co-ordinates and teaches on modules for the post-graduate taught Master's degrees. Her personal portfolio of research has had a forensic focus for more than the last decade. She is a well-known author of mental health and forensic nursing articles and books. Her research interests include assessment and therapeutic interventions, such as risk, observation and engagement.

Chris Knifton is Senior Lecturer in Nursing at the School of Nursing and Midwifery, De Montfort University, Leicester. He has particular interests in the care of people with dementia and learning disabilities.

Rebecca Lawday is a Chartered Forensic Psychologist, employed as the lead psychologist for women's services at Arnold Lodge Medium Secure Unit, Nottinghamshire Healthcare NHS Trust. She was previously employed as part of a small multidisciplinary team developed in order to pilot a regional service, working with violent individuals with a diagnosis of personality disorder who were approaching discharge from hospital or release from prison. She is an honorary lecturer and placement supervisor for the University of Leicester. Her areas of special interest include the impact of complex trauma, personality disorder and risk assessment.

Jerry Paul Ninnoni's focus is in health services and public policy research. He is currently completing a doctoral dissertation entitled: *Effective communication with people with learning disabilities with epilepsy and their carers* at the Robert Gordon University, Aberdeen.

Sukhbinder Panacer is a Clinical Team Leader at Arnold Lodge Medium Secure Unit, Leicester.

Stephen Pope was a student nurse at the School of Nursing and Midwifery, De Montfort University, Leicester at the time he submitted his contributions to this book.

Ryan, Stuart and Pete, amongst other roles, are experts by experience, and have used their experience as service users in teaching and writing.

Jay Sarkar is Consultant Forensic Psychiatrist, Personality Disorder and Secure Women's services, East Midlands Centre for Forensic Mental Health, Arnold Lodge, Leicester.

Ian Smith is currently Lecturer in Mental Health Nursing at Robert Gordon University in Aberdeen, Scotland. He taught learning disabilities nursing for many years prior to moving into the field of mental health nurse teaching. He has been involved in some nurse education research projects while teaching in this area.

Nicholas Taylor is Consultant Forensic Psychiatrist at Arnold Lodge Medium Secure Unit in Leicester. He has a background in medical education and has published a number of textbooks relating to psychiatric training. He has an interest in mental health law.

Julia Terry works as a Mental Health Nurse Tutor in the School of Human and Health Sciences at Swansea University. She is actively involved in both pre- and post-registration nursing programmes. She has recently researched mental health first aid instructors' experiences of programme delivery and is now developing research ideas related to service user involvement.

Glynnis Vann trained and worked in Leicester as a Community Psychiatric Nurse. Her experience covers working in psychiatric hospitals in multi-cultural Leicester, which includes acute care, services for people with eating disorders, and community psychiatric nursing. She then moved onto working in prisons, as a nurse manager in healthcare, primary and secondary mental health. She finally moved into a new service in the Criminal Justice Team, Northampton in the four police custody suites, and Courts. In conjunction with the above, she trained and worked as a Magistrate in Leicester.

Elizabeth Walsh qualified as a Registered General Nurse in 1995 and has worked for HM Prison Service in both clinical and practice development roles. She completed her PhD in 2007 and is currently in post as a Senior Lecturer in Offender Health in the School of Health Care, University of Leeds. Her research focuses on the support and development of the offender healthcare workforce through reflective practice and clinical supervision.

David Wilkinson qualified several years ago after a career change from electronics engineering. He has been working on a personality disorder unit since qualification and is currently working as a Clinical Team Leader.

Jane Wood lives with her husband. Her family includes her Mum and Dad and her brother. She was a primary school teacher, but is now at university, retraining.

Foreword

I was enticed to plunge into the depths of this book by the surface attractions of the subject matter. I emerged with a greater understanding of the most important ethical issues of concern, a wider vision, and an awareness of the hazards and possibilities for the future. Many of my assumptions have been challenged.

The publication of this book is timely as the Health Service is faced with unprecedented change and a national financial crisis, with potentially harmful impacts on healthcare. This comes at a time when there are policy and practice imperatives for closer working between health, social care and the criminal justice system. There will be some hard decisions to make. These will cause ethical and moral dilemmas which could have a serious and negative impact on practice standards and may hinder future progress.

In addition, the forensic speciality is further vulnerable to a public restlessly demanding safety and severe punishment for all offenders, without an understanding of the complex causative factors. Public opinion is often whipped up into a storm of prejudicial hysteria by the excesses of the tabloid media, who frequently vilify the professionals seeking to provide enlightened, personalised and safe care, often without the necessary resources, conditions, and national and local leadership.

The good news is that this book goes a long way to strengthen our ability to inform debates in a credible manner; to argue cogently in defending what has been achieved to date; to tackle resentments and fears; and to influence decisions about resource priorities.

If there is no place for the weak, abused and unloved they will suffer repeatedly, and ethical practice will be undermined and might disappear from our services and communities.

The editors have assembled an impressive body of expertise which brings fresh insights and weaves together their experiences and different perspectives. The chapter authors not only point to the inadequacies of the present system, but also provide authentic solutions and practical advice whilst, at the same time dispensing with some of the common myths which surround forensic care.

It seems to me that much human suffering stems from destructive emotions, ignorance or flawed assumptions. One of the basic responsibilities of care professionals is to alleviate suffering and provide well-being. In that mission we have to search for new ideas, increase our understanding and expand our knowledge and practice. I believe that the contributors to this book have paved the way for us. They have provided us with both the causes of and some of the cures for suffering and will encourage reflection on the many questions raised.

I envisage returning to the various chapters time and again as a source of information, advice and inspiration. I will use this book in the work I do in both investigating "service failures" and in service development initiatives. I also expect that I will use the insights I have gained in future presentations aimed at challenging existing thinking and encouraging different approaches.

I invite others to benefit from exploration of these pages, as I have.

Malcolm Rae OBE FRCN

In memory of Linda Hart

Forensic mental health services have and continue to be sites of contested identity for those using them. Identity is a multi-faceted aspect of all people but in some cases workers have been found to pay little attention to the full range of identity-relevant aspects of people (see, for instance, Norfolk, Suffolk and Cambridgeshire Strategic Health Authority 2003). In *Chapter 7* Mary Addo outlines a number of important issues in recognising and addressing the cultural, spiritual and diversity issues which are implicated in identities of users of forensic services. Mary concludes that these dilemmas may be resolved (or at least more successfully addressed) with recourse to fundamental values of mental health nursing based on respect and valuing of diversity rather than a focus on difference.

In *Chapter 8* Michael Coffey and Jeanette Hewitt address the safety versus autonomy debate in relation to community care of people with forensic mental health histories. They argue that balancing care with compulsion remains a difficult task and one which mental health nurses are increasingly being called upon to accomplish. One issue that continues to present problems is that of reciprocity or in other words the limitations placed on the liberty of clients for the purpose of providing treatments, which in some cases have poor evidence or are not actually available. Here again public protection and the prevention of risk behaviours may be deemed to outweigh any supposed benefits of treatment and compulsion but it should be remembered that these too are often cited as the rationale for treatment thus throwing into doubt the basis for professional claims. More thought and clarity is required here so that practice decisions are supported by fully thought-through arguments that are transparent and open to discussion.

One area of practice that has frequently presented workers and service users with dilemmas is the provision of care for women in the forensic system. Although proportionately making up a small section of the client group with mental ill-health and offending histories, women are nevertheless presented with a range of unique problems which services have often struggled to address. In her personal account Wendy Ifill (*Chapter 9*) indicates that a women's service provides a highly individual programme of care which is distinguished by providing choice on more communal mixing. This account and the personal difficulties that Wendy hints at are a useful prelude to Rebecca Lawday's chapter which follows. Rebecca provides a concise background to the development of women-only services and the needs of the client group. She makes the case for the importance of a consistent therapeutic relationship founded on trust, respect and honesty as the basis of a transtheoretical model of treatment.

Chapters 11 and 12 address the issue of prison healthcare. Firstly Liz Walsh presents some very interesting data from her study of prison healthcare nurses and identifies the importance of developing emotional resilience as a means for enabling continued work in this field. Glynnis Cooper and Richard Byrt follow this with an account and a response, respectively, to the experience of working as an in-reach nurse in prisons. Clearly the tensions presented by a system where security is promoted as fundamental, and treatment and care may be seen as secondary, can cause significant dilemmas and sources of challenge for forensic nurses.

The education and training of mental health nurses takes on a range of new challenges when considering forensic mental health practice. In *Chapter 13* Julia Terry considers the moral and ethical dilemmas presented by the need to improve service user involvement in education and the issues this suggests for forensic nurse education. This is followed by Alyson Kettle's chapter in which she highlights some of the aspects of ethical teaching that should be considered in this field. These two chapters mark another staging post in forensic nurse education as there is precious little written on the subject of ethics in forensic nurse education and even less on involving service users (and the ethical implications of this) in this enterprise. This is truly startling given the complexity of forensic nursing practice and the literally captive nature of the people who receive these services.

Stephen Pope's poem *Dark Light* is evocative of a type of hopelessness that must envelope people distressed by years of mental ill-health and detained for long periods with no sight of discharge. It is a fitting introduction to the chapter by Jay Sarkar and Tim Broughton exploring the fraught area of self-harm. This is an area for which mental health nursing can best be employed to good effect to achieve positive outcomes (Cremin et al 1995). A further important aspect of mental health nursing in secure facilities is how and when to use seclusion as an intervention. Richard Byrt and Satnam Kaur (*Chapter 16*) present a critical look at the use and misuse of seclusion. They note that despite the presence of ethical principles, which can easily be applied to use of seclusion, there remain many examples of services ignoring these. Clearly moving beyond the learning of lists of principles and towards methods of exploring values is an ongoing concern. Practitioners of all types must challenge themselves to reflect in their practice a values base that promotes respect and dignity for all people, and this is particularly pertinent when using seclusion as an intervention. Richard Byrt goes on to explore patient perspectives of seclusion in the following chapter and suggests some useful lessons from his analysis.

One recurring dilemma for many in forensic mental healthcare is balancing the impetus to involve service users more and gain insight into their experience with a concern to protect therapeutic integrity and provide the best protection against worrying risk behaviours. There is however a seemingly unstoppable movement towards more involvement and greater collaboration and, as Keith Halsall demonstrates, and later Paul Godin and

Jacqueline Davies show, it is not only desirable but also possible to engage service users in research. This will not only enable them to feel benefit from this engagement but also to achieve mutually advantageous goals. The use of moral reasoning in treatment approaches might also be considered a form of advanced engagement. As David Wilkinson and associates show, however, it presents an intriguing and potentially very useful treatment approach that is not without its own dilemmas.

In *Chapter 21* Tim Hardie usefully returns to notions of capacity and responsibility for criminal behaviours. Tim ranges wide in his use of the literature as he considers notions of free will and dualism between brain and mind that remain influential in current thinking. Tim urges caution as he notes that many clinical decisions are made based upon assumptions rather than knowledge of what is known and what is not known about available scientific evidence. This debate is perhaps further complicated when considering the implications of offending behaviours associated with various types of dementia. Chris Knifton presents in *Chapter 22* a very interesting and scholarly overview of the literature and complex dilemmas faced when attempting to work in this area. Chris points out that in an aging society, where increasing numbers of people are being diagnosed with different forms of dementia, there is likely to be more attention focused on offending behaviours in this group. Chris also notes that dementia is no protection from other types of mental illnesses and many people in this group will suffer with forms of depressive and psychotic conditions which further complicate the presenting picture.

In *Chapter 23* Tony Earp and Richard Byrt present an overview of the care programme approach and its application to forensic nursing practice. They highlight the legal and ethical issues that this presents and their analysis suggests that forensic services are not immune from the problems identified elsewhere with this approach to care planning (see, for example, Simpson 2005).

The penultimate chapter in this book is a personal account from "Billy B". Parts of it make chilling reading. The account, in its own way, makes an undeniable appeal as to the importance of awareness of legal and moral aspects of forensic nursing care and the very real necessity for debate and discussion in this area. As Billy B points out nursing staff have perhaps evolved ever-more subtle forms of punitive interventions and it is the lack of critical engagement and acknowledgement of this by the wider profession that makes a text such as this even more relevant.

In *Chapter 25*, Richard Byrt and "Billy B" note the very real concerns related to disempowerment and liberty deprivations associated with detention in high security hospitals and other closed facilities. They point to a concern too about how this contributes to reduced opportunities to listen to the

Box 1.2. The case for forensic mental health nursing (after Burrow 1993)

It can be argued that forensic mental health nursing is a distinct specialty for the following reasons:

1. The client group consists mainly of people with a mental illness who have offended or been diverted from custody.
2. Nurses care for the client population in the various settings in which they live, and contribute to the therapeutic care and treatment of the person and his or her illness and offending behaviour.
3. The care strategies follow the patient journey through detention/secure care to community-based services, in the variety of settings in which patients can find themselves.
4. Forensic mental health nurses have specific roles which differ from other mental health nurses. These differences relate to the following areas:
   - The complexity of patients' multiple pathologies
   - Individuals' criminal behaviours and recidivism in social/cultural systems,
   - Specific therapeutic/clinical competencies
   - Specific issues related to forging therapeutic relationships/interpersonal skills/boundary issues
   - Avoiding negative custodial care, but working safely in the reality of secure settings or measures to ensure safety in the community
   - Roles related to the criminal justice system and its workings
   - Legal issues such as the multitude of new laws, ethics and rights-based practice
   - Responsibility to and protection of the public
   - Probability/risk, offence-specific assessment and care
   - Meeting varying safety security needs applied through differing security levels.
5. Both advocacy and the delivery of culturally competent care differ from other areas of nursing, in view of the need to de-stigmatise and decriminalise the client group.
6. There are also specific needs to defend and maintain staff morale, as well as ensuring clinical supervision and other means to deal effectively with the emotional impact of caring for this client group.
7. The client group continues to have the potential for future dangerousness and requires the staff to have coherent and consistent risk assessment, management and probability measurement.

Box 1.2 cont/

8. Future challenges include:
   - Care which is increasingly holistic, in relation to the individual's safety, psychological, physical, interpersonal, spiritual, cultural, psychosexual, social, legal, advocacy, economic and other needs.
   - The provision of forensic services which increasingly both recognise individuals' shared humanity, and are sensitive to, and meet, the needs of individuals related to their diversity, including gender, age, culture, ethnicity, spirituality, varying intellectual, physical and sensory ability, sexual orientation and gender identity, in line with the Equality Act, 2010 (HM Government 2010) and related policy (Byrt and Hardie 2007).
   - Provision of new services for specific groups, such as women and adolescents; and services that are gender and culturally sensitive; and which cater for specific groups of people such as survivors/victims of domestic violence and facilities for people who are sex offenders.
   - New and/or extended roles: e.g. related to influencing relevant government policy and "public education and prevention" (Kettles et al 2006: 230).
   - Other challenges include the search for new knowledge and evidence through appropriate research, audit and assimilation.

Burrow 1993, Kettles and Robinson 2000, Kettles and Woods 2006, National Forensic Nurses' Research and Development Group 2006, 2007, 2008, Robinson and Kettles 1998

patient's "voice" and establish the "other". Social isolation and separation is indeed a telling feature of detention in forensic settings. However it would be wrong to fall into the trap of thinking that, once people move on to other settings or are discharged to community living, such deprivations cease. We must be cognisant of the very real but perhaps more subtle and hidden surveillance and monitoring that continues post-discharge and which in many cases continues to place limitations on the liberty of people with forensic mental health histories. We might argue that such approaches are a proportional and necessary response to risk behaviours of potentially dangerous people and this may be the case. However to simply accept this without question or attention to the effects of our actions places us in danger of replicating the problems of closed institutional practices in the new environment of community settings.

We hope that this text will provoke further debate and discussion about the role of forensic mental health nursing. If nothing else you should read it with a weather eye on your own practice and be prepared to challenge and question yourself in the delivery of your care. Mental health nursing can be a force for good, it can truly help people who are lost and distressed and do so in thoughtful and evidenced ways so that they leave care with a positive experience and a real sense of the potential for change. We believe that in this text you will find the beginnings of a range of ideas that will help inform this process.

Acknowledgement

The authors would like to acknowledge, with grateful thanks, Quay Books, MA Healthcare, Ltd for kind permission to reproduce material from Kettles, AM, Woods AK, Byrt R (2008) Introduction. In: National Forensic Nurses' Research and Development Group: Kettles AM, Woods P, Byrt R (eds) *Forensic Mental Health Nursing: Capabilities, Roles and Responsibilities*. Quay Books, MA Healthcare, Ltd: London.

References

Addo M (2006) Culture, spirituality and ethical issues in caring for clients with personality disorder. In National Forensic Nurses' Research and Development Group (eds) *Forensic Mental Health Nursing: Interventions with People with Personality Disorder* (pp.60–80). Quay Books, London

Adshead G (2010a) Principles of ethical reasoning in forensic psychiatry. In: Bartlett A, McGauley G (eds) *Forensic Mental Health. Concepts, Systems and Practice*. Oxford University Press, Oxford

Adshead G, Brown C (2003) *Ethical Issues in Forensic Mental Health Research. Forensic Focus 21*. Jessica Kingsley, London

Aiyegbusi A, Clarke-Moore J (Eds.) (2009) *Therapeutic Relationships with Offenders. An Introduction to the Psychodynamics of Forensic Mental Health Nursing*. Jessica Kingsley, London.

Bucky SF, Callan JE, Stricker G (eds) (2009) *Ethical and Legal Issues for Mental Health Professionals*. Routledge, Taylor and Francis Group, New York.

Burrow S (1993) An outline of the forensic nursing role. *British Journal of Nursing* 2(18): 899–904

Byrt R (1993) Moral minefield. *Nursing Times* 89(8): 63–6

Byrt R (2008) Power and participation in forensic services: An introduction. In: National Forensic Nurses' Research and Development Group: Kettles AM Woods P, Byrt R (eds) *Forensic Mental Health Nursing: Capabilities, Roles, Responsibilities*. Quay Books, MA Healthcare, London

Byrt R, Hardie T (2007) Cultural competence and patients' rights. In: National Forensic Nurses' Research and Development Group: Kettles AM, Woods P, Byrt R, Addo M, Coffey M, Doyle M (eds) *Forensic Mental Health Nursing: Forensic Aspects of Acute Care*. Quay Books, MA Healthcare, London

Chaloner C (2000) Ethics and morality. In: Chaloner C, Coffey M (eds) *Forensic Mental Health Nursing: Current Approaches* (Ch 14, pp. 269–87). Blackwell Science, Oxford

Chaloner C, Coffey M (eds) (2000) *Forensic Mental Health Nursing: Current Approaches*. Blackwell Science, Oxford

Coffey M, Bishop N (2000) Crisis plans in forensic mental health nursing. *Mental Health Practice* 4(4): 22–5

Coffey M (2006) Researching service user views of forensic mental health services: A literature review. *Journal of Forensic Psychiatry and Psychology* 17(1): 73–107

Coffey M, Jones R (2008) Forensic community mental health nursing. In: National Forensic Nurses' Research and Development Group: Kettles AM Woods P, Byrt R (Eds) *Forensic Mental Health Nursing: Capabilities, Roles, Responsibilities* (pp 259–71). Quay Books, MA Healthcare, London

Coffey M, Morgan J, Gronow T (2007) Forensic Aspects of Discharge Planning from Acute Care: Transition to Community In: National Forensic Nurses' Research and Development Group: Kettles AM, Woods P, Byrt R, Addo M, Coffey M, Doyle M (eds) *Forensic Mental Health Nursing: Forensic Aspects of Acute Care* (pp.175–85). Quay Books, MA Healthcare, London.

Cremin D, Lemmer B, Davison S (1995) The efficacy of a nursing challenge to patients: Testing a new intervention to decrease self-harm behaviour in severe personality disorder. *Journal of Psychiatric and Mental Health Nursing* 2(4): 237–46

Dale C, Woods P, Thompson T (2001) Nursing. In: Dale C Thomson T, Woods P (eds) *Forensic Mental Health: Issues in Practice* (Ch 3). Baillière Tindall/ Harcourt Publishers, London

Davies J, Godin P, Heyman B, Reynolds L, Shaw M (2008) Ecological validity and risk management in forensic mental health services. In: Petersen A, Wilkinson I (eds) *Health, Risk and Vulnerability*. Routledge, Taylor and Francis Group, Hove

Eastman N, Riordan D, Adshead G (2010) Ethical roles, relationships and duties of forensic mental health clinicians. In: Bartlett A, McGauley G (eds) *Forensic Mental Health. Concepts, Systems and Practice*. Oxford University Press, Oxford

Godin P (ed) (2006) *Risk and Nursing Practice*. Palgrave Macmillan, Basingstoke

HM Government. (1983) *Mental Health Act, 1983*. HMSO, London

HM Government (1984) *Police and Criminal Evidence Act, 1984*. HMSO, London

HM Government (1989) *The Children Act*. HMSO, London

HM Government (1998a) *Data Protection Act, 1998*. HMSO, London

HM Government (1998b) *Human Rights Act. Chapter 42*. HMSO, London

HM Government.(2003) *Criminal Justice Act, 2003*. HMSO, London

HM Government (2004a) *Civil Partnership Act, 2004*. HMSO, London

HM Government (2004b) *Gender Recognition Act, 2004*. HMSO, London

HM Government (2004c) *The Children Act, 2004*. HMSO, London

HM Government (2005a) *Disability Discrimination Act, 2005*. HMSO, London

HM Government (2005b) *Mental Capacity Act, 2005*. HMSO, London

HM Government (2006) *National Health Service Act*. HMSO, London

HM Government (2007) *Mental Health Act, 2007*. HMSO, London

HM Government (2008) *Health and Social Care Act*. HMSO, London

HM Government (2010) *Equality Act*. HMSO, London

HM Government, Scotland (2003) *Mental Health (Care and Treatment) (Scotland) Act, 2003*. HM Government, Scotland, Edinburgh.

Kettles AM, Byrt R, Woods P (2007) Introduction. In: National Forensic Nurses' Research and Development Group: Kettles AM, Woods P, Byrt R, Addo M, Coffey M, Doyle M (eds) *Forensic Mental Health: Forensic Aspects of Acute Care* Quay Books, MA Healthcare, London

Kettles AM, Robinson D (2000) Overview and contemporary issues in the role of the forensic nurse in the UK. In: Robinson D, Kettles AM (eds) *Forensic Nursing and Multidisciplinary Care of the Mentally Disordered Offender*. Jessica Kingsley, London

Kettles AM, Woods P (2006) A concept analysis of 'forensic' nursing. British *Journal of Forensic Practice* **8**(3): 16–28

Kettles A, Woods P, Byrt R (2006) Conclusions: Themes, action and research for the future. In National Forensic Nurses' Research and Development Group (eds) *Forensic Mental Health Nursing: Interventions with People with Personality Disorder* (pp.227–34). Quay Books, London

Kettles AM, Woods P, Collins M (2002) Introduction. In: Kettles AM, Woods P, Collins M (eds) *Therapeutic Interventions for Forensic Mental Health Nurses*. (Ch 1, p. 13–20). Jessica Kingsley, London

Kirby S (2000) History and development. In: Chaloner C, Coffey M (eds) *Forensic Mental Health Nursing: Current Approaches* (Ch 15, pp 288–305). Blackwell Science, Oxford

National Forensic Nurses' Research and Development Group: Woods P, Kettles AM, Byrt R, Addo M, Aiyegbusi A, Coffey M, Collins M, Doyle M, Garman., G., Watson C (eds) (2006) *Forensic Mental Health Nursing: Interventions with People with 'Personality Disorder.* Quay Books, MA Healthcare, London

National Forensic Nurses' Research and Development Group: Kettles AM, Woods P, Byrt R, Addo M, Coffey M, Doyle M (eds) (2007) *Forensic Mental Health: Forensic Aspects of Acute Care*. Quay Books, MA Healthcare, London

National Forensic Nurses' Research and Development Group: Kettles AM, Woods P, Byrt R (eds) *Forensic Mental Health Nursing: Capabilities, Roles and Responsibilities*. Quay Books, MA Healthcare, London

Norfolk, Suffolk and Cambridgeshire Strategic Health Authority (2003) *Independent Inquiry into the death of David Bennett*. NS&C SHA, Cambridge

Parker E (1985) The development of secure provision. In: Gostin L (ed) *Secure Provision* (Ch 1). Tavistock Publications, London.

Robinson DK, Kettles AM (1998) The lost vision of nursing. *Psychiatric care* 5(4): 126–9

Robinson D, Kettles A (eds) (2000) *Forensic Nursing and Multidisciplinary Care of the Mentally Disordered Offender*. Jessica Kingsley, London

Rowe D, Lopes O (2003) People with learning disabilities who have offended in law. In: Gates B (ed) *Learning Disabilities: Towards Inclusion* (4th edn), (Ch 14). Churchill Livingstone, Edinburgh

Simpson A (2005) Community psychiatric nurses and the care co-ordinator role:

Squeezed to provide 'limited nursing'. *Journal of Advanced Nursing* 52(6): 689–99

Swinton J, Boyd J (2000) Autonomy and personhood: The forensic nurse as a moral agent. In: Robinson D, Kettles A (eds) *Forensic Nursing and Multidisciplinary Care of the Mentally Disordered Offender*. Jessica Kingsley, London

Soanes C (ed) (2002) *Paperback Oxford English Dictionary*. Oxford University Press, Oxford

Wix S, Humphreys M (eds) (2005) *Multidisciplinary Working in Forensic Mental Health Care*. Elsevier, Edinburgh

Woods P (2004) The person who uses forensic mental health services. In: Norman IJ, Ryrie I (eds) *The Art and Science of Mental Health Nursing: A Textbook of Principles and Practice*. Open University Press, Maidenhead

CHAPTER 2

Ethical principles in forensic and prison nursing

Richard Byrt

This chapter provides an overview of ethical principles in forensic and prison nursing. For reasons of space and time, a limited number of topics will be considered. These include beneficence and non-maleficence related to the duty of care; autonomy; justice; respect for persons; confidentiality; and the application of absolutist and utilitarian ethical principles to the consideration of moral dilemmas.

Ethics is a branch of philosophy "concerned with what is good or bad... defining right and wrong" (Thompson et al 2006: 43); and principles used to decide this by individuals, and in social groups and societies (Adshead 2010a, Green and Bloch 2006, Thompson et al 2006). Ethics also involves individuals' duties and responsibilities, including what they should do or ought (or ought not) to do (Rumbold 1999). Codes of conduct, including the Nursing and Midwifery Council's (2008a) Code include ethical principles which health professionals are expected to follow.

Beauchamp and Childress (2009) formulated the "four principles approach" (Beauchamp 2006: 34) to ethics in healthcare, which is relevant to forensic and other areas of nursing, and to the work of other healthcare professionals. The four-principles approach includes beneficence (actions which result in good and that "balance benefits against risks": Beauchamp 2006: 34); and non-maleficence (avoiding harm). In forensic nursing, beneficence and non-maleficence are related to the duty of care (sometimes called duty to care (Hendrick 2000: 225) of forensic nurses and other healthcare professionals. This includes providing assessment, care and treatment which result in positive outcomes for each patient/client and avoiding actions that result in harm to her/him or to other people, including members of the public (Addo 2006, Addo and Smith 2008, Adshead 2010a). The Nursing and Midwifery Council's (2008a: 7) Code indicates nurses' duty of care related to "skills and knowledge" and reducing risk. "You must act without delay if you believe that you, a colleague or anyone else may be putting someone at risk" (Nursing and Midwifery Council 2008a: 6). Fry and Johnstone's (2002) comments can be applied to forensic and prison nursing:

> *In nursing, as…in other professional domains, the avoidance of harm is balanced by the provision of benefit, with acceptable ranges of both benefits and risks of harm established by standards of nursing practice and professional codes of ethics.*
>
> (Fry and Johnstone 2002: 22)

Florence Nightingale emphasised the importance of non-maleficence in her statement:

> *It may seem a strange principle to enunciate as the very first requirement in a hospital that it should do the sick no harm.*
>
> (Nightingale 1992: first published 1859)

Fry and Johnstone (2002) state that many ethicists have considered that within health services, professionals' duty to avoid harm is a more pressing moral imperative than the duty to be beneficent. It has been argued that the latter depends on the resources available (e.g. staffing), but "avoiding causing deliberate harm and injury to others...is…within [nurses'] individual capacity and resources" (Fry and Johnstone 2002: 22). Examples of harm in secure hospitals and ways to prevent this are considered in *Chapters 24 and 25*, respectively.

Autonomy is also identified in Beauchamp and Childress's "four principles approach" to ethics (Beauchamp 2006: 34). Autonomy refers to a person's capacity "to make informed decisions and choices, and take informed actions, unconstrained by both internal and external factors" (Byrt 2008b: 107, citing Thompson et al 2006). Internal factors that may affect individuals' autonomy include, for example, ingestion of large amounts of alcohol; biochemical changes resulting in symptoms of mental illness; or chromosomal differences resulting in severe learning disability (Collopy 2006). Examples of external constraints on autonomy include community treatment orders, compulsory admission to a secure hospital and its rules and policies (Thompson et al 2006, Adshead 2010a). Autonomy is an aspect of power, and patients of forensic and prison healthcare services have, in many respects, far less power than the professionals who work with them (Byrt 2008a). Patients' reductions in power relate to many areas, including lack of freedom, decisions about where and how to spend their time; control over decisions about their life, relationships and other desired goals; and "the ability to make other people do what you want them to do" (Masterton and Maslin-Prothero 1999: .212, quoted in Byrt 2008a: 78). Patients usually also have limited economic and political power, and a stigmatised status (Bartlett 2004, Byrt 2008a). Ethically, it can be argued that an important goal for forensic and prison nurses is to enable patients to increase their autonomy and empowerment (gains in power) within the parameters of safety (Byrt 2008b, Aiyegbusi and Clarke-Moore 2009). However, the extent to which this is possible depends on what is seen as "real" power: for example, the attainment of goals desired by the patient (Byrt 2008b). Whether true empowerment can be achieved relates, also, to the perspective of the individual. For example, a "consensus" sociologist would argue that staff can empower patients by assessing their views, increasing choice, and giving opportunities to put forward views to improve aspects of the service (Byrt 2008b, Byrt et al 2008). However, such "consumerist" participation (Braye 2000) has been criticised by theorists who adopt a "conflict" sociological approach, arguing that "real" power is impossible unless compulsorily detained patients can decide whether or not they accept prescribed "treatment" or leave the service (Szasz 2000, 2005). Related critiques of the ethical and other problems of "patient satisfaction surveys" are given by Coffey (2006) and in other chapters and in this book. A critique of consumerist approaches is neatly implied in the title of *Chapter 19*: "On a scale of one to five, how satisfied are you with the forensic mental healthcare service you receive?"

Free will and determinism are two ethical concepts of relevance to clients' autonomy, capacity and empowerment. Free will includes the ability of an individual to make rational choices, including deciding what is "good" or "bad", "responsible" or "irresponsible". Notions of free will have been important in many religions over many centuries; and this is true, for example, of Buddhism, Christianity, Hinduism, Islam and Judaism (Rumbold 1999). In contrast, determinism is the belief that an individual's thoughts, feelings and behaviours are caused (determined) by factors largely beyond her/his control, or outside conscious awareness. Spinoza (1955), a 17th Century French philosopher, wrote extensively about determinism, arguing that humans could not be seen as having total free will, in view of the many internal and external influences on their behaviour (Rumbold 1999). It has been argued that mental illnesses may "determine" individuals' thoughts, feelings and behaviours. Explanations range from abnormally functioning neurotransmitters to psychodynamic theory postulating that behaviour and thinking is influenced, to some extent, by unconscious neurotic conflicts (Stone 2006).

According to Beauchamp (2006: 34), justice, another of Beauchamp and Childress's (2009) four principles of healthcare ethics, refers to professionals' "obligations of fairness in the distribution of benefits and risks". This includes weighing up the relative benefits and risks of actions, in deciding for example, the granting of unescorted leave to a secure hospital patient, or whether or not a client of a community forensic mental health team should be compulsorily admitted. In both these examples, justice would partly involve ensuring that the client's restrictions on autonomy were the minimum necessary to ensure her/his safety and that of others, based on risk assessment (Department of Health 2007, Woods and Kettles 2009); although Eastman et al (2010) states, in relation to public safety, that it can be argued that the forensic psychiatrist's primary concern should be patient treatment.

The Nursing and Midwifery Council's (2008a: 2) Code states: "You must not discriminate in any way against those in your care". Another aspect of justice relates to central Government requirements of forensic and prison health services, as well as other public services, to ensure that all clients receive good quality assessment, care, treatment and service, without discrimination (Byrt et al 2007) in relation to the Equality Act, 2010 (HM Government 2010). Under this Act, public services, including secure hospitals, other forensic services, and prisons have a duty to avoid discrimination or abuse of individuals in relation to "age, disability, gender reassignment...race, religion or belief, sex [and] sexual orientation" (HM Government 2010: 1). Within all forensic and other health services, the implementation of the Equality Act, 2010 and related legislation and policy is monitored through a Single Equality Scheme. (At the time of writing, the most recent Single Equality Scheme is for the years 2010–2013: Department of Health 2010). Despite various efforts, in England and Wales, black patients are more likely than other people to be: compulsorily admitted under sections of the Mental Health Act; admitted to secure hospitals; be prescribed antipsychotic medication (Bhugra and Bhui 2006, Sewell 2009) and to be less satisfied with mental health services (Healthcare Commission 2009).

"Respect for persons"

"Respect for persons" relates to Beauchamp and Childress's (2009) "four principles approach" of beneficence, non-maleficence, autonomy and justice. Respect for persons involves beliefs that each client is a unique individual to be valued in her/his own right; and in need of care and compassion. The Nursing and Midwifery Council (2008a: 2) Code states: "You must treat people as individuals and respect their dignity." Respect for persons, as a concept, was articulated by the German philosopher, Kant, in his *Groundwork of the Metaphysics of Morals*, which was first published in 1785 (Thompson et al 2000: 16f). Kant argued that

> *...individual persons must always be treated as ends in themselves and never simply as instrumental means to an end..."Respect for persons"...* [requires] *us to respect the rights of* [patients], *and to avoid the exploitation or abuse of persons in our everyday practice.*
>
> (Thompson et al 2006: 31, citing Kant 1969 edition)

Carl Rogers' (1967, 1990) "core principles" of congruence, empathy and unconditional positive regard are related to respect for persons, although there appears to be limited literature on their application to forensic and prison nursing, particularly in relation to their application in response to some patients' violence and oppositional behaviours towards nurses (Ford et al 2010). This will be considered next.

Ethical values in forensic and prison nursing and "respect for persons"

Fulford (2004) argues that psychiatry should be based on ethical values as well as research evidence: a point which also has resonance for forensic and prison nurses (Byrt 2008b). Sadler (2005) considers the variety of meanings of "values"; and concludes that they are

> *...concepts we use to guide our actions, lead us to be deserving of praise or blame...Values are also concepts we use to describe such blame/ praiseworthy and action-guiding activities.*
>
> (Sadler 2005: 9).

Of particular relevance to forensic and prison nursing, and to the application of "respect for persons" (Thompson et al 2006), are Fulford's (2004) comments on values related to the need to listen to patients and appreciate their perspectives, including those that differ from those of the professional. Finding "common ground" is also emphasised (Fulford 2004). This involves forensic and prison nurses establishing therapeutic alliances (Kirby and Cross 2002) with patients, some of whom may be hostile, oppositional (Bowers 2002, Prins 2010) and understandably, reluctant to take on the role of "patient", perhaps preferring that of "prisoner" (Mason and Chandley 1990). Fulford (2004) emphasises, and some research findings suggest, that finding "common ground" is crucial in applying "respect for persons" and establishing a therapeutic alliance (Lowe 1992, McDougall 2000). In the author's experience, this can be facilitated through assessment of needs that the patient identifies as important; and providing practical help in response to the problems identified by them. (An example is given in *Box 2.1)*.

Common ground and respect for patients can also be furthered through active listening and the nurse's attempts to empathise (as in the example in *Box 2.1*). This includes attempts to appreciate the individual's perspectives and to convey that understanding to her/him through communication and practical action (Bowers 2002, Kunyck and Olsen 2001). It also involves the nurse's evaluation of both similarities and differences between her/his perspectives and those of the patient (O'Brien et al 2009). This is part of the

Box 2.1. Ian's new trainers

Respect for persons and finding common ground: An example

"Mr Ian Indigo" (a pseudonym) is a young man who is keen to maintain his relationships with his partner and their baby daughter, and who has a keen interest in keeping fit. He is transferred from a prison to a medium secure unit, with few clothes and no money. Not surprisingly, he is not happy with this transfer, as he does not agree with professional perceptions that he has a "mental illness". He decides not to engage with staff, and is hostile to Raj, his named nurse and to other staff.

Ian is very concerned that other young men on his ward will see him as "uncool" because his only pairs of trainers are very shabby. Raj is aware of this, and with Ian's agreement, approaches his social worker to obtain a clothing allowance and money from an emergency fund. Ian is able to order a pair of trainers from a catalogue. When they arrive, his self-esteem is considerably increased, as smart trainers are essential to his positive self-image and how he considers his partner and his peers will see him.

Raj did not make a judgement about the importance Ian attaches to the trainers, but accepts his perception of what is crucial for him, in order to improve his life at the time. Raj's assistance with an area that is important to Ian demonstrates to him that Raj is prepared to listen, and to respect him and his views. Ian concludes that Raj, "isn't too bad, really". Ian becomes slightly more willing to talk to Raj, and eventually feels able to ask for help in other ways.

assessment process in both the Tidal Model (Barker and Buchanan-Barker 2005) and the Betty Neuman Systems Model of nursing (Neuman and Fawcett 2010). In the author's experience, forging a therapeutic alliance and finding common ground often develop when patients find that they can have "ordinary" and "safe" conversations with nurses on topics such as music, football and current television programmes. In forensic hospitals and prisons, "respect for persons" can be manifest through such apparently "ordinary" conversations with nurses who present themselves as approachable, human, but able to provide a "holding environment" (Aiyegbusi and Clarke-Moore 2009. The latter includes safe, therapeutic relationships within professional boundaries (Peternelj-Taylor and Schafer 2008); the maintenance of physical security and respectful setting of limits to ensure safety; and a "structured day" with meaningful, fulfilling activities (Aiyegbusi and Clarke-Moore 2009, Dale and Gardner 2001). Bose (2009) indicates the forensic nurse's duty of care to ensure safe and therapeutic environments for patients:

> *The daily balance between security and treatment is often very challenging for any forensic mental health professional to maintain...The first responsibility*

> *of any forensic mental health nurse is that of providing a safe and secure setting for patients and staff. If patients do not have this fundamental safety, and their environment is chaotic and dangerous, treatment will have little impact. Subsequently, increased acting out and self-preservative or sadistic violence...occurs in a patient's attempt to survive. An unsafe environment is an exact replication of many patients' earliest experiences. If this is present in hospital, there will be little possibility of learning, change or maturation taking place in a treatment setting that mirrors the environment within which the original traumas occurred.*
>
> *The overall function of the "structured day" is to help nurses create and maintain an environment where patients feel held, and which is also safe to work in. Nurses can maintain a safe holding environment by appreciating the importance of boundaries that are defined and constant, but are balanced, with a flexibility to allow for patient and staff individuality.*
>
> (Bose 2009: 112f)

In contrast to such flexibility, and an empathetic approach which involves understanding the patient's view of the world and the extent that she/he wishes to change (Prochaska and DiClemente 1982), Fulford (2004) refers to "value myopia". An example of the latter is professionals' assumptions, for example, that an individual is prepared to accept the role of forensic patient, rather than that of "prisoner doing time" (Mason and Chandley 1990); or that she/he shares staff values that offending behaviours or "criminal thinking styles" are a "problem" (Byrt 2008b, Fox 1999). Fulford (2004) also describes "value blindness", which can include accepting without question that certain harmful attitudes and "rules, regimes and routines" (Byrt with James 2007: 36) must be ethically right, perhaps because everyone in the secure hospital or prison believes this to be the case. It can be argued that ethically, professionals working in these services have a duty of care to reflect on their attitudes and practice: for example, through effective use of clinical supervision.

Confidentiality

Ensuring confidentiality is another important aspect of ethical forensic nursing practice (Adshead 2010a). Confidentiality has been defined as:

> *A principle...*[that] *demands that information gained in a professional client relationship must be kept secret, even when its disclosure might serve a greater public good...Nevertheless, occasionally other important*

> *moral and legal considerations can oblige nurses to disclose information without a patient's consent.*
>
> (Hendrick 2000: 89, citing Johnstone 1989: 192).

Several texts refer to the nurse's duty to ensure confidentiality in relation to common law and within the Data Protection Act and other legislation. Common law in this area is based, not on specific Acts of

Box 2.2. Ethical questions for secure hospitals, other forensic health services and prisons

In relation to key ethical principles considered in this chapter, ethics applied to forensic mental health, forensic learning disability or prison health services could be concerned, for example, with the following ethical questions, many of which are considered elsewhere in this book and in other sources on forensic and prison nursing and services (Adshead 2010a, 2010b, Byrt 2008b, Chaloner 2000, Fulford 2004, 2008, Green and Bloch 2006, Walsh 2009).

- What are the ethical values of the service in relation to what are considered beneficent (creating good) and non-maleficent actions?
- What counts as good nursing and other professional practice in relation to promoting good and avoiding harm?
- How can abuses of power be recognised and avoided? In what ways can professionals meaningfully increase patients' power and participation?
- To whom does the service and its professionals have an ethical responsibility and a duty of care?
- In relation to the service provided, what are the rights of patients, carers, survivors/victims of offences, the public and forensic mental health professionals?
- What needs and rights of patients must the service meet? To what extent does the service aim to meet the needs, rights and requirements of other stakeholders (people with an interest in the service), including victims and survivors of patients' crimes (*Chapters 5 and 6*), patients' partners, spouses and other relatives, members of the public, patients' advocates, Government departments (such as the Ministry of Justice and Home Office) (Byrt with James 2007).
- Should patients, carers and members of the public be considered to have responsibilities (e.g. for their behaviour)? How does this relate to patients' capacity (in this context, meaning the ability to make informed decisions about their behaviours and aspects of their lives and health: Dimond 2009, HM Government 2005)?

Parliament, but on cases concerning breaches of confidentiality which have been considered in the Courts (Dimond 2008). The nurse's duty of confidentiality usually involves sharing information about the patient only with other professionals involved in her/his care and treatment, and, with the patient's consent (if she/he has capacity), with relatives or other people specified by her/him (Thompson et al 2006, Adshead 2010a). This is emphasised in the Nursing and Midwifery Council's (2008a) Code and in this regulatory body's leaflet, *What is Confidentiality?* (2008b). Relevant Acts of Parliament governing confidentiality in forensic and prison nursing and other aspects of healthcare and services, include the Data Protection Act 1998 (HM Government 1998a); the Freedom on Information Act 2000 (HM Government 2000); the Freedom of Information (Scotland) Act 2002 (Scottish Office 2002); and the Computer Misuse Act 1990 (HM Government 1990). In addition, Article 8 of the Human Rights Act 1998 emphasises the individual's right to confidentiality (HM Government 1998b, Nursing and Midwifery Council 2008b).

It is generally viewed as a disciplinary offence for Registered Nurses to give information about patients to individuals not involved in their care and without their permission (except in instances where divulging information is required by case law or legislation and serves the interests of the public: Nursing and Midwifery Council 2008b). Examples of unprofessional breaches of confidentiality include:

- Talking about named patients to partners or family or in public places.
- Failing to ensure the security of patients' records (e.g. a community forensic psychiatric nurse leaving records in an unlocked car; or in a room accessed by patients or staff who are not involved in the care of the individuals concerned).
- Giving information on request, face to face or over the telephone, without checking, or being aware of, the identity of the caller. An example is informing an ex-spouse or relative that an individual is a patient in a secure hospital or prison healthcare service when she/he has asked that this information is not divulged, and there are no legal or other reasons to do so.
- Divulging information about a patient to the media without the permission of the individual concerned and of managers (Castledine 1999). Details may be given unwittingly, as the nurse may not be aware that the caller works for the media. Secure hospitals and prisons sometimes admit individuals whose crimes have been widely publicised, with considerable media interest. Phillips (2003) describes the role of the media in reporting events at Ashworth, a high secure hospital, and indicates the ethical issues involved.

Castledine (1999) reported that a nurse in a secure hospital divulged information to the media about a patient to whom he had been primary nurse. This patient had previously generated publicity because of his offence, and the nurse complained to the press about the luxurious lifestyle supposedly enjoyed by the patient in the hospital (Castledine 1999).

Making the limits of confidentiality clear to clients

Pritchard (2001) pointed out that professionals do not always make the limits of confidentiality clear to mental health clients. Her comments on confidentiality in social work are applicable, also, to forensic and prison nursing:

> *It is crucial at the beginning of any involvement with a client that the social worker explains what is meant by confidential. The client's understanding of the term confidential may be very different to that of the social worker…*
>
> *Social workers should be upfront and honest about the fact that they cannot keep information to themselves. Each worker is accountable to a manager and to the department as a whole…The client must be made aware that the worker discusses* [clients] *with the line manager and that records are kept.*
>
> (Pritchard 2001: 120)

Pritchard (2001) goes on to suggest that professionals need to be aware of the boundaries of confidentiality and the extent that the client knows who has access to information about him/her.

"I've murdered an old lady": Limits to confidentiality

"I've murdered an old lady". This was the first thing that a patient said to the author on meeting him for the first time in a non-forensic mental health service. Limits to patient confidentiality were immediately explained, and the on call manager and the patient's responsible medical officer contacted in the first instance. After assessment and discussion with the patient and clinical team members, his statement was reported to the police. Fortunately, it was found that he had not committed the murder (which had actually occurred several years previously). (Some details have been changed to ensure confidentiality.)

As indicated in the above example, the usual legislation and policy regarding confidentiality excludes disclosure to the police of a serious offence (e.g. killing or rape) which a patient says she/he has committed, or will commit, and which is not known to the constabulary (Cordess 2001,

Dimond 2002, Eastman et al 2010). In such instances, case law indicates that professionals should disclose serious offences to the police (Eastman et al 2010):

> *Non-consensual breach of confidentiality is permissible where there is significant risk of serious harm to others in the absence of such a breach.*
>
> (Eastman et al 2010: 318)

A court case in California in 1974 (the Tarasoff case) influenced subsequent requirements for disclosure by mental health professionals of patients' reports of serious offences that they had committed, or were planning to commit. In the Tarasoff case, a client disclosed to a psychologist that he was going to murder his (the client's) girlfriend. He did so, and the young woman's parents successfully sued the service concerned.

> *The court held that the therapist owes a legal duty of care not only to his patient, but also to* [the] *patient's would-be victim.*
>
> (Dimond 2002: 157)

In addition, specific child protection legislation (HM Government 1989, 2004) and policy requires that offences against children, including physical, sexual and emotional abuse and neglect are reported by professionals (Dimond 2008).

Eastman et al (2010) state that, although the Criminal Justice Act 2003 (HM Government 2003) does not state that mental health professionals are required to share information with multi-agency public protection panels (MAPPs), there will probably be clear expectations to do so. Eastman et al (2010) state that these can conflict with many forensic psychiatrists' perceptions that their main duty is to provide treatment for patients, rather than concentrating solely on reducing risk. In relation to the expectations of MAPP members, a professional would be faced with a moral dilemma if she/he experienced a conflict of interests related to the patient's right to confidentiality versus disclosure in the public interest.

Moral dilemmas

Identifying ethically correct actions does not necessarily provide professionals with clear answers about the "right" actions to take. A moral dilemma exists when a professional is unable to decide which action is ethically correct in a particular situation. She or he is faced with alternative courses of action, and finds it hard to choose which one to take because each of the alternatives appears equally bad or equally desirable or could result in benefit to one or more people (e.g. the patient) but harm to others: for example, the general public (Chaloner 2000, Thompson et al 2006). In some moral dilemmas, two ethical duties conflict (Adshead 2010a): e.g. the need to "tell the truth" and to ensure safety in situations where a patient's risk to others may increase if she/he is given information that is difficult to cope with. Fry and Johnstone (2002: 166) state that, in moral dilemmas, "two or more ethical principles seem to apply to the situation, but they support mutually inconsistent courses of action for the nurse. Faced with this type of situation, the nurse is truly in a 'dilemma' in terms of choices of action".

Another type of moral dilemma involves conflicting roles of the forensic and prison nurse: for example the "security (or custody) versus therapy" debate. This concerns the extent that nurses in secure hospitals and prisons should be involved in aspects of physical security, such as searching patients or their rooms, checking that doors and windows are safe, and using handcuffs when escorting patients. Part of the debate about this concerns the extent that the nurse's participation in these tasks interferes with her/his therapeutic role (Clarke 1996, Burrow 1998, Collins et al 2006). There is a need for the Nursing and Midwifery Council to issue ethical guidelines regarding physical security aspects of the nurse's role (Byrt 2005): an area which is not covered in pre-registration texts on mental health nursing (e.g. Barker 2009, Norman and Ryrie 2009).

Absolutism informing ethical practice

Deontology and consequentialism are two sets of ethical theories that can be used to inform ethical nursing and multidisciplinary practice, and in some instances, to resolve moral dilemmas. In the next part of this chapter, deontology and consequentialism will be considered in relation to absolutist and utilitarian ethical theories, respectively.

Deontological ethics

> *...maintain that the morality of actions is to be judged in terms of their conformity with moral rules, duties, obligations [and] rights...rather than in terms of their consequences.*
>
> (Parker and Dickenson 2001: 324)

Absolutism, an aspect of deontological ethics is an ethical position that a value, belief or action is always right or wrong, regardless of the consequences (Thompson et al 2006). Absolutist beliefs include those based on conscience or certain religious faiths; and include the ethical principles of beneficence, non-maleficence, respect for autonomy, and justice (Beauchamp and Childress 2009). An example of an absolutist belief is Carl Rogers' (1967, 1990) statement that the core principles of congruence, empathy and unconditional positive regard should be maintained in all therapeutic relationships. Thomas Szasz's belief that people who offend should never be "treated" in secure hospitals also appears to be an absolutist belief (Szasz 2003, 2005). Other examples include fixed beliefs which help the forensic or prison nurse cope with the job: e.g. "patients with personality disorder are always manipulative."; "patients' aggression never makes me anxious". Bowers (2002) gives examples of both positive and negative beliefs and attitudes towards individuals with personality disorder diagnoses; and Mercer et al (1999) consider some forensic nurses' apparently absolutist beliefs that some patients were "evil" and could never change.

It can be argued that absolutist values and beliefs about the nature of sound ethical and clinical practice enable nurses and other professionals to be aware of the need to base interventions on beneficence and non-malificence and other clearly stated ethical principles. Absolutism also involves clear beliefs and statements about what is ethically right or wrong (Thompson et al 2006: 341). However, absolutism is said by some writers on nursing and psychiatric ethics to have disadvantages (Adshead 2010a). These include the imposition of rules that are "too...rigid and insensitive" (Hendrick 2000: 21); and a failure to appreciate the complexity of many difficult ethical decisions in practice (Adshead 2010a). A forensic nurse or other professional may be faced with conflicting moral imperatives: for example, the need to ensure a patient's safety and well-being versus that of others. This would be the case if it is known that a patient experiences trauma from seclusion, but this appears to be the only way to ensure other people's safety. (See *Chapters 16 and 17*.) It has also been argued that absolutism does not give enough consideration to the outcomes or consequences of actions (Hendrick 2000). For example, action based on an absolutist belief that patients should "always be told the truth", could result in increased risk if a patient is unable to cope with this "truth" and responds with violence (Adshead 2010b). An example of an ethical approach to this problem is given later in this chapter.

Utilitarianism

In contrast to absolutism,

> *Consequentialist ethical theories maintain that the morality of actions is to be judged according to their foreseeable outcomes.*
>
> (Parker and Dickenson 2001: 324)

Utilitarianism, an example of a consequentialist ethical theory, holds that it is the consequences or outcomes of particular actions or beliefs that matter: the ethically correct action is seen to be the one that results in the greatest good or happiness, or is in the best interests of the individual patient, and, often, in forensic and prison nursing, of other people likely to be affected by the action (Adshead 2010a). This consideration of consequences for individuals, besides the patient, is reminiscent of John Stuart Mill's description of utilitarianism in relation to "things that count as contributing to the greatest happiness for the greatest number...measured by the criterion of the greatest benefit to all" (Thompson et al 2006: 353, citing Mill 1972: first published in 1861).

The advantage of applying utilitarian ethical principles is that they can assist patients, carers and professionals with the process of weighing up the relative advantages and disadvantages, ethically, of particular courses of action. In the author's experience, doing so can aid reflection on difficult and complex ethical situations. However, a problem with utilitarianism is that actions taken may not take sufficient account of the absolutist principles of certain people involved in, or affected by decisions that are made. What if the patient or a professional finds a decision ethically objectionable when everyone else involved in the decision agrees with it? In addition, utilitarianism is less applicable in emergencies where decisions have to be made quickly, or in situations where it is clear that action should be guided solely by absolutist principles (Adshead 2010a, Collopy 2006). For example, the maintenance of safety and reduction of risk would generally be seen as an essential absolutist principle in all forensic and prison health services (Dale and Gardner 2001). However, utilitarianism could inform how this principle is applied in practice, in relation to other ethical imperatives such as enabling patient autonomy (Adshead 2010a).

Ethical decision making, using utilitarian principles, may be informed by considering the views and perspectives of the patient, her/his carers at home (usually with the patient's consent if she/he has capacity) and members of a multidisciplinary team. Thompson et al (2006: 279) point out that an advantage of multidisciplinary team involvement in ethical decision making is that discussion between different health professionals may enable an understanding of varied perspectives of the nature of the moral dilemma and possible resolutions. It may be of value to consider the views of, not only the patient and professionals, but also those of members of the public and of critics of forensic and prison services. This is considered in relation to "Roy Red's" transfer from a prison healthcare service to a high secure hospital (*Table 2.1*), which is relevant to an example from practice considered in *Chapter 12* in this book.

The application of absolutist and utilitarian ethical principles: Some examples

The next part of this chapter considers how ethical decision making can be enhanced by:

Table 2.1. Roy Red's transfer from a prison healthcare service to a high secure hospital

Perspective of patient	*Perspective of staff*	*Perspective of "Person in the street"*	*Perspective of anti-psychiatrist/critical sociologist*
I don't want to go to a high secure hospital because this will increase the time I spend locked up	We agree that this may be the case, but feel that, at present, you need admission to the high secure hospital for your health and well-being and the safety of others	No one perspective, but many people would say: People like that are a danger and should be locked up	One of many perspectives: Mental health professionals should not be involved in treating people who are prisoners against their will (Szasz 2003, 2005)

- Consideration of absolutist ethical principles underpinning professional action.
- Using utilitarian principles to weigh up the arguments for and against two or more different courses of action.

In each example, only some of the relevant ethical issues have been considered.

Should Mr Gladstone Gold receive antipsychotic medication against his will?

Mr Gladstone Gold has a generally happy family life with his partner and their three young children. After a period of initial assessment, he was recently admitted to a low secure unit under Section 37 of the Mental Health Act, 1983 (HM Government 1983), with a diagnosis of schizophrenia, following an assault on a passer-by in the street. Risk assessment by the clinical team indicates that Gladstone is seriously at risk, not only of assaulting others, but also of harming himself in response to abusive auditory hallucinations (voices) telling him he is wicked.

Mr Gold has declined medication, rightly referring to research evidence that antipsychotics are over-prescribed for black people such as himself (Sewell 2009). He has also expressed concern that medication may adversely affect his ability to concentrate on his Open University history studies, which he is trying to continue in the low secure unit.

However, most of the professionals involved in Gladstone's care consider that without this medication, his level of distress is likely to worsen, and that he is at considerable risk of harming or neglecting himself, as well

Table 2.2: Utilitarian principles informing nursing/ multidisciplinary decisions concerning Mr Gold	
Points for Mr Gold being given medication against his will	*Points against Mr Gold being given medication against his will*
The need to ensure Mr Gold's and other people's safety is the paramount clinical and ethical consideration. To rely on methods other than medication could increase risk.	The safety of Mr Gold and others could be ensured through other means such as intensive nursing care, engagement and observation (Cutcliffe 2009) – and through psychosocial interventions, which have been found to work for some people with schizophrenia, sometimes without medication (Raguram et al 2002, Keen and Barker 2009).
The duty of care to ensure safety and health has to be a higher ethical and clinical imperative than ensuring patient autonomy.	Giving medication against Gladstone's will is a serious infringement of his autonomy (Szasz 2000).
Whilst we need to ensure that care and treatment is not inherently or overtly racist, we should also be aware that for many patients, including some who are black, there is evidence that antipsychotics can relieve distress, and in some instances, prevent neglect and ill health, and decrease risk (Maden 2007, Keen and Barker 2009).	Research findings have shown that psychoactive medication is over-prescribed for black people (Sewell 2009).
Side-effects of antipsychotics can be carefully monitored and discussed with Gladstone and drugs/doses can be changed to minimise side-effects.(Healy 2010). Are side-effects worse than increasing distress for long periods (perhaps over a life time) and serious risk of ill health if Gladstone does not receive antipsychotic medication?	Antipsychotics often have serious side – effects including loss of sexual libido, obesity, and drowsiness (Healy 2010). (Would you, or the professionals working with Gladstone agree to them)?
Research findings demonstrate the efficacy of certain drugs in reducing symptoms of schizophrenia and the considerable distress associated with them (Healy 2010).	You're only suggesting medication because of the immense influence of global drug companies making huge profits (Hogg 1999) and overly influencing what professionals see as the correct method for treating schizophrenia. Some research has found relatively high recovery rates for individuals with schizophrenia who do not take medication (Leff 2001).

as assaulting others. Staff believe that if Gladstone were well, this would not occur. His consultant psychiatrist considers that a "Second Opinion Appointed Doctor" be consulted and that, with the agreement of this psychiatrist and other professionals, Gladstone should be given antipsychotic medication against his will under Section 58 of the Mental Health Act, 1983, as modified by the Mental Health Act, 2007 (HM Government 2007).

Absolutist principles informing nursing/multidisciplinary decisions concerning Mr Gold

The absolutist principles are as follows:

- Duty of care: Ensure Mr Gold's health, safety and well being, and other people's safety – whether this is achieved through antipsychotic medication and/or other means.
- Respect for persons: Listen actively and attempt to empathise with Mr Gold's perspectives and experiences, and respond to them.
- Awareness of differences in power between Gladstone and staff: Attempt to reduce power imbalances.
- Respect Mr Gold's identity and experiences as a black man – with a willingness to learn from his perspectives.
- Make a commitment to providing a service that takes account of the cultural and other specific needs of Gladstone and of other clients/ patients.
- Make a commitment to enabling Mr Gold's autonomy as much as possible – within the parameters of safety.

When should Roy Red be told about his transfer? A moral dilemma involving truth-telling

Tuckett (2004) has considered the ethics of truth telling in healthcare, and the next example is concerned with this area, which is also considered in *Chapter 12*.

Mr Roy Red is a single man of 23, who is currently an inpatient receiving care in a prison health service. He has had a variety of interesting jobs in industry, enjoys carpentry, and is a keen follower of a premier division football team.

Roy has a diagnosis of antisocial personality disorder, and finds it very hard to trust others, partly because of considerable abuse and neglect as a child, with subsequent considerable trauma and distress (Adshead and McGauley 2010). Roy also finds it difficult to manage his impulsive aggression towards others. Before his remand to prison, he killed a man whom he suspected of planning to murder him. Since admission, Roy has attempted to physically assault other prisoners and staff, and on one occasion, caused serious physical injury.

Following their detailed assessments, professionals at a high secure hospital have agreed to his admission. It is felt that this would more effectively meet his needs, and prevent harm to others.

The prison nurses wonder if they should tell Roy about his transfer immediately, or on the morning of his move in a week's time. Roy has previously stated: "If I'm transferred, I'll smash up this place and everyone in it."

This example poses a number of moral and clinical dilemmas. One which faces staff is: When should Roy Rudd be told about his transfer?

Table 2.3. Should Roy Red be told imediately about his transfer to a low secure unit? Consideration of ethical reasons for and against, according to utilitarian principles

Points for Mr Red being told immediately	*Points against Mr Red being told immediately*
There are many ways we can help Roy, whether or not he is violent after we tell him about the transfer.	We may not have the resources to help Roy if he is violent, or to easily prevent his harming others. The high secure hospital, with its higher staffing ratios and facilities, is better equipped in these respects.
Staff's honesty is essential in establishing trust and building up therapeutic relationship with patients.	Being totally "honest" is (a) impossible, and (b) may harm some patients who cannot accept, or do not want, the "truth".
If Roy is told about the transfer now, he is more likely to trust staff, both on his present ward, and in his new service.	Roy may find it so hard to cope with the truth that he may prefer not to be told until the last moment.
The staff's openness and honesty may help Roy to creatively share his own feelings and fears.	Roy could find it very hard to acknowledge or cope with his feelings and may, as a result, become seriously distressed and aggressive or violent, causing harm to himself or others.
Roy may ask staff if he is soon to be transferred and the staff could be put in a position of having to lie or be evasive.	There may be occasions when evasiveness or telling a lie is justified, if telling the truth results in a greater evil.
Other patients may wonder if staff are likely to keep the truth from them.	They may well appreciate the reasons for the staff's decision in this instance.

Should Roy Red be told immediately about his transfer to a low secure unit? Underlying absolutist ethical principles

These include:

- Professionals' duty of care to ensure the safety of Mr Red and other people.
- Professionals' duty of care to evaluate effects of the decision on the autonomy of Mr Red and other people.
- The establishment of therapeutic relationships, based on "respect for persons" (Kant 1969), so that Mr Red can gradually begin to trust staff.
- Making a decision which is beneficent (creating as much good as possible) and non-maleficent (resulting in the least possible harm) in the short-term and the long-term – for Roy and for other people.

Ms Greta Green's leave: Freedom versus safety

This last example concerns Ms Greta Green, aged 29, the mother of two children in care. She enjoys cooking, is a keen indoor football player and enjoys sessions in the multigym. Greta is also a talented artist, and has won two Koestler awards for her work. At present, she is a patient in a medium secure ward for women. She was admitted two years ago, after setting fire to buildings on two occasions. A child sustained slight physical injury during one of these incidents.

Greta, who has a diagnosis of paranoid schizophrenia, says that she set fire to the buildings in response to command hallucinations telling her to do so.

Members of the clinical team are considering whether to apply to the Ministry of Justice for unescorted leave for Ms Green. Some staff feel she is ready for this, as does Greta herself. Others point out that her arson has constituted particularly serious dangers to the public, and advise caution.

The moral dilemmas facing staff relate partly to balancing Greta's needs for freedom and responsibility against her own and others' needs to be protected from harm.

Should an application be made for Greta Green to have escorted leave? Absolutist principles to inform ethic decision making

The absolutist principles would include the following:

- A duty of care to ensure:
    - The safety of Ms Green and of others: e.g., members of the public

Table 2.4. Should an application be made for Greta Green to have escorted leave? Examination of factors for and against, according to utilitarian principles	
For Greta's Leave	*Against Greta's Leave*
Careful risk assessment suggests that, according to various criteria, Greta presents less risk than when she was admitted.	Caution in granting this leave is needed in view of Greta's former risky behaviours. Any predictors of future risk to others may have limited reliability.
Greta has needs for autonomy and freedom, and to be treated like an adult.	She also has needs to be protected from harming herself and others.
Greta's progress will be enhanced if she is given opportunities to develop her own controls, and take responsibility for herself. This would be achieved, in part, through granting the leave.	Because of the need for Greta and other people to be protected from harm, there are arguments for beneficent control by staff and the provision of a secure, structured environment.
Greta has basic rights, including autonomy, adequate rehabilitation, including recovery principles, and provision of the maximum amount of freedom with which she can cope.	Greta's rights need to be balanced against the rights of the public to be protected from her possibly harming them.

(although some critics, e.g. Szasz 2000, have questioned whether the latter should be part of mental health professionals' role).
  - Prevention of behaviours related to Greta's lack of capacity, and which she may later regret.
- Consideration of issues concerning the autonomy of Ms Green and other people.
- Awareness of the rights of Greta to have the least amount of restrictions commensurate with her assessed level of risk.
- The rights of members of the public to be protected from harm.

This chapter has provided an overview of ethical principles related to forensic and prison nursing. The next chapter considers mental health legislation.

References

Addo MA (2006) Culture, spirituality and ethical issues in caring for clients with personality disorder. In: National Forensic Nurses' Research and Development Group (eds) *Forensic Mental Health Nursing: Interventions with People with 'Personality Disorder'*. Quay Books, Mark Allen Healthcare, London

Addo MA, Smith I (2008) Equality and diversity: Respecting the person with a learning disability. In: National Forensic Nurses' Research and Development Group: Kettles AM, Woods P, Byrt R (eds) *Forensic Mental Health Nursing: Capabilities, Roles and Responsibilities*. Quay Books, MA Healthcare, London

Adshead G (2010a) Principles of ethical reasoning in forensic psychiatry In: Bartlett A, McGauley G (eds) *Forensic Mental Health Concepts, Systems and Practice*. Oxford University Press, Oxford

Adshead G (2010b) Ethical issues in secure care. In: Bartlett A, McGauley G (eds) *Forensic Mental Health Concepts, Systems and Practice*. Oxford University Press, Oxford

Adshead G, McGauley G (2010) Caring for individuals with personality disorder in secure settings. In: Bartlett A, McGauley G (eds) *Forensic Mental Health Concepts, Systems and Practice*. Oxford University Press, Oxford

Aiyegbusi A, Clarke-Moore J (eds) (2009) *Therapeutic Relationships with Offenders. An Introduction to the Psychodynamics of Forensic Mental Health Nursing*. Jessica Kingsley, London

Barker P (ed) (2009) *Psychiatric and Mental Health Nursing: The Craft of Caring* (2nd edn) Arnold, London

Barker P, Buchanan-Barker P (2005) *The Tidal Model. A Guide for Mental Health Professionals*. Brunner–Routledge, Taylor and Francis Group, Hove

Bartlett A (2004) Fashions in psychiatric care: Implications for sense of self. In: Crisp AH (ed) *Every Family in the Land: Understanding Prejudice and Discrimination Against People with Mental Illness*. Royal Society of Medicine Press, London

Beauchamp TL (2006) The "four-principles" approach. In: Green SA, Bloch S (eds) *An Anthology of Psychiatric Ethics*. Oxford University Press, Oxford

Beauchamp T, Childress JF (2009) *Principles of Biomedical Ethics* (6th edn) Oxford University Press, New York

Bhugra D, Bhui K (2006) Racism in psychiatry: Paradigm lost – paradigm regained. In: Green SA, Bloch S (eds) *An Anthology of Psychiatric Ethics*. Oxford University Press, Oxford

Bose S (2009) Containment and the Structured Day. In: Aiyegbusi A, Clarke-Moore J (eds) *Therapeutic Relationships with Offenders. An Introduction to the Psychodynamics of Forensic Mental Health Nursing*. Jessica Kingsley, London

Bowers L (2002)*Dangerous and Severe Personality Disorder: Response and Role of the Psychiatric Team*. Routledge, London

Braye S (2000) Participation and involvement in social care: An overview. In: Kemshall H, Littlechild R (eds) *User Involvement and Participation in Social Care: Research Informing Practice*. Jessica Kingsley, London

Burrow S (1998) Therapy versus security: Reconciling healing and damnation. In: Mason T, Mercer D (eds) *Critical Perspectives in Forensic Care: Inside Out*. Macmillan, Basingstoke

Byrt R (2005) *Forensic Mental Health Nurses' Involvement in Physical Security: Points for Consideration*. Unpublished paper sent on behalf of the National Forensic Nurses' Research and Development Group as a response to the Review on Mental Health Nursing

Byrt R (2008a) Power and participation in forensic services: An introduction. In: National Forensic Nurses' Research and Development Group: Kettles AM, Woods P, Byrt R (eds) *Forensic Mental Health Nursing: Capabilities, Roles, Responsibilities*. Quay

Books, MA Healthcare, London

Byrt R (2008b) Negative control or life saving? Perspectives on power. In: National Forensic Nurses' Research and Development Group: Kettles AM, Woods P, Byrt R (eds) *Forensic Mental Health Nursing: Capabilities, Roles, Responsibilities*. Quay Books, MA Healthcare, London

Byrt R, Aiyegbusi A, Hardie T, Addo A (2007) Cultural and diversity issues. In: National Forensic Nurses' Research and Development Group: Kettles AM, Woods P, Byrt R, Addo MA, Coffey M, Doyle M (eds) *Forensic Mental Health Nursing: Forensic Aspects of Acute Care*. Quay Books, MA Healthcare, London

Byrt R, Hart L, James-Sow L (2008) Patient empowerment and participation: Barriers and the way forward. In: National Forensic Nurses' Research and Development Group: Kettles AM, Woods P, Byrt R (eds) *Forensic Mental Health Nursing: Capabilities, Roles, Responsibilities*. Quay Books, MA Healthcare, London

Byrt R, James L (2007) Towards therapeutic environments: Challenges and problems In: National Forensic Nurses' Research and Development Group: Kettles AM, Woods P, Byrt R, Addo MA, Coffey M, Doyle M (eds) *Forensic Mental Health Nursing: Forensic Aspects of Acute Care*. Quay Books, MA Healthcare, London

Castledine G (1999) Psychiatric nurse talks about a client to a newspaper and radio. *British Journal of Nursing* **8**(12): 767

Chaloner C (2000) Ethics and morality. In: Chaloner C, Coffey M (eds) *Forensic Mental Health Nursing. Current Approaches*. Blackwell Science, Oxford

Clarke L (1996) Participant observation in a secure unit: Care, conflict and control. *Nursing Times Research* **1**(6): 431–41

Coffey M (2006) Researching service user views in forensic mental health: A literature review. *Journal of Forensic Psychiatry and Psychology* **17**(1): 73–107

Collins, M, Davies S, Ashwell C (2006) The assessment of security need. In: National Forensic Nurses' Research and Development Group: Woods P, Kettles AM, Byrt R, Addo M, Coffey M, Collins M, Doyle M, Garman G, Watson C (eds) *Aspects of Forensic Mental Health Nursing: Interventions with People with 'Personality Disorder.* Quay Books/MA Healthcare, London

Collopy BJ (2006) Autonomy in long term care: Some crucial distinctions. In: Green SA, Bloch S (eds) *An Anthology of Psychiatric Ethics*. Oxford University Press, Oxford

Cordess C (ed) (2001) *Confidentiality and Mental Health*. Jessica Kingsley, London

Cutcliffe J (2009) Engagement and observation of people at risk In: Barker P (ed) *Psychiatric and Mental Health Nursing: The Craft of Caring* (2nd edn) Arnold: London

Dale C, Gardner J (2001) Security in forensic environments: Strategic and operational issues. In: Dale C, Thompson T, Woods P (eds) *Forensic Mental Health: Issues in Practice*. Bailliere Tindall/Royal College of Nursing, Edinburgh

Department of Health (2007) *Best Practice in Managing Risk*. Department of Health, London

Department of Health (2010) *Single Equality Scheme, 2010–2013*. Department of Health, London Available from: www.dh.gov [Accessed 4 June, 2010]

Dimond B (2002) *Legal Aspects of Patient Confidentiality*. Quay Books/Mark Allen Publishing, Dinton, Salisbury

Dimond B (2008) *Legal Aspects of Nursing* (5th edn) Pearson Education, Harlow

Dimond B (2009) *Legal Aspects of Consent* (2nd edn). Quay Books, MA Healthcare, London

Eastman N, Riordan D, Adshead G (2010) Ethical roles, relationships and duties of forensic mental health clinicians. In: Bartlett A, McGauley G (eds) *Forensic Mental Health Concepts, Systems and Practice*. Oxford University Press, Oxford

Ford K, Byrt R, Dooher J (2010) *Preventing and Reducing Aggression and Violence in Health and Social Care: A Holistic Approach*. M & K Publishing, Keswick

Fox KJ (1999) Changing violent minds: Discursive correction and resistance in the cognitive treatment of violent offenders in prison. *Social Problems* 46(1): 88–103

Fry S, Johnstone M-J (2002) *Ethics in Nursing Practice A Guide to Ethical Decision Making* (2nd edn) Blackwell Science, Oxford

Fulford KWM (2004) Facts/values: Ten principles of values-based medicine. In: Radden J (ed) *The Philosophy of Psychiatry: A Companion*. Oxford University Press, Oxford

Fulford KWM (2008) Values-based practice: From the real to the really practical. *Philosophy, Psychiatry and Psychology* **15**(2): 183–5

Green SA, Bloch S (eds) (2006) *An Anthology of Psychiatric Ethics*. Oxford University Press, Oxford

Healthcare Commission (2009) Cited in: Parish C (2009) Mental health services are failing people from ethnic minorities. *Mental Health Practice* 12(5): 3 (Full citation not given in Parrish 2009)

Healy D (2010) *Psychiatric Drugs Explained* (5th edn) Elsevier Churchill Livingstone, Edinburgh

Hendrick J (2000) *Law and Ethics in Nursing and Health Care*. Stanley Thornes, Cheltenham

HM Government (1983) *Mental Health Act, 1983*. HMSO, London

HM Government (1984) *Police and Criminal Evidence Act, 1984*. HMSO, London

HM Government (1989) *The Children Act, 1989*. HMSO, London

HM Government (1990) *Computer Misuse Act, 1990*. HMSO, London

HM Government(1998a) *Data Protection Act, 1998*. HMSO, London

HM Government (1998b) *Human Rights Act Chapter 42*. HMSO, London

HM Government (2000) *Computer Misuse Act, 2000*. HMSO, London

HM Government (2003) *Criminal Justice Act, 2003*. HMSO, London

HM Government (2004) *The Children Act, 2004*. HMSO, London

HM Government (2005) *Mental Capacity Act, 2005*. HMSO, London

HM Government (2007) *Mental Health Act, 2007*. HMSO, London

HM Government (2010) *Equality Act, 2010*. HMSO, London

HM Government, Scotland (2002) *Freedom of Information (Scotland) Act, 2002* HM Government, Scotland, Edinburgh

Hogg C (1999) *Patients, Power and Politics: From Patients to Citizens*. Sage: London

Kant I (1969) *The Moral Law: Kant's Groundwork of the Metaphysics of Morals*. Hutchinson, London (Translated by Paton HJ; First published 1785) Cited in: Thompson IE, Melia KM, Boyd KM, Horsburgh D (eds) (2006) *Nursing Ethics* (5th edn) Churchill Livingstone/Elsevier, Edinburgh

Keen T, Barker P (2009) The person with schizophrenia. In: Barker, P (ed) *Psychiatric and Mental Health Nursing: The Craft of Caring* (2nd edn) Arnold, London

Kirby SD, Cross D (2002) Socially constructed narrative interventions. A foundation for therapeutic alliances. In: Kettles AM, Woods P, Collins M (eds) *Therapeutic Interventions for Mental Health Nurses*. Jessica Kingsley, London

Kunyck D, Olsen JK (2001) Clarification of conceptualisations of empathy. *Journal of Advanced Nursing* **35**(3): 317–25

Leff J (2001) Cultural Influences in Schizophrenia. In: Lieberman JA, Murray RM (eds). *Comprehensive Care of Schizophrenia. A Textbook of Clinical Management*. Martin Dunitz, London

Lowe T (1992) Characteristics of effective nursing interventions in the management of challenging behaviour. *Journal of Advanced Nursing* **17**: 1226–32

McDougall T (2000) Violent incidents in a forensic adolescent unit: A retrospective analysis *Nursing Times Research* **5**(2): 87–98

Maden T (2007) *Treating Violence: A Guide to Risk Management in Mental Health*. Oxford University Press, Oxford

Mason T, Chandley M (1990) Nursing models in a special hospital: A critical analysis of efficacy. *Journal of Advanced Nursing* **15**: 667–73

Masterson A, Maslin-Prothero S (1999) Power, politics and nursing. In: Mastersonson A, Maslin-Prothero S (eds) *Nursing and Politics. Power Through Practice*. Churchill Livingstone, Edinburgh

Mercer D, Mason T, Richman J (1999) Good and evil in the crusade of care. *Journal of Psychosocial Nursing and Mental Health Services* **37**(9): 13–17

Mill JS (1972) *Utilitarianism, Liberty, and Representative Government* Acton, HB (ed) Everyman, Dent, London (First published 1861) Cited in: Thompson IE, Melia KM, Boyd KM, Horsburgh D (2006) *Nursing Ethics* (5th edn) Churchill Livingstone, Elsevier, Edinburgh

Neuman B, Fawcett J (2010) *The Neuman Systems Model*,(6th edn) Appleton and Lange: Norwalk, CT

Nightingale F (1992) *Notes on Nursing: What It Is and What It Is Not*. Skretkowicz V (ed) Scutari Press, London (First published 1859)

Norman I, Ryrie I (eds) (2009) *The Art and Science of Mental Health Nursing. A Textbook of Principles and Practice*. McGraw Hill Open University Press, Maidenhead

Nursing and Midwifery Council (2008a) *The Code: Standards of Conduct, Performance and Ethics for Nurses and Midwives*. Nursing and Midwifery Council, London

Nursing and Midwifery Council (2008b) *What is Confidentiality?* Nursing and Midwifery Council, London. Available from: www.nmc-uk.org [Accessed 5 June, 2010]

O'Brien AJ, Morrisoni E, DeSouza R (2009) Providing culturally safe care. In: Barker P (ed) *Psychiatric and Mental Health Nursing: The Craft of Caring*. Arnold: London

Parker M, Dickenson D (eds) (2001) *The Cambridge Medical Ethics Workbook*. Cambridge University Press, Cambridge

Peternelj-Taylor C, Schafer P (2008) Management of therapeutic boundaries. In: National Forensic Nurses' Research and Development Group: Kettles AM, Woods P, Byrt R (eds). *Forensic Mental Health Nursing: Capabilities, Roles and Responsibilities*. Quay Books, MA Healthcare, Ltd, London

Phillips R (2003) The good, the bad and the ugly: The role of local radio as a medium for overcoming prejudice. In: Dooher J, Byrt R (eds) *Empowerment and the Health Service User.* Quay Books, Mark Allen Publishing, Dinton, Salisbury

Prins H (2010) *Offenders, Deviants or Patients? Explorations in Clinical Criminology* (4th edn). Routledge, Taylor and Francis Group, Hove

Pritchard J (2001) The myth of confidentiality: A social work view. In: Cordess C (ed) *Confidentiality and Mental Health*. Jessica Kingsley, London

Prochaska J, DiClemente C (1982) Transtheoretical therapy: Towards a more integrative model of change. *Psychotherapy: Theory, Research and Practice* 19(3): 276–88. Cited in O'Carroll M, Park A (2007) *Essential Mental Health Nursing Skills*. Mosby Elsevier, Edinburgh

Raguram R, Ventakeswaran J, Ramakrishna J, Weiss MG (2002) Traditional and community resources for mental health: A report of temple healing from India. *British Medical Journal* 325(7354): 38

Rogers C (1967) *On Becoming a Person: A Therapist's View of Psychotherapy.* Constable, London

Rogers C (1990) A client-centred/person-centred approach to therapy. In: Kirschbaum, Hand Henderson VL (eds) *The Carl Rogers Reader.* Constable, London

Rumbold G (1999) *Ethics in Nursing Practice* (3rd edn) Bailliere Tindall/Royal College of Nursing, Edinburgh

Sadler JZ (2005) *Values and Psychiatric Diagnosis*. Oxford University Press, Oxford

Sewell H (2009) *Working with Ethnicity, Race and Culture in Mental Health A Handbook for Practitioners*. Jessica Kingsley, London

Spinoza BDE (1955) *Ethics*. Gregory TS (ed) JM Dent, London. Cited in: Thompson, IE, Melia KM, Boyd KM, Horsburgh D (2006) *Nursing Ethics* (5th edn) Churchill Livingstone, Elsevier, Edinburgh

Stone AA (2006) The ethics of forensic psychiatry. In: Green SA, Bloch S (eds) *An Anthology of Psychiatric Ethics*. Oxford University Press, Oxford

Szasz T (2000) The case against psychiatric power. In: Barker P, Stevenson C (eds) *The Construction of Power and Authority in Psychiatry.* Butterworth Heinemann, Oxford

Szasz T (2003) Psychiatry and the control of dangerousness. The apotropaic function of the term "mental illness". *Journal of Social Work Education* **39**(3): 375–81

Szasz T (2005) Should psychologists be coercive agents of the state? *Current Psychology* **24**(92): 77–9

Thompson IE, Melia KM, Boyd KM, Horsburgh D (eds) (2006) *Nursing Ethics* (5th edn) Churchill Livingstone, Elsevier, Edinburgh

Tuckett AG (2004) Truth-telling in clinical practice and the arguments for and against: A review of the literature. *Nursing Ethics* **11**(5): 500–9

Walsh L (2009) The emotional labour of nurses working in Her Majesty's (HM) prison service. *Journal of Forensic Nursing* **5**:143–52

Woods P, Kettles A (eds) (2009) *Risk Assessment and Risk Management in Mental Health Nursing*. Wiley–Blackwell, Chichester

CHAPTER 3

Ethical and legal aspects of the Mental Health Act 2007 and related legislation

Nicholas Taylor

Introduction

Mental health law has always been a complex and highly contested area. There is an inherent tension between the duty of mental health professionals to provide safe care, which often involves restricting the liberty of patients, and the wishes of many patients to be released entirely from detention or supervision. These difficulties are most prominent in forensic mental health services.

Mental health law has evolved almost as rapidly as the theory and practice of mental healthcare have evolved. As is often the case, the law has often changed reactively, with a lag-time behind conceptual or practical changes. This lag has been particularly evident in recent years as the much-delayed revision of the Mental Health Act 1983 has dragged on, leaving the old law somewhat stalled, whilst expectations have been raised about the forthcoming legislation (Butcher, 2007).

This particular hurdle has now been cleared and, even by the historical standards of mental health law, we are in a particularly dynamic era. The new Mental Health Act has recently commenced, the new Mental Capacity Act has brought significant change, and the full implications of the decade-old Human Rights Act are still becoming clear. To add to the turmoil, judge-made common law has continued to evolve.

It is easy to feel somewhat lost in the midst of all this change, and this chapter aims to provide guidance regarding the legislation which governs mental health nursing and to examine in detail some of the more challenging areas.

The main areas of law which are of interest include domestic statute law, particularly the Mental Health Act 2007 and the Mental Capacity Act 2007. The European Convention on Human Rights, enshrined in United Kingdom law by the Human Rights Act 1998, is also increasingly relevant. The third area is judge-made common law.

It is important to understand these recent changes in legislation in the wider political and cultural context. The devolution of power to Scotland, and, to a lesser extent, Wales, has become a reality in recent years, and this is reflected in new mental health legislation. Scotland has the Mental Health (Care and Treatment) (Scotland) Act 2003 whereas England and Wales have the Mental Health Act 2007. Although England and Wales share the same Act, they have different Codes of Practice, issued by Westminster and the Welsh Assembly Government in Cardiff, respectively. There is the possibility that Northern Ireland will also develop its own Act (Zigmond 2008).

The law relating to detention and treatment of children is a more specialist area, requiring detailed treatment of its own and will not be covered here.

Legislation

Mental Health Act 2007

As readers will be aware, the main legislation dealing with compulsory treatment of people with mental disorders is the Mental Health Act 2007. This takes the form of an amendment to the Mental Health Act 1983.

The Act specifies who can be detained and treated and in what circumstances, as well as the procedures which must be followed. A fundamental principle underlying the Mental Health Act and the detention of patients is the concept of "entitlement". This idea was first articulated in this way by the Richardson Committee:

> *If you take compulsory powers over an individual then they are entitled to a certain minimum quality of care.*
>
> (Department of Health 1999)

Additionally, they are entitled to information about why their liberty has been restricted and about rights of appeal.

Main amendments to the Mental Health Act 1983

The Department of Health identifies nine main changes brought about by the Mental Health Act 2007 (Department of Health 2007).

1. The old categories of mental disorder have been abolished and a new, single, "catch-all" definition has been introduced (Department of Health 2007)

Under the 1983 Act, there were four categories of mental disorder. These have now been abolished and a new single category of mental disorder (defined as "any disorder or disability of the mind") has been introduced.

An exclusion has effectively been made for alcohol and substance use. Although these can constitute mental disorders (for example, according to the ICD-10 system), they do not constitute mental disorder under the new Act. If alcohol or substance use leads to a mental disorder, however, then it will be possible to detain a patient for treatment of the resulting disorder, such as delirium tremens.

Alcohol or substance use cannot therefore be the sole reason for detention and treatment. Treatment can be given for alcohol and substance use problems under the Act whilst a person is detained, however, if this treatment is "an appropriate part of treating the mental disorder which is the primary focus of the treatment" (Department of Health 2008).

The previous exceptions for promiscuity, immoral conduct and sexual deviancy no longer apply. The net effect of this is to remove significant legal barriers to the detention of sex offenders in hospital.

2. *The old "treatability test" has been abolished and a new test, of "appropriate medical treatment" has been introduced for all the longer-term powers of detention (Department of Health 2007)*

The "treatability test" made it clear that treatment for a patient must have been "likely to alleviate or prevent a deterioration of his condition". This is now the "appropriate treatment test" which requires that "appropriate medical treatment is available". "Medical treatment" is defined as "medical treatment, the purpose of which is to alleviate, or prevent a worsening of, the disorder or one or more of its symptoms or manifestations" (Mental Health Act 2007).

This change is significant. Previously, the treatment had to be "likely" to be effective. Now, there is no such requirement. It must simply be the "purpose" of the treatment to be effective. This may remove some barriers to the detention of dangerous people with personality disorder (and possibly sexual offenders) on a long-term basis, regardless of their involvement in treatment or the effects of treatment on them. It may be, though, that long-term non-engagement in treatment will be found to cause the treatment not to be "appropriate". If this is found to be the case, ongoing detention will be unlawful and this legislative change will have had little effect.

3. *The old restrictions on Responsible Medical Officers (RMOs – who had to be doctors) and Approved Social Workers (ASWs – who had to be social workers) have been abolished and replaced by Responsible Clinicians and Approved Mental Health Practitioners (Department of Health 2007)*

The changes made in this regard have implications for forensic services but will primarily be of interest in community services and in general psychiatric settings.

The new category of Approved Clinician (AC) has been introduced by the 2007 Act. This grants some of the powers previously reserved for doctors to a wider range of professionals who receive further training. ACs can give evidence in Court about a patient's mental state and about bed availability when a patient is remanded. Of less relevance to forensic settings, ACs can detain in-patients for up to 72 hours if they believe that an application for admission should be made. The overwhelming majority of in-patients in forensic settings are already detained under the Act, so this change is likely to be of limited significance.

Patients are now under the care of Responsible Clinicians (RCs), who are ACs who have undergone further training. RCs assume overall responsibility for a patient's care. They can be from a range of professions and can include doctors, nurses, psychologists, occupational therapists and social workers. Although two doctors are still required for the initial detention of a patient under Sections 2 or 3 of the Mental Health Act, the RC has a range of powers over a patient once the patient has been detained. These include the power to control Section 17 leave, recommend Supervised Community Treatment (SCT), recall a patient from SCT, renew detention under Section 3 or Section 37, and to discharge all but restricted patients, with the approval of an Approved Mental Health Professional (AMHP).

Strategic Health Authorities now have responsibility for granting approval for Responsible Clinicians. It is expected that this will be delegated to primary care trusts in many cases.

A range of competencies have been set out which it is expected that potential ACs and RCs will possess prior to being submitted for approval. In effect, it will be the responsibility of primary care trusts working with NHS or foundation trusts to implement this. Little indication has been given to date of how this is likely to work in practice.

AMHPs will be appointed by local Social Services Authorities. They can come from a range of professional backgrounds including social workers, nurses and psychologists, but not doctors. They are required to have appropriate skills. Their role includes applying to admit patients for assessment or treatment. They also have to concur with RCs before patients can be discharged or made subject to SCT.

4. *The antiquated and traditional nearest relative provisions of the 1983 Act have been brought up to date, allowing patients to displace their nearest relative. Civil partnerships are now recognised (Department of Health 2007)*

The nearest relative provisions have been recognised as outdated for some time. Some of the many problems included the potential for a previously abusive relative to have the power granted by the nearest relative over the patient/victim's care and treatment. The patient had no power to object to this and displace their nearest relative. This has been addressed in the new Act. There is also now additional scope for professionals to displace the nearest relative if they consider them to be unsuitable. Civil partnerships did not exist at the time of the 1983 Act and were not recognised by it. This has changed, so that civil partnerships are now fully recognised as equivalent to marriage for the purposes of the nearest relative provisions.

5. Supervised Community Treatment has been introduced in order to provide for effective care of patients in the community with a history of disengagement with mental health services (Department of Health 2007)

Supervised Community Treatment (SCT) has been introduced as an option for unrestricted detained patients (particularly those under Sections 3 and 37) with a history of "revolving door" admissions. The SCT must be planned in advance whilst the patient is an in-patient, and involves the patient becoming subject to a Community Treatment Order (CTO). Once in the community, patients can be recalled to hospital by the Responsible Clinician, under the same Section under which they were previously treated as an in-patient. If they are not discharged within 72 hours, the CTO must be revoked. The patient then has the right to apply to a tribunal. CTOs have conditions; one condition of all of them is that patients make themselves available for examination.

6. Mental Health Review Tribunal (MHRT) arrangements have been significantly altered (Department of Health 2007)

A wide range of procedural changes have been made to the tribunal system, which are not of direct relevance to most staff attending tribunals to give evidence.

From the nursing perspective, the most significant change to the tribunal system is that a written report is now required from a nurse. Usually, in the past, nurses presenting evidence to the tribunal have been asked in fairly general terms about a patient's presentation on the ward, level of compliance, motivation and so on. This is likely to continue, but if the nursing report contains information or opinion about other areas, such as diagnosis, prognosis and so on, then it is possible that the nurse will be examined on these. It is therefore advisable for nurses before tribunals to be mindful of the contents of reports.

7. *A requirement is now made for "age-appropriate services" for patients under 18 years of age (Department of Health 2007)*
8. *Independent mental health advocates are required to provide help to patients (Department of Health 2007)*

Advocacy services have been provided to patients previously on a variable basis, dependent on local policy and resources. The provision of advocacy has now been expanded, with the requirement that Independent Mental Health Advocates (IMHAs) are available to all "qualifying patients". The advocates have the right to see the records of consenting patients who have capacity to agree to this, and the right to meet with patients in private, as well as the right to interview anyone involved in the patient's treatment. Patients have their correspondence with their IMHAs protected from interference by hospital managers.

9. *New safeguards relating to the use of electroconvulsive therapy (ECT) have been introduced (Department of Health 2007)*

The 1983 Act provided very little scope for a detained patient to refuse treatment. This was the case regardless of whether or not the patient had capacity to make decisions about treatment. This remains the case in the amended Act, but the situation has changed where electroconvulsive therapy (ECT) is concerned. Patients who have capacity to refuse ECT cannot now be given ECT against their wishes. The only exception to this is when ECT is given as an emergency (under Section 62) to a patient who has capacity but refuses.

Seclusion

The Code of Practice to the 2007 Act deals with seclusion in some detail. It defines seclusion as:

> *...the supervised confinement of a patient in a room, which may be locked. Its sole aim is to contain severely disturbed behaviour which is likely to cause harm to others.*
>
> (Department of Health 2008)

It warns against keeping patients in seclusion and trying to avoid the paperwork and procedures associated with seclusion by giving it a different label, such as "segregation". The requirements for reviews of patients in seclusion are provided.

The sometimes difficult issue of self-harm and seclusion is addressed directly. Seclusion is primarily used to manage risk of harm to others. It should not be the primary means of managing the risk of self-harm. It is possible to manage a patient in seclusion who has a history of self-harm or current self-harm, but the additional risk of self-harm in seclusion needs to be balanced against the benefits of seclusion in terms of reduced risks to others in such cases.

Mental Capacity Act 2005

As with the new Mental Health Act, the Mental Capacity Act contains guiding principles that are of paramount importance. These dictate that people are assumed to have capacity unless proven otherwise, that people must not be found to lack capacity until "all practicable steps" (Mental Capacity Act 2005) have been taken to help them to regain capacity. Other principles make it clear that patients cannot be found to lack capacity simply because they make a decision which staff consider to be unwise, and that patients must be treated in the least restrictive manner.

Capacity is, as always, decision specific. It is defined as the ability to understand the information relevant to a decision, to retain that information, to use or weigh that information as part of the process of making the decision and to communicate the decision. Importantly, the communication can be by speech, sign language, writing or any other means. The greater the implications of a specific decision, the more capacity is required.

In many respects, the introduction of the Mental Capacity Act simply codified existing law in new statute law.

An example of this is the introduction of Advance Decisions and Advance Statements, previously known as Advance Directives or "Living Wills". These are essentially refusals of treatment, made in advance. They are made when the patient has capacity to make a decision which is intended to be put into practice after the patient becomes unwell, loses the capacity to make a decision and is in need of treatment. They are aimed mainly at patients at the start of a degenerative process, particularly dementing or degenerative illnesses, in order to give patients some choice about treatment options later in their illness.

Advance Decisions can only be made by those over 18 years of age who have capacity to make the specific decision(s). They must be voluntary and made by patients who have been properly informed about the treatment they are refusing in advance. Advance Decisions give patients the power to refuse even life-saving treatment and they are absolutely binding on healthcare staff if they can be shown to be valid.

They sound like very powerful instruments, but early cases demonstrate that it is difficult to show clearly that the Advance Decision is valid. How can it be demonstrated that the patient had capacity at the time that the Advance

Decision was made? How do we know that patients were properly informed about their decision to refuse a treatment? Who informed them about the options available? Solicitors are often involved in drawing up Advance Decisions but they do not have the knowledge to give sufficiently informed information about treatment and the consequences of refusing treatment.

A major challenge for Advance Decisions in forensic settings is that they are not binding on staff if a patient is detained under the Mental Health Act.

Advance Statements are essentially lesser forms of Advance Decisions. They do not have to fulfil the requirements set out above for Advance Decisions and are non-binding.

It is important to note, however, that Advance Decisions that are found not to be valid, or Advance Statements, may still hold important information about a patient's wishes and can be very helpful in informing treatment decisions.

The principles underlying the Mental Capacity Act 2005 involve supporting people in making decisions whenever possible. When this is not felt to be possible, actions must be taken in the person's best interests and in the least restrictive manner.

The Mental Health Act 2007 amends the Mental Capacity Act 2005 in that it sets out procedures by which individuals who lack capacity to consent to treatment can have their liberty restricted. It also provides safeguards (the Deprivation of Liberty Safeguards, or DOLS) which protect people in this position. This addresses the longstanding issue of "the Bournewood gap" (the need to prevent arbitrary detention in hospitals of those lacking capacity to consent to treatment, Allen, 2010). Patients in the Bournewood gap are, by definition, not detained under the Mental Health Act. DOLS are therefore of only limited relevance to forensic settings and will not be covered in greater detail here.

Duties and powers of a nurse

Nurses, in common with many other healthcare professionals, have a range of specific legal powers over others and various duties to those in their care. The new Mental Health Act extends many powers previously reserved for doctors to a wider range of professionals, including nurses, who have undergone special training. This section deals with generic issues for all mental health nurses.

Power to prevent a patient from leaving hospital: S5(4)

The vast majority of in-patients in forensic mental health services are detained under the Mental Health Act. In many services, this is a necessary pre-requisite for admission. A few patients are not detained, however, and the work of forensic mental health services often involves liaison with other services in giving advice and support regarding the management of more challenging patients, who may be informal.

The Mental Health Act 2007 grants the same Holding Power to nurses as was available under Section 5(4) of the Mental Health Act 1983. Nurses of the "prescribed class" may detain current voluntary hospital in-patients who wish to leave, as long as the nurse considers that:

- The patient is suffering from a mental disorder to such a degree that it is necessary for the patient to be immediately prevented from leaving the hospital either
  - for the patient's health or safety or
  - for the protection of other people, and
  - it is not practicable to secure the attendance of a doctor or approved clinician who can submit a report under Section 5(2) (Mental Health Act 2007).

The (non-renewable) Holding Power lasts until a doctor or Approved Clinician with the power to use Section 5(2) arrives or until 6 hours has elapsed. The Approved Clinician or doctor is expected to arrive as quickly as possible, and not simply wait until the Holding Power is about to expire.

The power comes into effect as soon as the nurse makes the appropriate record that it is to be used. This is entered onto the relevant form, copies of which should be stored in an accessible location within the hospital. Once the form is complete and the Holding Power has been invoked, the form should be passed to the hospital managers as quickly as is practical.

Once the patient has been detained, the reason for the use of the power should be entered into the patient's records. Staff then have a duty to inform the detained patient of his or her rights, as required by Section 132 of the Mental Health Act 2007.

As with the old 1983 Act, the power is designed to act as an emergency measure, and is expected to be used relatively infrequently and for the shortest possible time, until arrangements can be made for a fuller review.

Clearly, the absence of a nurse of the prescribed class does not mean that all patients should be allowed to leave hospital, however unwell, confused and vulnerable they are. If a nurse who was not of the prescribed class was present, a patient could be detained under common law in certain circumstances (see *Box 3.1*). In order for this power to be used, the person would have to be a voluntary in-patient in hospital already and would lack capacity to make the decision about staying in hospital. It must also be necessary in the patient's best interests for the patient to be prevented from leaving (Fennell 2004).

Box 3.1. Detention of an informal patient by a nurse

Mr Smith is an elderly man with dementia. He has been admitted voluntarily to hospital after an alleged sexual assault on his elderly wife. They have been married for 54 years and have recently been struggling to manage living independently due to illness.

Mr Smith is confused and does not realise that he has been admitted to hospital. He declares, late on a cold January night, that he, "needs to go and get a paper", wearing only his pyjamas, and demands to be allowed to leave, despite discouragement from staff.

The duty doctor is busy in the accident and emergency department and will not be able to attend for two hours.

How can Mr Smith be prevented from leaving?

If a nurse from a prescribed class is present, he can be detained under Section 5(4) of the Mental Health Act 2007. This can only be done once the reasons for it have been recorded on the appropriate documentation. The doctor must attend as soon as possible.

If the only members of the nursing staff present are not of the prescribed class, he can still be detained, this time under common law, until a nurse from the prescribed class becomes available (when he can be detained under Section 5(4) as above) or until the doctor becomes available.

Once the doctor arrives, detention can be authorised under Section 5(2) of the Mental Health Act, allowing time for a full assessment.

Clearly, due to the risks involved, it is critical that Mr Smith is not allowed to leave, and this is where common law is useful.

Duty of care

Nurses have a duty of care to their patients. This is a common law duty and nurses are obliged not to cause their patients harm by either acts (wrongful acts) or omissions. If nurses breach this duty of care and, in doing so, injure a patient, they have acted negligently if their conduct is not supported by a reasonable body of professional opinion, which a judge believes to be "supported by logic" (see *Box 3.2*).

Other issues

A proportion of patients already detained under the Mental Health Act 2007 will perpetrate acts of violence to staff or commit other illegal acts. Unfortunately, "Zero Tolerance" policies are often hard to enforce

Box 3.2. The Bolam/Bolitho test

The Bolam test was originally set out in the case of *Bolam v Friern Barnet Hospital Managment Committee* as long ago as 1957.

Essentially, it dictates that a healthcare professional's actions will not be considered negligent if they are supported by a responsible body of professional opinion. In practice, this has involved a professional accused of negligence finding another professional to support their case in court as an expert witness.

This test was modified in the more recent case of *Bolitho v City and Hackney Health Authority* in 1998. In this case, the judge stated that the professional opinion needs to be "supported by logic" in order to be effective in supporting a defence against negligence.

in psychiatric hospitals, where it is difficult to refuse treatment to or bar patients whose behaviour would not be tolerated in other healthcare settings and who are often detained by law.

In these cases, the police are often contacted to provide assistance. They are sometimes reluctant to take appropriate action in terms of interviewing alleged victims and perpetrators. This may be due to a perception that the alleged perpetrator is already detained and that there is therefore no benefit in public protection terms in proceeding vigorously with a view to prosecution. Mental disorder is clearly an issue in such cases, and this muddies the waters further.

There are potential benefits relating to prosecution, however, in terms of ensuring that patients (ill or otherwise) are held to account for their (illegal) actions; that the crime is properly recorded for the information of future services and carers; and, in some cases, ensuring that the patient is appropriately detained, for example under Section 37/41 of the Mental Health Act 2007.

Covert administration of medication

Administering medicines without a patient's knowledge is clearly a difficult area and the 2001 UKCC *Position Statement on the Covert Administration of Medicines – Disguising Medicine in Food and Drink* provides welcome guidance.

Clearly, this constitutes treatment without consent, and so must be carried out under common law if the patient lacks capacity to consent, or under the provisions of Section 58 of the Mental Health Act 2007, if the patient has capacity to refuse medication.

The position statement makes it clear that it is only in the first of these cases (the patient lacking capacity) that medicine is likely to be administered covertly. In practice, this occurs most frequently in the care of the elderly, with dementing illnesses, or the learning disabled, who lack capacity and are unlikely to develop or recover capacity.

Clearly, local safeguards in terms of policies, multidisciplinary discussions and careful documentation must be in place to support covert administration of medication, which must only be done after appropriate discussion and consultation.

Conclusion

Forensic mental health services must have regard to a wide range of statute laws which have been much altered in recent years. Additionally, case law is developing at a rapid pace. It is critical that staff act lawfully at all times in providing the very best care for their patients, whilst acknowledging that not all patients will thank them for this.

At the same time, forensic mental health services are under more legal scrutiny than any other area of healthcare. Solicitors are frequent visitors to secure hospitals, and tribunals take place regularly.

A chapter can only offer the briefest of introductions to such a complex area, and staff are strongly encouraged to make sure they keep their practice up to date by taking advantage of appropriate training and professional development opportunities.

When in doubt about any area of work, particularly where such important principles as patient safety, autonomy and liberty are at stake, all members of staff have a responsibility to seek appropriate advice. This can be provided by managers, staff from other disciplines, or by trust solicitors or other lawyers where appropriate.

References

Allen N (2010) The Bournewood Gap (as amended?). *Medical Law Review* **18**(1): 78–85

Butcher J (2007) Controversial Mental Health Bill reaches the finishing line. The Lancet 370: 117–18

Department of Health (1999) Report of the Expert Committee. Review of the Mental Health Act 1983. London: Department of Health

Department of Health (2007) The Mental Health Act 2007. Department of Health, London. Available from: http://www.opsi.gov.uk/acts/acts2007/ukpga_20070012_en_1

Department of Health (2008) Mental Health Act 1983: Revised Code of Practice. Stationery Office, London

Fennell P (2004) The Law and Ethics of Mental Health Nursing. In Norman I, Ryrie I. (eds) *The Art and Science of Mental Health Nursing*. Open University Press, Buckingham

HM Government (2005) *Mental Capacity Act, 2005*. HMSO, London

HM Government (2007) *Mental Health Act, 2007*. HMSO, London

Zigmond T (2008) Changing Mental Health Legislation in the UK. *Advances in Psychiatric Treatment* **14**: 81-83.

The Wall

Andrew Higgins, Mandy Laird, Monica Elaine Mantey, Phineas Mapfumo, Tapiwa Mugabe and Folorunso Olubukola with Giotto Bonomaully

The wall, erected by ancestors; seen from afar, seen by many.
They too have troubles, seeing it from within.
Marginalised youth, brutal rebels over years.
How long can the wall be ignored?
How long before its frustrations explode?

Do we build a wall?
We need a hammer and a chisel to bring it down.
But they offer psychotherapists...they too are dangerous.
I see a gap in the wall...visualisations.
What we are they say is an abstract thing:
A rehabilitation centre called The City of Rest.

The wall has dedicated itself to saving
An unsaveable and believes that
"Nobody is beyond help".
Possibilities for going over the wall will remain illusory.
Vulnerability manifested with horrific effect.
Needles and tablets, our everyday nutrition
For us, and not for them.
Those outside the wall, who say
"The power of the oppressed person cannot
Be underestimated in the desire to create disturbances".

(Both quotations from: Jones F (2007) West Africa's forgotten generation. *The Demon: the Official Newspaper of the Students of De Montfort University* **60**: 8–9).

CHAPTER 4

The promotion of autonomy in clients with learning disabilities

Ian Smith, Mary Addo and Jerry Ninnoni

This chapter explores some of the ethical and legal issues surrounding the promotion of autonomy when providing care in a forensic setting for people who have a learning disability. It is important to note that learning disabled clients in these types of settings may experience many problems other than their disabilities in learning. For example, they may experience stereotyping and unhelpful attitudes on the part of staff which could result in them being on the receiving end of discriminatory treatment. This means that staff in these units need to take extra care to ensure that clients' rights are not denied and that people with learning disabilities get the same quality of care as non-learning disabled people. This can be achieved by paying close attention to the structure of the service and how it promotes the client's rights and welfare through good decision-making processes that take account of the client's perspective. The elements of an effective forensic service for this client group are outlined in *Box 4.1* on page 68 and reference will be made to many of these elements throughout the chapter.

Examples of ethical principles and legal issues in forensic settings

The key ethical principles that may be involved in providing a forensic service for people with learning disabilities include autonomy, respect for person, beneficence, non-maleficence, justice and fidelity. Legal issues in the same situation could include those related to capacity/competence, informed consent, client understanding, duty of care, advocacy, nurse accountability, and detention-related issues, such as the restrictions imposed by compulsory orders.

One of the key ethical principles currently employed in the care of people with learning disabilities is autonomy which can be regarded as the right to self-govern or self-determine one's own actions or behaviour. Autonomy is a major component of consumer empowerment. The consumer empowerment movement developed, in part, in response to the rights infringements of devalued groups including people with learning disabilities. The plight of many thousands of people with a learning disability living in institutions in the UK and other European countries came to light in the 1960s and resulted in the development of the potentially empowering philosophy of normalisation. Early versions of normalisation (Nirje 1969) promoted unconditional acceptance of people with learning disabilities while later versions, such as Wolfensberger's social role valorisation (Wolfensberger 1983), encouraged services to enhance the social image of the client group. Later versions, such as John O'Brien's five service accomplishments (O'Brien and Lyle 1987), married the two approaches and in this version normalisation is regarded as an empowering approach in which the promotion of client autonomy is a key element. The promotion of client autonomy was meant to be a counterbalance to services which were based primarily on a medical model and which were professionally driven. Currently most NHS units for people with learning disabilities in the UK are likely to include autonomy in their philosophy or mission statement.

So how do you employ an empowering principle such as autonomy within the potentially restrictive ethos of a forensic unit? To help service providers in Scotland in their decision-making the Mental Health (Care and Treatment) (Scotland) 2003 emphasises the need for services to employ the principle of "least restrictive practice" (Scottish Government, 2004). The need to apply the least restrictive option is further supported by the Adults with Incapacity (Scotland) Act 2000. This Act states that all decisions made on behalf of an adult with incapacity must:

- Benefit the client.
- Adopt the least restrictive option.
- Take account of the adult's present and past wishes if these can be ascertained.
- Take account of the nearest relatives, primary carer or relevant other.
- Restrict the adult's freedom as little as possible.

Scottish Government (2009)

The English Mental Capacity Act 2005 and Mental Health Act 2007 have similar principles within them. So what do the concepts of capacity and incapacity mean and how do they apply to the principles of autonomy and client choice in forensic settings? Legally, in both Scotland and England capacity is assumed and people with learning disabilities are expected to be able to make their own decisions. One can only employ legislative frameworks if one has doubts about a person's capacity. For example, in

Scotland under the terms of the Adults with Incapacity (Scotland) Act 2000 an adult is considered to be covered by the Act if he or she is incapable of making decisions, understanding those decisions, or communicating those decisions to others. A view which is commonly expressed in legislation is that capacity and incapacity are not at fixed levels for individuals but vary according to the decision. This means that capacity is decided on a decision by decision basis in those situations where capacity may be an issue. For example, some clients may be able to make relatively simple choices, such as what to eat and what to wear, but may have more difficulty in more complex choices, such as varied treatment options. But even then it is not as easy, as simple choices equal capacity and complex choices equal incapacity for most clients. It can be argued that the onus is on forensic unit staff to present ideas and options in such a way as to facilitate decision-making.

Effective communication will significantly determine the extent to which service users can exercise autonomy and be involved in the decision-making process. People with learning disabilities as a sub-group of the general population may have different communication needs and therefore may need appropriate support and facilities to enable them to make consumerist decisions regarding their care. People with learning disabilities may communicate using a wide range of different methods. These include both verbal and non-verbal forms of communication; others may require the use of augmentative and alternative methods, such as pictures and photographs, to supplement spoken words and also to keep the communication focused on key issues (Ninnoni 2010). Therefore, there may be the need to individualise communication and identify strategies that will facilitate it.

It important that staff working with people with learning disabilities make an effort to identify the communication needs of the service user to facilitate communication (Royal College of Nursing 2006, Ninnoni 2010). Ninnoni and colleagues yielded a range of strategies that facilitate communication. These include: identify a suitable communication environment; use accessible language; reinforce the message and check for understanding; and use alternative communication methods, such as pictures and photographs, to supplement the spoken word (Ninnoni 2010).

When people are denied the opportunity to express their views due to poor communication it may lead to management problems. Moreover, poor communication has been reported as a recipe for "challenging behaviour" (Kevan 2003). "Challenging behaviour" is said to be socially mediated; people use challenging behaviour when other more conventional forms of communication fail (Kevan 2003, van der Gaag 1998). People with learning disabilities may be candidates for forensic care due to perceived aggression or "challenging behaviours", however, certain behaviours may be expressions of unmet needs and sometimes they are used as communication strategies

(Ninnoni 2010). Poor communication may lead to denial of the individual's rights to autonomy, and clients in the forensic setting may well be unduly victimised due to lack of opportunities for them to express their views.

Paternalism

Given the nature of the client's perceived index offence, there may be times when the nurse feels that he or she has to override client choice for the protection of either the client or the public. This is fine if it is based on an adequate assessment of the risk posed in the situation. However, the decision to restrict the client's autonomy may be based on the nurse's general assumption that all forensic clients pose an increased risk to themselves or others or both. Such thinking may be based on unchallenged assumptions and may be reinforced by other staff members in the unit who hold similar views. Intervening in this way can become a habitual and routinised mode of operating for nurses in the unit.

Such actions may be viewed as paternalistic and this form of paternalism is often equated with institutional behaviour from the past and often reflects a medical model of care. This may be seen as undesirable in contemporary healthcare services where the emphasis is on social models of care in which autonomy and respect for clients are promoted. Furthermore, research findings suggest that people with learning disabilities will value more discursive relationships with their healthcare professionals where they can input on issues affecting their care rather than being told what to do (Ninnoni 2010). Such a view may be regarded as fitting with the collaborative model of care promoted in many contemporary health services. Paternalism does have its place in protecting clients and staff where concerns have a solid foundation, but in some cases it is difficult to justify its use. To avoid the sometimes excessive and unthinkingly applied paternalism of the past, staff need to be non-judgemental and view each situation holistically with an open mind. A thorough consideration of the unit's purpose combined with a clear decision-making framework might allow staff to more confidently make decisions which protect clients while allowing for maximal expression of client autonomy within the unit.

Encouraging autonomy and client development, including the promotion of client self-awareness and self-control, will involve risk taking on the part of clients and staff. Conversely, a lack of risk taking might have an adverse effect on autonomy and development. Hessler and Kay (1993) argue that there may be a lack of risk taking in services for people with learning disabilities. They argue that the client group may be viewed as having a fixed incompetence or lack of capacity, despite what legislation might say, and, as a result, may not be provided with developmental opportunities with associated risk. They also argue that this client group may be assessed at a higher standard before risks are offered, that is, they may have to "prove" that they can understand the concepts involved and the risks attached to a given activity before they are allowed to do it whereas people without a learning disability do not have to do so. Related to this, the Royal College of Nursing (2006) points out that some staff have a tendency to assume clients with a learning disability do not have capacity if they make a decision which the staff member does not agree with. Perhaps this might best be regarded as an extension of the "Doctor/nurse knows best" form of paternalism. When working with clients staff may need to ask themselves the question, "Does the client not understand the risks in the situation or is it the case that I simply don't like the thought of them doing this thing (whatever it is)?" To reduce the possibility of staff biases hindering client choice and autonomy, it may be useful to consider more formal risk assessment processes where a greater attempt is made to achieve objectivity. Also, staff may need to reflect upon their own views of the competence of this client group and compare these with the current philosophies of care. To summarise so far, we have seen that there are a number of factors that can impede the promotion of client autonomy.

Factors hindering promotion of client autonomy

- Fixed view of capacity and competence
- Need for a higher level of proof of competence
- Ineffective communication strategies
- Unchallenged assumptions of staff
- Routinised, non-critical modes of staff operation
- Staff biases

At this point it is useful to consider how effective risk assessment can be used to protect the client's autonomy. Risk assessment in a forensic unit might more usually be undertaken to assess the risk of violence and aggression posed by clients to themselves and others. However, it can be argued that it should be used equally vigorously to protect clients from those factors that can hinder their development as human beings. Indeed, Inglis et al (2003) recognise that criminal justice systems and therapeutic professionals, such as nurses, typically have opposing priorities, such as risk minimisation and risk taking. These are the two sides of the risk assessment coin. In this case we need to ensure that the service we provide benefits the client and does no harm, that is, we need to apply the ethical principles of beneficence and non-maleficence in aiding client development in forensic settings.

Promoting autonomy via positive use of risk assessment

Firstly staff may need to consider their current approach to risk assessment. Learning disabilities services, like mental health services, may be under political pressure to reduce the perceived dangers clients might pose to other people. There is the possibility of moral panic ensuing should a client, currently within the care of an NHS or local authority unit, harm a member of the public during a trip to a community setting aimed at facilitating client development. This might lead to a negative approach where the bulk of policies and procedures within a unit are aimed at reducing the risk of such events to the exclusion of more liberating and positive policies and procedures. The management ethos of the organisation is particularly important here. Reason (2000) argues that health organisations tend to take a person approach to the management of perceived errors, that is, if harm comes to a client or, in this case, a client action results in harm to others then management is likely to assign blame to the individual staff members deemed to be responsible for that person's care rather than look to the system in which the care is provided. Reason argues that most errors result from system factors such as inadequate staffing, poor training, lack of safe systems, inadequate consideration of things that can go wrong and consequent lack of pre-emptive action by management, and so on, rather than being purely the result of individuals failing to discharge their responsibilities correctly. If the organisation has a "blame culture" resulting from this type of approach then individual staff members may be concerned that they will be blamed if things go wrong so they may refuse to promote risk taking with clients. This may lead to the development of a culture of risk aversion within the unit. Management needs to ensure that staff are properly trained in the area of risk management and it then needs to support staff in the promotion of risk taking in order that client development can be encouraged.

As already indicated, staff may need to explore their own views towards people with learning disabilities generally. In addition to the unchallenged assumptions of dangerousness mentioned earlier, staff may hold low expectations of people with learning disabilities. This may lead to reduced learning opportunities and consequently reduced client development which, in turn, will reinforce the view that these people are not capable of learning. This leads to the creation of a vicious circle that is hard to break. Rogers (1995) argues that this kind of self-fulfilling prophecy can be very damaging to clients' self-esteem. So having high expectations of the possibility of client development and of positive changes in their behaviour would seem to be an important attitude to cultivate within staff. The Scottish Recovery Network (2008) set out a number of factors that influence the judgements we might make in risk-taking with clients. We can apply these to working with people with learning disabilities as follows:

- *Existing knowledge of the risk*: Is it sufficient or do we need more information?
- *The circumstances in which the risk will be taken*: How much preparation and support will the client need?
- *Prejudices and preconceptions*: We might think clients will not manage or that they will panic in response to stress.
- *The degree of control you have over risks*: The more control you have over the risk the more likely you are to encourage that risk. The challenge is to find the balance between control and giving the client freedom to learn.
- *Previous experience*: If a client has had a bad experience in your care in the past you are less likely to take a similar risk. Maybe you could review why things did not go well and change things next time?
- *Are others affected?* This might influence risk taking adversely. Do clients need more support in this case?
- *Skills, confidence and self-esteem*: Possession of confidence by nurse and client will promote positive risk taking. Consider how you can both become more confident.

The framework suggested above will aid decision-making with regard to risk. The client should be involved in this process, wherever possible. As we have seen capacity is not an "either/or" thing, rather it is a much more fluid concept. You do not know how a client will respond to involvement unless you try, so a useful working principle is to always try to include clients at all stages of decision-making using the communication principles outlined earlier. Initially, it may be the case that clients are hesitant about getting involved and may even resist it if they have been used to people making decisions for them or if their views have previously been discounted or trivialised. Also, Seawood and Rees (2001) have found that many learning disabled clients in forensic settings come from a poor background, have poor social skills and have a history of social and financial difficulties within the family. It is not hard to imagine that some of these clients may have come from chaotic or unsupportive family backgrounds and may be unused to stable, supportive trusting relationships. This might mean that you need to work on developing a mutually trusting relationship to begin with.

Once trust has been established you may be surprised at how well clients respond to someone showing faith in them and trusting them. This can be seen as the flip side of the self-fulfilling prophecy. Similarly, if you believe that clients can benefit from a range of valued experiences then you will try hard to present these experiences in such a way that the chances of clients responding positively are much increased. The client's self-esteem can grow in an environment where there is opportunity to learn and where support is offered by staff within a trusting relationship. Wolfensberger (1972) highlighted the importance of the self-fulfilling prophecy in a normalisation-based service. He argued that services should always try to create conditions where success is likely so that the client will then be viewed more positively and a helpful role circularity can then be created. This is especially important with a client group that has two unhelpful labels attached to it, i.e. learning disability and forensic patient. It can be argued that this group is even more likely to be viewed negatively than people with learning disabilities alone. Promoting client autonomy and viewing clients' abilities in a positive light may be regarded as essential elements in countering the effects of these negative labels.

Having considered effective organisational approaches and helpful staff attitudes in working with this client group we need now to consider how we could support clients in expressing their autonomy. Falloon et al (2007) used a problem-solving approach used with people with a mental illness which can be modified to suit the needs of this client group.

Decision-making framework for the promotion of autonomy

Identify the goal to be achieved

You could begin by asking clients what they would like to do or achieve. If the client is unable to say what he or she would like then you could offer choices appropriate to the setting and the client's legal status. The principle of normalisation may be used to help identify valued options which could be offered to the client. Examples might include going to the beach for an outing, watching a favourite football team, etc. If the client chooses a negatively valued option then you could discuss the potential effects this may have on how people view the client; that is, the client can make an informed choice. If the choice of activity is not normally offered to clients then staff may need to reappraise their unit philosophy rather than reject the idea out of hand.

Identify the different courses of action to achieve this goal

Here you can encourage the client to think of who would be involved and of all the steps needed to achieve the goal. This can help clients to develop skills in making responsible decisions which take into account the effects of their decision-making upon others. This may help the client develop a sense of responsibility and respect for others, both of which may be useful developmental goals.

Consider the benefit and possible risks associated with each action

Decide on which course of action looks most promising to try first

This can be achieved by looking at the lists of benefits and risks and seeing which might have the greatest benefits and the least risks.

Think about how risks can be minimised if things do not work out as expected.

Make a decision whether or not to proceed

The nurse and client need to make a decision whether or not to proceed. There may be practical issues such as finance or staff support which may influence the decision. However, if the service is serious about meeting client needs then these issues are likely to be less of a barrier as ways around them would be explored.

Make detailed plans for proceeding with that chosen option

This involves agreeing what the service will do to support the client.

Review and further action

Review of the success of the activity from both the client and service perspective is important. What worked well for the client and what did not work so well should be identified. If things did not work out well, then what can be learned from the situation for next time? Experiencing disappointment is a learning experience and a necessary part of life; clients should be encouraged not to see it as a sign of their failure. In this case the client should be encouraged to try again or to try something different. If things go well it is just as important to identify why this was, as these positive lessons may actually be remembered more effectively than negative ones.

The above decision-making framework could be used as part of a person-centred planning approach to care. Many services now employ this type of approach and there is no reason why it cannot be employed in a forensic setting. Indeed, it could be argued that such a setting may need the positive focus of a person-centred planning approach to ensure that the client's continued development as a human being remains within the consciousness of staff. In support of this the British Institute of Learning Difficulties (2002) acknowledges that person-centred planning helps build a shared commitment to action that recognises a person's rights. In addition to decision-making frameworks and person-centred models the unit needs staff that have the requisite knowledge and skills. Alaszewski et al (2001) found that less than one-quarter of staff felt that initial nurse education prepared them for their first role. It can be argued, though, that initial nurse preparation cannot be expected to cover all specialities and that trained nurses need to develop their knowledge and skills when they start work in a speciality such as forensic nursing. If that is the case then effective continuing professional development would be required to develop and maintain an appropriate knowledge and skill base. This, in turn, requires good leadership and supportive management to both allow staff to be released for development and to motivate them to engage in learning activities. These requirements, along with a number of others, are set out in *Box 4.1*.

Service requirements for the effective promotion of autonomy

As can be seen in *Box 4.1* there are a number of important requirements which, it is argued, need to be in place before a service can promote the autonomy of its client group. If such requirements are present then the service will be in a stronger position to assure clients that they will receive a safe and effective service that allows them to exercise their right to as much autonomy as practicable within the restrictions of the setting and within the client's capacity to self-determine.

Box 4.1. Service requirements for the effective promotion of autonomy in forensic settings

- Robust staff selection procedures
- Good induction and orientation of staff
- Adequate staff knowledge base regarding learning disability and issues related to the care of this client group – capacity and communication
- Specific skills in relation to forensic nursing such as safety, security, aggression management, as well as specific therapies (UKCC 1999)
- Clear philosophy of care which is under continual review
- Effective risk assessment and decision-making frameworks
- Good staff awareness of common pitfalls in nursing forensic clients
- Reflective model of practice
- Person-centred planning approach to care

References

Alaszewski A, Gates B, Motherby E, Manthorpe J, Ayer S (2001) *Education preparation for learning disability nursing. Research Highlights No 47*. English National Board for Nursing, Midwifery and Health Visiting, London

British Institute of Learning Disabilities (2002) *Factsheet: Person centred planning*. BILD, Kidderminster

Falloon IRH, Barbieri L, Boggian I, Lamonacal D (2007) Problem solving training for schizophrenia: Rationale and review. *Journal of Mental Health* **16**(5): 553–68

Hessler I, Kay B (1993) Ethical issues. In Shanley E, Starrs T (eds) *Learning disabilities: A handbook of care*. (2nd edn) (pp 293–306) Churchill Livingstone, Edinburgh

Inglis P, Robinson M, Thornton P, English P (2003) *Partnerships in nursing and education: Enhancing the role of the specialist RNLD in forensic settings*. Available from: www.ldoffenders.co.uk/conferences/3rdCon2004/.../04partEIGHToi.doc [Accessed 26.3.10]

Kevan F (2003) Challenging behaviour and communication difficulties. British *Journal of Learning Disabilities* **31**: 75–80

Ninnoni J (2010). *Effective communication with people with learning disabilities with epilepsy and their carers*. PhD thesis (unpublished). Robert Gordon University Aberdeen

Nirje B (1969) The normalization principle and its human management implications. In Kugel R, Wolfensberger W (eds) *Changing patterns in residential services for the mentally retarded*. Washington, DC: President's Committee on Mental Retardation

O'Brien J, Lyle C (1987) *Framework for accomplishment*. Responsive System Associates, Lithonia, GA

Reason J (2000) Human error: Models and management. *British Medical Journal* **320**: 768–70

Rogers J (1995).Work is the key to recovery. *Psychosocial Rehabilitation Journal* **18**: 5–10

Royal College of Nursing (2006) *Meeting the health needs of people with learning disabilities: Guidance for nursing staff*. RCN, London

Seawood S, Rees C (2001) Responding to people with a learning disability who offend. *Nursing Standard* **15**(37): 36–9

Scottish Government (2004) *Mental Health (Care and Treatment) (Scotland) Act 2003*. Available from: http://www.scotland.gov.uk/Publications/2004/01/18753/31686 [Accessed 24.3.10]

Scottish Government (2009) *Evaluation of the Adults with Incapacity (Scotland) 2000 Part 4*. Available from: http://www.scotland.gov.uk/Publications/2009/12/18144540/4 [Accessed 24.3.10]

Scottish Recovery Network (2008) *Realising recovery: Learning materials* (p 127). NHS Education Scotland, Glasgow

UKCC (1999) *Nursing in secure environments*. UKCC, London

Van Der Gaag A (1998) Communication skills and adults with learning disabilities: Eliminating professional myopia. *British Journal of Learning Disabilities* **26**: 88–93

Wolfensberger W (1972) *The principle of normalisation in human services*. York University, Ontario

Wolfensberger W (1983) Social role valorisation: A proposed new term for the principle of normalization. *Mental Retardation* **21**(6): 234–9

CHAPTER 5

My personal tsunami: Surviving assault

Frances Barrone

The present

Ten years on: Late January 2010 travelling on a train

I am dressed in black as I want to blend into the blur of commuters and not draw attention to myself. I silently congratulate myself for taking this trip to do a one-day training course for professional development, away from the safety of my familiar work environment.

My journey had been meticulously planned. I booked the train tickets in advance and was armed with Google route map, directions, and the address and telephone number of the hotel that was hosting the event. All this would support me if my second worst fear occurred, that of getting lost and wandering into a dangerous area. I also had the train timetables and my mobile at the ready should my plans go awry. To minimise the risk of my worst fear, being attacked or in any way under threat of such, I was wearing square-heeled boots that would allow me to sprint, yet still be strong enough to hurt someone should I need to use my legs and feet to kick out. The boots were fit for purpose yet still looked semi-fashionable and went well with my sombre, yet roomy professional attire. I needed comfort and manoeuvrability in what I wore so I could cope with whatever cropped up during the day.

The night I was attacked I was wearing strapless summer sandals. They were easy to get on and off quickly so I could avoid spending too much time in the miniscule changing rooms swamped by children and sweaty adults pouring in and out of their exercise classes. Back then in 2000 I loved going to the Dojo. For the first time since playing basketball at school I had learned to love sport again, in particular an exercise called Te Geri. This is a form of non-contact martial arts and kickboxing. I was at peak physical fitness then and have never before or since achieved that. Ironically this is what perhaps saved my life but also, by virtue of pursuing this sport, was paradoxically what nearly cost me it.

As the train started to fill up with passengers I remembered that it was exactly 10 years since the most incredible, traumatic and life-altering night in my 40 plus year history. I have to trust that it influenced me in choosing a path to greatness rather than one of destruction, which I have dallied with in the interim period. I always wanted to be a writer and here I am writing this for you, yet I never planned to be writing for quite this reason. I would like this account to be not just an impact statement but, more importantly, my survival story. From the early days of recovery it had to be a survivor's journey rather than a victim's story.

Sitting back comfortably into my seat I let out a small sigh of relief, feeling breathless and fatigued from the brisk 15 minute walk from the hotel to the station. The exercise was good for me but perhaps what was not so healthy was me operating in fight or flight mode. I now know this reaction causes the increased production of adrenalin, which was floating around my system and wearing me down. I have huge swings of energy levels for this very reason, but as a certified lifeskills consultant for the last two and a half years I know how to combat it – but only after actually burning myself out.

I started to reflect on my day, remembering that morning when, despite the map, I still had to ask two people for directions. I had chosen those people carefully, realising it is always best to follow the crowd even if it does take me a little off the path I need.

I would text my husband when we passed the station just before my destination, so I would not have to wait outside the train station. I always feel uncomfortable hanging around anywhere in case someone approaches me; being inconspicuous in public is what I aim for. Yet, I am naturally confident, a bit of a performer at heart. I used to love attention and being able to speak up, the feeling of putting myself out there and making what I hoped would be a positive and inspiring influence. I had been a lecturer and had ambitions to become a public speaker before 2000. Little did I know that that ambition would unwittingly be made real when I was asked to speak of my attack at two political party conferences in London and Brighton 10 months after I had been stabbed.

I was sponsored to speak by Lilly (makers of anti-depressant and other prescribed drugs) who had contacted me through the Zito Trust. The Zito Trust was mentioned to me by my cousin's husband in response to my desperation and near madness at trying to understand this crazy stabbing episode in my life. The Zito Trust gave me purpose through my recovery and helped me to make some meaning of what had happened to me. I had fought to save my life that January night and I needed to continue to fight for something bigger – to raise the importance of mental health issues and the safety of us all in the midst of it in an attempt to look at why supports were failing so many families. I realise as I read this back to my family for editing and my voice is breaking and my tears starting to flow, that it is a fight I still continue to make.

Normally I get dropped off at work and collected by my husband of 5 years; my marriage at the time of my big life-affecting event had ended some 7 years previously. If my husband wasn't on standby to drop me anywhere I would drive myself as long as I had already worked out the details of where to park and how to walk safely to my destination with minimum risk. I used to be such an independent and adventurous woman and realise even now that I have curbed this natural spirit. This realisation is a bit of a revelation as it took me a long time to reach a good level of confidence following my own childhood ordeals and teenage angst. I realise that the 2000 event knocked a massive amount of that confidence out of me and I am still in the re-building phase whilst remaining on red alert for an incident or less enlightened or considerate person to shake it for me again! I understand this fragile confidence needs strengthening every day, so my work in lifeskills serves me well.

Back to my train journey. I was just about to plug my headphones into my mobile phone to listen to something soothing and relaxing and to slow the pace of my heart and regulate my breathing when I was momentarily distracted by the loud and assertive voice of a belligerent sounding man on crutches who wanted someone to move their bags from an empty seat. I was glad to be one row further up the aisle towards the exit in front of this noisy, dishevelled and unpleasantly odorous man. I was glad he wasn't sat next to me and was at least one seat to the side of me, as I did not want him directly behind me (I had been attacked from behind and was always watching my own back so to speak!). I carried on with my relaxation and recovery plan and someone much cleaner, fresher, anonymous and female took the vacant seat next to me – perfect! As the train pulled into the next station the anonymous lady left. I sent a text to my husband and settled back into my seat again.

All of a sudden the belligerent man pipes up,

"Oh you want to go to the toilet? Well I suppose I have to move then!"

With that I find the same odorous man leaning into the space created by the woman who had left. He was asking permission to sit next me. My stomach contracted and my heart sank as I heard myself say,

"You're welcome to sit there."

As per my lifeskills training I remember my stress combat techniques to focus on my breathing and smile to look calm and to ease tension. I quickly re-frame my panic-inducing thoughts aiming to compose myself and appear non-plussed on the outside. The image of a duck sprang to mind; I was apparently gliding along on the surface whilst paddling like mad underneath the water. This is my coping mechanism and much more useful than the previous ones that caused me to avoid and avert rather than live through such experiences successfully. I laughed inside at the image of me being a duck, since my maiden name is Swan, so I upgraded my mental image to the more graceful one, which reaped yet more dividends as I began to be more graceful. This was particularly effective as the man beside me struck up a most poignant conversation.

He told me that he had just been in court as his brother had been killed in a knife attack. He himself was frightened to be in the town where the case was being heard and felt under threat of attack at the court. He was feeling unsure of how to get to his destination as he did not know the train timetable and which platform he needed to change trains. He was supposed to be going to London the next day for an official matter but was weary from life and his disability which necessitated the crutches. He was also just recovering from the shock of his sister dying from cancer and had already lost other siblings to this disease. This man, who told me he was 60 years old, was obviously battling his way through his day and his life. It seemed obvious to me then that he felt he had to shout for his seat for his voice to be heard; he wanted someone to care and offer him support. I felt aghast at what he told me as this was my first venture out into the wider world since returning to the town where I lived only a few short months ago. For the previous five years I had been living in a self-imposed exile in the West of Ireland to stabilise my life.

This was a reminder that knife crime still remains a real threat, people still struggle to get much needed support, and to many, life seems bleak. This man was proud of his age and actually thought he looked younger than his years. I suspect the fact he had the attention of a seemingly kind, smiling lady, with a softly spoken voice who gave him a listening ear, encouraged conversation with interested questions and offered a mild compliment, boosted him a little after his tough day. I was stunned to perceive that he looked 20 years older than his years and bore all the hallmarks of a man who had endured prolonged hardship. He was actually younger than my parents, both of whom have had it tough, but he looked a lot older than them. I am of the opinion that how well we wear our age has generally got something to do with the support we have to help us in life, the ability to distract ourselves from the downward spiral of negative rumination, and the making of a conscious choice to be positive rather than negative. I am not convinced I could have been so sure of this before, but experience is a great teacher if you allow it to be.

The past

So this is the bit that I have procrastinated over writing! It is not that I am "not over it", it is just that since that evening in January 2000, I have spent so much time stuck in the incident, when I was nearly murdered, that I am a little reluctant to re-visit it yet again. It is still so surreal yet I know that it was me in the nightmare of that night.

I truly thought it was my final night on this earth and that thought was most distressing to me as I lay in the ambulance having been rescued from a large pool of blood that spurted and flowed like fountains from my multiple knife wounds. I watched this happen as I lay on the ground kicking out at my attacker, unable to get to my feet as he had pulled me down from behind in an attempt to slash my neck. At first my racing brain thought I was being mugged for my handbag. When I saw the glint of the knifepoint in the glare of the streetlamps I screamed, but the shock somehow contorted the sound into something barely audible as human.

I was terrified, not just for me and the potential loss of my life, but also as the mother of my eldest child. I so wanted to be there for her, she needed me; I had waited so long to become a mother after my failed pregnancies. Now I had got there I was about to be cheated of the chance to fulfil that ambition. Thankfully, I am here and am so very grateful for that. Quite simply it was millimetres that made the difference as the knifeman was intent on murder. He was going for main arteries but missed by the tiniest amount. My daughter, who was then four and half years old, turned up at the scene with her dad to find the pool of blood, the ambulance and the police. We were new to our area and did not know anyone well enough to leave her with, otherwise she would have been spared this trip. It is a memory that caused her to be almost hysterical for years whenever she saw the slightest amount of blood. Thank God, she seems to be growing out of that now as she has matured into a young teenager.

The knife nicked my toes and fingers as I used them to defend myself and I could see people in the restaurant across the road and at the fast food outlet a few feet away from me looking on motionless. I was spinning and rocking on the ground, unable to co-ordinate my movements to get up whilst keeping the attacker within my sights. It was like some weird break-dance routine, and all the while my brain was calculating, anticipating and plotting the most effective course of action. I soon realised that my attacker was not giving up on his mission and I was the only one who could make him stop before he killed me. I grabbed him by the balls and squeezed as though my life depended on it, shouting for help. I finally let go when I saw some men running towards us from the restaurant and the Dojo, where I had been, as he proceeded to run away. My eyes never left him, even when he was caught by my instructors who were martial arts champions, and who held him until the police arrived.

The wife of the man from the restaurant knelt on the ground next to me and put my head in her lap as she tried to soothe me. I was hysterical and, seeing the huge blood loss, felt sure I would die right there and then. Someone arrived with tea towels from the restaurant to stem the blood and the husband of my comforter held my legs up to try to reduce the flow. I started feeling my consciousness slipping and wanted to be kept awake, terrified that if my eyes closed they would never again open. My rescuers were doing a magnificent job of talking to me and asking me lots of questions to keep me alert as a first-aider gave instructions down a mobile phone. All the while I was petrified that the loud squealing knifeman who was struggling with his captors might break free and come back to finish the work he had started. This fear remained with me for many months afterwards as the flashbacks and lucid dreams persisted.

I was whisked off to hospital to the sound of wailing sirens. My wounds were examined, bathed and cleaned as they checked how long it was since eating for the anaesthetic and surgery. The wounds needed packing and stitching and I had to have a routine battery of tests. My husband was distraught and in disbelief; he knew the tragedies that had befallen me before. Part of me felt so sorry for having to put him through this again, and I felt exactly the same for my poor parents who had also suffered with me before and would no doubt have to find the money to get from Ireland to see me in the midst of their own health and financial challenges. Still I was alive and, once I was suitably patched and covered up, my little girl would be able to come and see me to feel reassured that I was okay. What a bloody night, no pun intended, what a bloody life; it was just one thing after another!

The next day it was all action stations; police, radio and news reports, medical visits to explain my care plan, work colleagues, family calls, appointments missed and notifications to be made and, oh my God, my car! That would surely get a parking ticket. All useful in the scheme of distraction and positive motivation but so draining too; yet more things to organise and have energy for. I did not ask for this drama or diversion but yet here it was and I had to work out, why me? As it happens I was able to answer that later as I realised it was not personal, but it was significant insofar as it has influenced the rest of my life.

The man who had tried to kill me was under orders that night to kill a woman, any woman, to please the love of his life! This young man, who was in his 20s, lived in a community home round the corner from where I trained and was a registered mental health patient who had had increasingly delusional episodes. He was convinced that, by committing this murderous act, the voluptuous, blond, bathing beauty from a popular TV show would become his girlfriend, if he made this sacrifice for her. The message was given to him through his television set by a well-known actress. I later discovered that this man was known for his activities. He had previously attacked at least one other woman. This information came to me as hearsay and apparently sectioning had been considered but due to staffing challenges and bureaucracy was just left to go unaddressed by the near retirement house manager, despite the serious concerns of his care team. This was later corroborated in the recommendations from the ensuing internal report. An independent enquiry was requested but as I was not dead this was not supported.

The detectives came two days later to take my statement. I felt under scrutiny, uncomfortable and vulnerable in my nightdress and dressing gown in a small room with these large, authoritative and assertive men. I was glad to have my husband with me as at least I could trust him. I was later to develop a slight paranoia about men, but then started to challenge that in a perversely daring way by meeting Internet dates when my first marriage broke up. It was through the Internet that I met my current husband, although we did have friends in common, so I could check him out to some extent.

My recovery from the night of the knife attack was fraught with difficulties. My house had been on the market since Christmas and our respective families were aware that we had agreed our marriage was over. This made things harder psychologically as catholic guilt was upon us. We were already feeling wretched at breaking our vows and failing our young child, despite all the attempts we had made to save the marriage prior to that fateful night. Now I felt like God was punishing me yet again. As part of my treatment, anti-depressants were prescribed to help me be less emotional. I understand the need to reduce nervous arousal but it is not actually what I believe works effectively and they only served to make me feel less like myself and more like a patient with compromised insurance premiums and future job prospects. Perception is, after all, reality. I called on victim support to help me through the first few months.

The Crown Prosecution Service contacted me just as I was making progress and was on a reduced hours return-to-work programme. They wanted blood samples and I remember feeling absolutely distraught and angry that they had not asked for these at the hospital. I was being interfered with again and had had enough discomfort.

One day as I was getting dressed my young daughter saw the damage to my legs which were black, blue and purple. She stopped in her tracks and said,

"Oh mummy, I am so, so sorry that the naughty man hurt you so much."

I wondered what kind of impression this lovely young mind, my child, had of the world; it ripped at my heart. The Crown Prosecution Service was in touch on a regular basis to update on the progress of the hearings. On more than one occasion the attacker was deemed unfit to attend court. I must admit at first I believed it to be a ploy and that it was simply a strategy to allow an evil person to evade justice. I had heard of many cases before that had claimed mental illness as a reason for such attacks and like many thought that this was a well-worn excuse. Having seen the man in question at a hearing a year later I believe if he was not mentally ill at the time of the attack then he sure was not well at court. He seemed to have gained a lot of weight, with big bulging eyes and did not seem to be quite there. All the terror was with me seeing him flanked by guards, as I had heard of a case in court where someone had jumped the dock and attacked a witness. The next big court case was heard about 18 months later. This was the one that I had been waiting for; it would bring some closure to the event that had disrupted my life. Until that time I felt that I was dominated by the attack and fearful that my attacker could escape any time, even though I was told he was being detained in a secure unit.

The day in court was nerve-wracking. I knew my evidence was crucial; the one thing that I was grateful for was that I had not taken my eyes off him that night until the police had arrived and taken him. If I had had to rely on description only I am not sure how well I would have been able to do that. If I had had to point him out, even in court, his appearance had changed to such an extent that I would not have felt 100% sure. I see why cases can be hard to prove. I tried to imagine how his family felt in court that day and felt sad for them. I thought if it had been a son of mine I would have apologised to the victim for the pain and anguish caused.

The outcome was that the attacker was sent to a secure hospital until deemed fit by the Home Secretary to leave. There was no feeling of celebration, just deep sadness for us all to have walked this path. Who knows where he is now. I hope that wherever he is, he is well and that people around him are safe.

From here on in

That night in January 2000 left its mark. My job went downhill as I struggled to cope with the pressures of having to take on a new role. Also my marriage break-up and moving out of my house took longer than we had planned due to the impending court case and my recovery time. I was seeing a counsellor and eventually felt better when I asked for referral for post-traumatic stress. I also saw a psychiatrist as I felt I was somewhat out of control and was beginning to take ridiculous risks. Thankfully this was short-lived and the post-trauma session helped me to gain an understanding about why people on the scene that night appeared to be standing back and not helping me.

I decided that I needed to get back to teaching again and somehow managed to re-train to be a specialist in literacy. All the while I had a fascination with understanding people with mental illness. I needed to do some teaching work experience and ironically was offered a slot teaching "special needs" adults with learning difficulties, many of whom were intellectually, mentally and physically challenged. To my surprise I found the work very rewarding and this eased my curiosity. I was later offered a lecturer's post working with disadvantaged young adults with emotional and behavioural issues. I learned that we all need love, support, understanding and encouragement to be all that we can be. I learned that we can promote goodness and happiness and show that we care. I learned too that mental illness will touch nearly all of us in our lifetime, if not directly then at least someone close.

The years in between brought other challenges for me that included me witnessing, reporting and experiencing bullying at work; more miscarriages; and three more house moves as I struggled to gain stability for myself. I went through a few more episodes of being prescribed anti-depressants and other drugs to help me recover from grief and post-natal depression. The journey has allowed me wonderful opportunities to work on myself as well as allow others to do the same with counselling, massage therapy, personal development workshops, cognitive-behavioural therapy, and physical therapy in various forms. I have benefited from them all, apart from the anti-depressants. For me drugs failed to meet my emotional needs; I believe that human connections and emotional re-connection with "self" does that to best effect.

In 2007 the best turn of events happened when I realised I had come so far but needed to sustain my stability and that is when I trained in lifeskills consultancy. The wonderful thing is that it has enabled me to work with others and to see them strengthen and grow forwards into their life challenges. I facilitate groups, training and workshops as well as one-to-one consultations with the express aim of stress reduction and goal orientation. I am a firm believer that this holistic approach serves us best as we are all individual and need to be treated as such. This work has brought me face-to-face with the most fragile of people, some of whom are in the mental healthcare system. I think that if Lifeskills were on the school curriculum and were supported by the NHS then the mental health of the nation would improve. Of course on the other hand, there would be the decline in the prescription of drugs; sadly, it seems that the health of the nation lies firmly in the hands of the pharmaceutical industry.

I actively seek to work with people who are depressed, dejected, frightened, angry, defeated, disillusioned, despairing, desperate and often self-destructive or at least self-deprecating. I want to somehow show them that there is comfort, hope and laughter left; there is untapped talent and potential for greatness latent in us all; that life can be fulfilling and less painful. I love that there is such a great variety of people, places and adventures to be had in this world. I want to continue to promote well-being and offer and develop appropriate supports that enable and empower us to be more independent yet considerate of others. I want to live and let live, yet ease the struggle that we can all encounter in this life with an open heart and mind. I am conscious that underlying it all is my experience that informs me that danger lurks amidst all the wonder and beauty upon which I choose to focus. I am left with the knowledge that life and people are very fragile and the understanding that my life and yours is precious. I can say this because not only have I nearly lost my life in this decade but also in the previous one. I have also lost five babies through miscarriage and a brother from an asthma-related death when I was nine years old. The point is, it is all cumulative and when the Big One hits, it really can be like a Tsunami, smashing everything in its path.

CHAPTER 6

From hero, to hospital, to hope: A carer's experience

Jane Wood

We were an ordinary family, two parents, my brother and I. My brother was my hero, all who met him loved him; his personality was warm, kind and generous, he was fun to be with as well as intelligent and talented. There was rarely a dull moment when he was around and he could always make me laugh when I was sad. We had a shared interest which resulted in us spending time and studying at university together, graduating at the same time and cementing our adult relationship as friends. I trusted him, respected him, yet worried about his "live life to the full" philosophy. Whilst our lives took different paths, mine fairly conventional, his anything but, we remained close and enjoyed each other's company.

Over a period of 12 months, a few years later, my family and I became extremely concerned about his health, not really understanding what was happening. He became more distant, was hospitalised for self-harm, and eventually diagnosed with schizoaffective disorder. Although we had experienced other family members with mental health issues, it was a shock to receive the news that he had schizophrenia. After a few months in hospital, escaping overnight and not wanting to see us, he was placed on medication and discharged to a half-way house having been categorised as "homeless". He was placed in a YMCA, a large and isolating place with minimal supervision from a social worker and psychiatrist. He was just left to get on with it.

Later that year I left to go travelling for several months but kept in touch via email. About a month before I was due back the tone of his email alerted a "sixth sense" that things weren't right. It wasn't what he said; it was the language he used. I rang my mother expressing concern and she said she'd spoken to him; he had explained and seemed OK.

After I had returned from travelling we were due to go away for a weekend to mark a family celebration. Over the weekend he displayed some strange behaviour; my mother, father and I sat discussing it in the hotel bedroom. My brother had told my mother that he wasn't feeling well and was due to visit his psychiatrist at the end of the week. It transpired that he had been reducing his medication under the psychiatrist's supervision and was told to contact her if he needed to. A patient with a serious mental illness was given responsibility to monitor his condition and seek help if necessary. As a family, we knew small bits about the condition, little about the signs and symptoms and almost nothing about the risks.

We returned to my parent's house and I went to bed, I awoke to find I was being violently attacked by my brother who had a knife and was trying to cut my throat. I screamed and, with the help of my parents, wrestled the knife off him, pinned him down, and phoned the police. It was like my brother was possessed and had superhuman strength. Eventually the police arrived, cuffed and arrested him. My father and I went to hospital to have our wounds treated, which luckily were not life-threatening, but it would not be over-dramatic to say I had had a near death experience, inflicted by the person I cared for most in the world. That night our "normal" family life ended and a nightmare began.

My memory of the next two months is hazy, my brain's way of protecting me from the emotional pain. In summary, my brother was under a different health authority to the one my parents lived in, therefore the local authority was not willing to section a clearly very ill man until an appropriate bed was found by his own health authority (the police told us there was no bed in the whole country). He was therefore detained in the hospital wing of the local prison. As a family we knew he needed help desperately, all we wanted was for him to be treated in a psychiatric hospital. The next few weeks consisted of my parents undertaking prison visits, and a daily ritual of several hours on the phone between health, social and police services, trying to ensure that he received the treatment he so desperately needed. Eventually his health authority found a suitable forensic hospital placement. Before he moved, I found the courage to have a single visit with him in prison. Whenever I drive past those prison walls my heart still lurches at the thought of what transpired. How many other mentally ill patients, who don't have families to support and fight for them, are locked behind those walls?

Finally, he was transferred to the forensic hospital and on reflection the rehabilitation and treatment he received was of a very high standard, but I am plagued by the question; why did I have to nearly lose my life before he received the necessary care? Why does someone have to commit a serious offence to be given the treatment they deserve?

After my brother reached the forensic hospital and gave permission for our family to be kept informed about his medical treatment, the hospital and professionals began to see us as an integral part of his rehabilitation and we were able to contact the staff, attend Care Programme Approach meetings and begin to understand what was going on. The police, wishing to pursue the court case, asked my father and I to make statements. We could get no legal advice due to our familial relationship with the "accused" and so had no one to advise us. This is where my support from the forensic hospital became vital, I rang and spoke to my brother's psychiatrist who advised me that to have him charged would ensure that he received the best treatment and would not get "lost in the system", as he required lifelong supervision. It is disgraceful that you have to prosecute someone to ensure they receive adequate medical care, but I took the advice. This was incredibly traumatic for all the family as it seemed until the last moment that I would be called to give testimony against my own brother in the crown court. Thankfully, I didn't have to. I decided not to attend the trial because, although I was trying to support my brother, I didn't want that lasting memory of him being brought into court in handcuffs.

Things settled down and it has taken three years of rehabilitation for my brother to be well enough to undertake the next move to supervised accommodation, where he is now. During that time my family and I have participated in family therapy provided by the hospital and this has been invaluable in allowing us to discuss the traumatic event and how we could move forward as a family. The hospital staff included us and informed us and were there to help support us emotionally. Without this I would not have been able to rebuild my relationship. I still have accompanied visits with a nurse and have yet to decide when I will feel able to be with my brother on my own.

Victim Support was a life-line through the initial trauma; I was unable to work for five months, so suffered financially. Although I wouldn't want my brother to have had poorer treatment, I, as the victim, had to seek support through my GP. I had to wait five months prior to receiving any initial counselling, which unfortunately I did not find helpful. After a further assessment I was eventually referred on for psychotherapy after 18 months, which was helpful. While I waited for NHS counselling, the support we were given by the forensic hospital allowed our family to re-form, in a different way. We have still not all been together after four years, but would not be where we are had we not been included by the forensic hospital staff.

I have been through hell and back; I was the victim of a violent attack; I lost the trust in someone I cared for, someone who was my hero; but I desperately wanted to support my brother too. I have been putting my life back together and things are looking up; I am getting married shortly, but even this happy event has been affected, as I have had to take the painful decision to exclude my brother.

I want to dedicate this short story to the courage of my family, who have all been brave, and as a result have something to celebrate. I have the utmost admiration for my brother's acceptance of his situation and illness, I couldn't have suffered the loss of freedom and indignities he has had to face with such grace. I hope you can still feel my continued admiration, although our relationship will never and can never be the same carefree one it was once. This has only been made possible by the hard work of the forensic hospital staff. Do not underestimate the importance of your role, not just to the patient, but also to their family and victims.

Acknowledgements

The Editors would like to thank Michael Howlett, Director of the former Zito Trust for allowing us to use this organisation's website to request contributions from survivors/victims of offences; and to Frances Barrone and "Jane Wood" for kindly contributing their experiences.

CHAPTER 7

Ethical and legal issues of culture, spirituality, diversity and equality in forensic nursing

Mary A Addo

Introduction

The culture of nursing refers to the learned and transmitted life ways, values, symbols, patterns and normative practices of members of the nursing profession of a particular society (Bjarnason et al 2009). This implies that to serve the unique and diverse needs of clients in the forensic nursing context in the United Kingdom, it is essential that all stakeholders have knowledge and an understanding of the importance of culture, spirituality, diversity and equality (CSDE). This requires the recognition and valuing of CSDE by nurses, including examining their own health-related values and beliefs, in addition to those of the health organisations in which they work. Without this values clarification awareness, it will not be possible to champion the principle of respect for persons and the ideals of transcultural care (Blofeld 2003, Addo 2006a, Byrt et al 2007, Bjarnason et al 2009).

The attention being drawn to the impact of CSDE is to ensure that bad forensic nursing practice based on ignorance through lack of underpinning knowledge, discrimination and unfair treatment, as experienced by clients, is prevented in the context of care provision (Department of Health and Home Office 1992, Blofeld 2003, Addo 2006a, Byrt et al 2007, Addo and Smith 2008). These are important factors that need to be considered in the design, commissioning, provision, and delivery of forensic services to persons from diverse socio-economic, cultural, ethnic, religious and political backgrounds (Fernando 2002, Scottish Executive 2006a, Byrt et al 2007, Mental Welfare Commission of Scotland 2007). Embedding these values in practices shows respect for clients' perspectives and their rightful participation as equal partners in the decision making process regarding their care and treatment (Millan Principles 2001, HM Government Equality Acts 2006, 2010, Scottish Executive 2006b).

This chapter presents some of the ethical and legal issues involved in CSDE, through promoting client autonomy, choice and confidentiality, seeking informed consent, and involving clients in the decision-making process. An argument is posited that addressing the CSDE issues in forensic nursing practice can only serve to raise the public profile of this specialised field, and contribute to excellent care and treatment experiences of all clients and their families. In this chapter, strategies are suggested to help maximise the therapeutic efficacy of stakeholders' actions. This involves respecting their clients' needs, where CSDE are critical components of their existence as fellow humans, in order to enable scarce health resources to be used more efficiently.

Context

Culture, spirituality, diversity and equality are issues that challenge the philosophies underpinning contemporary forensic nursing. They are influenced by professional ethical and legal codes to guide professional practice, which place a high premium on respect for persons, and this respect occurs regardless of the diversity issues present. These ethical and legal codes directly or indirectly impact on the treatment and care outcome for forensic clients (International Council of Nurses Code of Ethics 2006, HM Government Equality Acts 2006, 2010, NMC 2008). CSDE are concepts that challenge forensic nurses and service providers to reflect and examine their values base. This does not sit comfortably with the multi-dimensional elements of diversity in professionals' assessment of clients' psychopathology and pathophysiology issues. Neither does it accord with various social and political problems of service provision and delivery, and the treatment and care practices that do not take into account the total personhood of the client (Swinton 2000, 2001, Swinton and Boyd 2002, Addo 2006a, Mohr 2006, NHS Education for Scotland 2009). As forensic nurses are called upon to conduct assessments that enable decisions to be made about appropriate interventions for care and treatment provision for clients, it is prudent that they have a current working knowledge of the legal framework and ethical codes that should underpin their actions.

Respect for expansion in client autonomy is seen as one of the fundamentals of healthcare ethics (Gillon 1986, Downie and Calman 1994). Issues of autonomy, informed consent, and promoting choice immediately come to mind when we consider the Nursing and Midwifery Council (NMC) (2008) Code of Conduct for nurses, the mental health legislation and in examining the ethical dimensions of clinical practice (Scott et al 2003). The focus on partnership working in healthcare delivery and engaging with the client's perspective in the planning and delivery of care are also indicated in policy documents (Human Rights Act 1998, Millan Principles 2001, Department of Health 2001a, 2001b, Scottish Executive 2006a, 2006b, NMC 2008).

In fact, Wallace (2000) maintains that policy developments, extended roles within healthcare practice, clinical governance, and human rights legislation have brought further obligations for nurses to ensure that the client is an active and informed participant in the process of consent. The UK is one of the most diverse countries in the world, and although such diversity gives us the opportunity for social inclusion and cultural interactions, this opportunity can also at times pave the way for poor healthcare practices experienced by minority ethnic client groups (Fernando 2002, Blofeld 2003, Cortis 2004, HM Government Equality Act 2006, Byrt et al 2007, NHS Health Scotland 2010).

The human condition described as a mental disorder has no respect for an individual's economic, social, cultural, or socioeconomic standing in society; sexual orientation; race; ethnicity; or language. This disorder knows no boundaries, colour or creed. No amount of fame, social standing and wealth will protect an individual from its reach, whether young or old, beautiful or ugly (Addo 2001). All humans in any given society have the same right for shelter, warmth and food, and the same opportunities for leisure and recreation, meaningful work and effective support in order to take control and live a fulfilling life as a fellow human being (Human Rights Act 1998, Millan 2001, HM Government Equality Act 2006, Mental Health (Care and Treatment) (Scotland) Act 2003, Scottish Executive 2006a, 2006b).

The context and methods of practice guidelines used within the forensic environments to prevent bad practice, client abuse and exploitation; protect client's rights; empower; and prevent harm are matters of concern (Gallop 1998, Human Rights Act 1998, Blofeld 2003, Millan 2001, HM Government Equality Act 2006). The NMC (2008) Code of Professional Conduct states: "You must not discriminate against those in your care". This statement makes clear the value position of the NMC on matters of CSDE in contemporary nursing practice.

Nurses' work with clients is not based on just the principles of duty, altruism or necessity, but also on an employment contract for which they are paid. At the same time, nurses do not relinquish their individual character, personal beliefs and values in their perception of self when they adopt the professional nurse role (Addo 2006b, Mohr 2006). It is the co-existence of these personal values and the professional expectations required of forensic nurses that present legal and ethical challenges for them in their work. It is therefore essential that nurses explore the ethical and legal issues of relevance to CSDE. This includes, firstly, the client within the forensic service; secondly, the approaches to assessment and how care and treatment interventions are undertaken from admission to discharge and follow-up support; and, thirdly, the forensic service provider (HM Government 1992, Blofeld, 2003, Mental Welfare Commission 2009). Any aspect of these three areas can be negatively impacted upon if the concepts of CSDE are not given due regard in the decision-making process of service design and delivery for forensic clients.

Culture care: "Knowing me knowing you"

There are culturally embedded ideas regarding the interpretation of causes of illness and disease which may differ widely from medical and nursing aetiologies. Symptoms of mental illness have cultural meanings which individuals will interpret and respond to differently (Marsella 1980, Chalanda 1995, Fernando 2002). It is therefore important for forensic nurses to understand the knowledge and complexity of CSDE and their relevance to care and treatment outcomes for clients. CSDE issues have been widely acknowledged in the forensic nursing literature and policy documents (Swinton 2001, Swinton and Boyd 2002, Department of Health 2005a, 2005b, Mohr 2006, Addo 2006a, Byrt et al 2007, Addo and Smith 2009, NHS Education for Scotland 2009). The impact of CSDE on illness, health, and healthcare delivery in any given context cannot be overlooked as these are important aspects of any individual human being, and evidence shows that lack of attention in helping clients to meet these areas of their "being" can impact negatively on their health and well-being (Post et al 2000, Mohr 2006, NHS Education for Scotland 2009). However, not all cultures subscribe to the Western notion of "autonomy" and therefore it is important for the care provider to understand the client's cultural world view, for it is through this cultural "lens" that understanding through interpretation of the client's perceptions occurs as to his or her "ontological being" in the nursing care context.

In a recent scoping exercise undertaken by NHS Scotland (2008) with black and minority ethnic groups on perceptions of mental well-being in Scotland, it was reported that there are differences within cultures in conceptualisations of what mental health and mental illness is. The report provides insights into how this view is inextricably linked to family well-being, spiritual well-being and material well-being, with emphasis on the importance of social roles and connectedness. Having knowledge about what an individual is dealing with, it can be argued, empowers that individual, and, in the context of nursing work, it is the knowledge of the nurse that gives nurses the self-confidence in their role, that they translate into their interactions with clients. When that knowledge is not present, it means the interaction with forensic clients will not be based on sound professional knowledge and judgement (Addo 2006a).

Non-maleficence, the ethical principle that requires prevention of risks of treatment and harm to patients, can at times be challenged by the belief that good treatment effects outweigh the bad effects. This is evident in the over-use of major neuroleptic drugs in the treatment of clients of African-Caribbean origin placed in forensic care settings, a situation of concern to many (Department of Health and Home Office 1992, Blofeld 2003, Addo 2006a, Byrt et al 2007). Perspectives reflect the need for values clarification of all stakeholders involved in forensic service provision for clients from different cultures, whose belief systems and practices appear inconsistent with the care providers' own (HM Government 1992, Fernando 2002, Blofeld 2003, Addo 2006a, Byrt et al 2007). Respecting the client's cultural perspective and rights is one of the key ways of enabling clients' autonomy to be operationalised in the context of healthcare (Scott et al 2003).

Communication styles within cultures varies and while some cultures encourage outward expression of both positive and negative emotions openly, other cultures practise restraint in showing negative emotions publicly, and others value harmony, and therefore adopt a more indirect non-verbal communication (Chalanda 1995, Johnstone and Olga 2009). This means that the communication styles adopted by stakeholders in the clients' care and treatment, are crucial. There has to be an awareness of language use and linguistic meanings, communication styles, age, gender and the perceived quality of the relationship with the client, as all these can influence the negotiation process (Peplau 1991, Chalanda 1995, Arnold and Boggs 2003, Barker 2009). Issues of providing information for clients and opportunities to get involved in decision-making regarding their care are crucial elements in promoting client autonomy in working with CSDE, in order to make a positive difference to their lives (Scottish Executive 2006a, 2006b).

Chalanda (1995) asserts that familiarity with a particular culture facilitates negotiations through the process of culture-brokering, which is defined as the act of bridging, linking or mediating between groups or persons for the purpose of reducing conflict or producing change (Jezeweski 1990, 1993). Cultural-brokering's potential lies in helping to shift the dimensions of care the client is given and promotes the connection between the client and his or her cultural supportive networks, and further enhances the client's coping skills in how he or she reacts to the illness experience. To achieve this with the client will draw on the knowledge, clinical wisdom and values of stakeholders as service providers and on how they enact the mental health legislation and ethical codes of practice to make a positive health and social difference to the forensic client's situation (NMC 2008,

Box 7.1. Understanding the legislation

- Have up-to-date knowledge and understanding of the workings of the Act
- Know the patient's rights and responsibilities in relation to the particular detention order as applied
- Be familiar with and understand the documentation and recording processes and channels of communication involved
- Know the roles of members of the multi-disciplinary team and their contribution to this process
- Know the implications of the Act to engaging and providing care for the patient/ family, and working in partnership with other agencies
- Support the patient/family to gain an understanding of the implications of the Act in providing care for the relative
- Know and understand the 10 Essential Shared Capabilities for engaging and working with people diagnosed with mental health problems in Scotland.

Adapted from Scottish Executive (2003)

Scottish Executive 2003a, 2006b, HM Government Equality Act 2006, NHS Education for Scotland 2009). For the forensic nurse this can be achieved through the understandings listed in *Box 7.1*.

Making the gift of time (Barker 2001, 2003) to listen to the client's world view is the cornerstone in helping to lay the foundations for cultural brokerage where mutuality of understanding on both sides can be achieved. This is important as the client's world view needs to be identified and discussed with him or her, prior to any informed consent for proposed treatment interventions proceeds (Chalanda 1995). According to Jezeweski (1990, 1993) cultural brokering makes important contributions to client care (see *Box 7.2*).

Box 7.2. Benefits of cultural brokering

- Break barriers that cause misunderstanding between client and care provider
- Assist the nurse in adopting more culturally appropriate communication and intervention styles
- Nurse should have the respect of both parties
- Nurse should have knowledge of both systems
- Nurse should be able to introduce and translate ideas into a language understood by both parties/systems

Quoted from Jezeweski (1990; 1993)

Values clarification

Equality and diversity: "my values", "your values", "our values"

The Dalai Lama (2002) gives a thoughtful assertion on how values clarification can enable humanistic engagement when he asserts that knowledge is important, but more important is the use towards which it is put; that the use of knowledge depends on the heart and mind of the one who uses it. Equality and diversity are about the whole person. They are about treating people fairly according to their needs, and making this normal practice and behaviour in what we do as nurses. Diversity is about respecting and working positively with differences (HM Government Equality Acts 2006, 2010, NHS Education for Scotland 2009); and being non-judgemental is one of the key professional attributes expected of the registered nurse (NMC 2008) in any given context.

Forensic nurses are individuals with their own beliefs and value systems, having been socialised by the culture from which they originate, with further socialisation coming through joining the nursing profession, to think and conduct one's self in a particular manner in the chosen field of specialised practice (NMC 2008, Bjarnason et al 2009). In the socialisation process some nurses are able to maintain a check between the "self" they know and the "self" as a nurse, this showing how self-aware the person is (Rawlinson 1990, Mohr 2006). Cameron (2003) asserts that nurses with good character traits would not exploit others for personal gain; therefore each nurse has a moral responsibility to know his or her ethical self.

However, a conflict of interest arises when the professional self cannot harmonise with the opposing views originating from the personal self in engaging with forensic clients. This can lead to ethical dilemmas, resulting in the forensic nurse asking questions, such as, "What is the right thing to do in this situation?", when the client's world views and value systems are different from that of the nurse (Cameron 2003, Mohr 2006).

Liaschenko (1994) asserts that nurses do recognise such conflict situations as an ethical concern which calls into question the moral standing of the individual nurse, a situation that, if not managed carefully, can contradict what the Code of Professional Conduct (NMC 2008) expects of nurses in working with clients, regardless of any differences that exist. Austin (2001) provides an answer to this dilemma, asserting that, within the nurse–client relationship, there are the issues of non-maleficence, beneficence, autonomy and justice which the nurse must use to guide moral practice within the professional relationship.

Furthermore, how nurses perceive forensic clients, whether as individuals, patients, perpetrators or prisoners, will inevitably influence how they engage with them (Addo 2000). This inevitably will create tensions in individual nurses, therefore the quality and intensity of their engagement with clients in the therapeutic alliance can be precarious. The ability of nurses to develop and maintain professional relationships with their clients is a competence expected of every nurse (NMC 2008). The nature and quality of the nurse–client relationship is generally perceived as essential for the helping relationship, and the need to establish trust with clients is a core principle for nursing and a pre-requisite for therapy. Woods et al (2002) assert that the essence of forensic nursing is in the essential foundations of the nurse–patient relationship, the vehicle by which all interventions proceed.

Arnold and Boggs (2003) contend that an essential component of the successful implementation of the therapeutic relationship between the nurse and client is self-knowledge which, they argue, is the precursor to professionalism. This means that as individuals we are what we have become in terms of our personalities and the world views we hold which are a product of our early socialisation and other experiences encountered in life. Therefore, how the nurse relates to the client in the care situation is influenced by the perception of the self of the nurse (Rawlinson 1990, Addo 2000). Unless nurses are aware of who they are, recognise personal and cultural beliefs, and understand intrapersonal strengths and limitations, it will be difficult for them to attend to the clients' needs and maintain a therapeutic relationship (Boyd 1998). Thus, nurses' self-concept, their personality, and how self-aware they are, can all impact on how they engage and interact with CSDE with clients to whom these concepts are central to their very "being" as fellow humans (Hammer 2000, Addo 2006a).

The therapeutic use of self is an important aspect of client care and requires nurses to have a level of self-awareness of who they are (Barker 2003, 2009). Without this, the nurse's engagement with the client becomes fraught with difficulties, as there will be aspects of the nurse's self which are unknown to him or her, but are unveiled in interactions with clients, which may prove difficult to manage. Such aspects of the nurse's own history may emerge as can any unfinished business in the nurse's personal life. In this situation nurses are confronted with a dilemma of having an unmet need yet being expected to function effectively in their role through therapeutic interactions in their work. This position is what challenges contemporary forensic nurses to reflect on their values clarification in order to fulfil the responsibilities and accountabilities vested in the legal title of registered nurse given to them by the professional regulatory body (NMC 2008).

As nurses we each are accountable for our actions and omissions in practice (NMC 2008), therefore a registered nurse lacking knowledge and understanding of the value and impact of CSDE on a client's health and well-being, raises professional, ethical and legal concerns in relation to clinical effectiveness, assessment and intervention provided to enable the client's recovery process (Scottish Executive 2003a, 2006a, 2006b).

Spirituality

Spirituality includes the acceptance of the whole person (NHS Education Scotland 2009). Spiritual needs of patients are well recognised as enabling the recovery process, giving comfort to patients when faced with the vicissitudes of life struggles. The Royal College of Nursing (2010) supports the promotion of holistic care and asserts that spirituality is important in client care, but that it is a complex area in the diverse field of nursing practice. Nonetheless, despite the recognition of spirituality as an aspect of the human dimension that applies to all of us, it can also be a taboo and misunderstood topic for others in society.

Post et al (2000) maintain that clinical studies have helped to clarify that spirituality and religion can contribute to the coping strategies of many patients with severe, chronic and terminal conditions. Pargament (1997) adds that the key to emotional coping with serious illness and disability is frequently found within the realms of patient spirituality as this provides an interpretive framework for clients in managing the stress of illness. Furthermore, promoting equality rests on promoting spirituality, because it is evidenced that inequality and discrimination can impact on the client's spiritual needs and fulfilment (NHS Education Scotland 2009).

The ethical and legal challenge is whether forensic nurses can attend to the spiritual dimensions of the clients' experiences through discussing spiritual issues raised by the client, and if so, what are the boundaries between the nurse and the client in this context? As mentioned earlier, practising ethically (Millan 2001, Scottish Executive 2006, NMC 2008) means respecting and acknowledging diversity, and working in ways that validate the worth of the person.

As members of communities or groups in society we enter into hospitals with particular spiritual needs which are not shed prior to arriving (Ross 1994). Cameron (2003) indicates that there are important elements underpinning spiritual values (see *Box 7.3*).

The NMC (2008) requires each nurse to treat each client as a unique individual and to foster hope and meaning through collaborative working with the client. Equality, respect for clients' rights and autonomy cannot be achieved in this context if forensic nurses fail in their duty to appreciate the multi-complex and dimensional aspects of diversity, including spirituality. Failing to enable the fulfilment of the client's spiritual needs because the nurse does not share the client's perspective constitutes neglect and omission.

Box 7.3. Spiritual values

- *Compassion*: a good heart filled with loving kindness, humility, forgiveness, patience, and altruism
- *Happiness*: well-being, self-actualisation, human flourishing, and joy
- *Meaning*: seeing one's life as a part of a bigger, purposeful picture
- *Meditation/prayer*: contemplation promoting awareness of self, others, the sacred, and the interconnectedness of everything
- *Peace*: harmony, contentment, and tolerance
- *Spirituality*: evolving towards wholeness and experiencing what is higher, deeper, and greater than self
- *Sacred*: God, infinite, life force, underlying order, higher power, unmoved mover

Quoted from Cameron (2003)

Autonomy and informed consent

The concept of autonomy involves any attempts made to enable choice with reference to the treatment plan, having involved the client in the decision-making process through discussion of the benefits, risks and possible care outcome expected. According to Beauchamp and Childress (1994) respect for autonomy is based on general recognition that individuals have unconditional worth, with capacity to determine their own destiny. Autonomy relates also to respect of individuals' sense of "self", which, when undermined, impacts on self-efficacy and self-directing behaviours and clients' ability to exercise their rights (Scott et al 2003).

When care providers do not pay due regard to involving clients in the decision-making process relating to CSDE this affects their very existence as fellow humans (Downie and Calman, 1994). Informed consent is at the core of the ethical principle of respect and nurses are legally bound and implicated in the process (Draper 1998, NMC 2008). The legal aspect of informed consent requires ensuring that clients have been given information to guide their decision-making based on respect for their autonomy. Such information should be offered verbally and in enough detail to enable the client's understanding of issues discussed, especially when CSDE issues are present. Gaining such understanding of the client's family structure, traditional beliefs and practices, including cultural assessment, are other ways through which forensic nurses and service providers can get to know clients from diverse cultural backgrounds when seeking their informed consent.

The decision-making process is flawed when clients are made to agree and sign a form giving consent, when, in fact, they have not been enabled by the nurse to understand the issues surrounding their treatment. This shows a

Box 7.4. The three principles to achieve cultural understanding

- Clients have the right to have their sociocultural background understood
- Care givers should respond to those needs and use that knowledge
- It is unsafe and unscientific to treat clients alike

Quoted from Chalanda (1995)

lack of respect to the client, and denies him or her the opportunity to exercise self-autonomy and to seek support from advocacy. Such an example can lead to a practice where the client's CSDE needs are not effectively addressed. Research evidence shows the impact of CSDE on clients' reaction to, and coping with, health-related situations (Chalanda 1995, Post et al 2000, Mohr 2006, NHS Education Scotland 2009). Chalanda (1995) argues that clients and practitioners employ different cognitive systems for understanding illness and disease, and proposed three principles to adhere to (see *Box 7.4*).

These three principles indicate that truth-telling by being honest, transparent, sincere and open and with clients is an important ethical principle that forensic nurses should promote in practice to ensure clients' trust in the totality of the forensic service. Truth-telling as part of showing respect to the client requires nurses to show active listening skills and genuineness in their responses to clients' needs. It is therefore unethical for the forensic nurse to be present with the client while the nurse's attention is focused elsewhere (Peplau 1991). The requisite knowledge of whether the client has legal capacity or not, and if considered competent, to make a decision about his or her treatment and care under the mental health legislation, must be considered in relation to: (a) whether or not the client is able to understand and retain information about the proposed treatment, and (b) whether the client is able to weigh the information given to arrive at a choice (Scott et al 2003).

Addo et al (2010) report their research finding of the lack of client involvement in the decision-making process relating to patient observation in acute care and intensive psychiatric care unit settings. A key finding from their study shows informed consent seeking was not routine practice when decisions were made to increase or reduce levels of observations implemented for clients. This demonstrates that working in partnership with clients and promoting their involvement in the decision making process about their care and treatment is an area that needs further championing. The provision of information to clients and/or family members, and their comprehension of the information given, alongside voluntary participation are paramount in the consent seeking process. The lack of client involvement in the decision making process raises concerns regarding the cultural and social context of care and treatment provided. This finding highlights the

Box 7.5. Millan Principles

- *Non-discriminatory*: an individual with a mental disorder retains the same rights and entitlements as a person with any health need
- *Equality*: there should be no direct or indirect discrimination on the grounds of age, gender, sexual orientation, ethnic group or religion
- *Respect for diversity*: all care treatment and support should be given respectfully and with equity in mind
- *Reciprocity*: it is the obligation of health and social services to provide safe and appropriate services
- *Informal care*: if possible, care, treatment and support should be without recourse to compulsory measures
- *Participation*: all service users should be involved in all aspects of care and given information and support to enable them to participate fully
- *Respect for carers*: informal carers should be treated with respect for their role and experience, given information and have their views taken into account
- *Least restrictive alternative*: all necessary treatment and support should be given to service users in the least invasive and restrictive manner and within a compatible environment
- *Benefits*: any intervention should produce a benefit to the service user that cannot be achieved otherwise
- *Child welfare*: welfare of the child is emphasised in relation to any interventions imposed by the Act

Quoted from Millan (2001)

lack of enactment in working with diversity in relation to the Millan (2001) Principles (see *Box 7.5*), which are embedded in the Mental Health (Care and Treatment) Scotland Act (2003) and are viewed as a "blueprint" that will guide the practice of mental health practitioners in their work with clients (Scottish Executive 2003a). This also contradicts further the values-based principles embedded in the Ten Essential Shared Capabilities (see *Box 7.6*) (Scottish Executive 2006b) which promote values-based practice in the delivery of mental health services.

Swinton and Boyd (2002: 136) assert that a dilemma confronted by forensic nurses working with clients relates to being faced with the difficult reality of having to respect the personhood of individuals who show little respect for themselves or for others, who are frequently aggressive and violent, sometimes dishonest, often deceitful, and who may appear to have little or no remorse for the antisocial acts they have perpetrated. Austin (2001) maintains that, within the nurse–client relationship, ethical issues of non-maleficence, beneficence, autonomy and justice need to be used by the nurse to guide moral practice within the professional encounter with clients.

Box 7.6 The 10 Essential Shared Capabilities

- *Working in partnership.* Developing and maintaining constructive working relationships with service users, carers, families, colleagues, lay people and wider community networks. Working positively with any tensions created by conflicts of interest or aspiration that may arise between the partners in care
- *Respecting diversity.* Working in partnership with service users, carers, families and colleagues to provide care and interventions that not only make a positive difference but also do so in ways that respect and value diversity, including age, race, culture, disability, gender, spirituality and sexuality
- *Practising ethically.* Recognising the rights and aspirations of service users and their families, acknowledging power differentials and minimising them whenever possible. Providing treatment and care that is accountable to service users and carers within the boundaries prescribed by national (professional), legal and local codes of ethical practice
- *Challenging inequality.* Addressing the causes and consequences of stigma, discrimination, social inequality and exclusion in service users, carers and mental health services. Creating, developing or maintaining valued social roles for people in the communities from which they come
- *Promoting recovery.* Working in partnership to provide care and treatment that enables service users and carers to tackle mental health problems with hope and optimism and to work towards a valued lifestyle within and beyond the limits of any mental health problem
- *Identifying people's needs and strengths.* Working in partnership to gather information to agree health and social care needs in the context of the preferred lifestyle and aspirations of service users, their families, carers and friends
- *Providing service user-centred care.* Negotiating achievable and meaningful goals; primarily from the perspective of service users and their families. Influencing and seeking the means to achieve these goals and clarifying the responsibilities of the people who will provide any help that is needed, including systematically evaluating outcomes and achievements
- *Making a difference.* Facilitating access to and delivering the best quality, evidence-based, values-based health and social care interventions to meet the needs and aspirations of service users and their families and carers
- *Promoting safety and positive risk taking.* Empowering people to decide the level of risk they are prepared to take with their health and safety. This includes working with the tension between promoting safety and positive risk taking, including assessing and dealing with possible risks for service users, carers, family members, and the wider public
- *Personal development and learning.* Keeping up-to-date with changes in practice and participating in life-long learning, personal and professional development for one's self and colleagues through supervision, appraisal and reflective practice

Quoted from Scottish Executive (2006b)

Box 7.7. Conditions essential for informed consent

- Receive adequate information
- Understand this information
- Consent voluntarily

Quoted from Schachter et al (1994)

These require the nurse to do no harm in any way to clients; to promote good and do good towards them; promote respect and give the right to choose; and make decisions and be fair in engagement with them.

In addition, Hodge and Renwick (2002) assert that there is a need for practitioners to consider the complex interplay of factors underpinning the client's motivation for engagement and participation in the treatment process. Hodge and Renwick state that failure to examine the client's world view and perspective as a person and the external factors that impact on the client as a person, including the context of the environment in which they are cared for, can influence care outcomes. Therefore, forensic nurses should heed clients' perspectives otherwise they will not be in a position to understand clients' motivation or lack of motivation to engage and participate in the treatment process (Addo 2006a). According to Schachter et al (1994), central to informed consent is information, and they provide three conditions that have to be met (see *Box 7.7*).

Scott (1998) maintains that autonomy is influenced by internal and external constraints. Within the context of healthcare practice the position of autonomy is to ensure that clients are respected as human beings, and that their rights as human beings are promoted and protected (Johnstone and Olga 2009). In this context respecting clients implies that treatment and care are not provided without first involving them in decision-making, and ensuring that they are well informed about the process of how consent is sought regarding their treatment and care plan.

Evidence base

Equity and excellence in forensic healthcare practices can only be achieved by the expertise and professionalism of forensic nurses based on their underpinning knowledge, understanding and application of the concepts of CSDE in their day-to-day engagement with forensic clients. This will require forensic nurses to have background socio-cultural knowledge of the clients and their world views on their health and illness; and interact with them in ways that show recognition and accommodation of clients' differing cultural world views by adopting the use of validated culturally sensitive assessment tools.

Evidence-based practice is a concept that is used widely within the healthcare literature to demonstrate approaches to care and treatment interventions based on the conscientious, explicit and judicious selection and application of the best evidence available (Sackett 1996, Drake et al 2001). This requires forensic service providers and nurses to integrate clinical expertise with available forensic nursing knowledge derived from research findings and other kinds of evidence to help address the CSDE needs agenda. In this regard forensic nurses' individual expertise can be perceived as their own proficiency and judgement that they acquire through clinical practice experience.

Evidence-based forensic nursing practice of CSDE care brings into play issues of autonomy, informed consent, shared decision making, respect, fairness, and legal issues regarding professionalism (Registered Nurses' Association of Ontario 2007, NMC 2008). A persuasive argument is that evidence-based forensic mental health nursing practice promotes scrutiny and allows for the best evaluated approaches of nursing interventions, including the identification of harmful approaches that do not address the ethical and legal issues surrounding CSDE.

CSDE in forensic mental health nursing practice can be managed effectively if practice is evidence-based. However, having the evidence alone is not enough to tackle the ethical and legal issues inherent in CSDE in clinical decision-making. Guyat and Rennie (2002) assert that knowing the tools of evidence-based practice is necessary but not sufficient for delivering the highest quality of patient care. They also advocate that apart from the clinical experience of the clinician, he or she is required to have compassion, show sensitive listening skills, and have broad-based perspectives from the humanities and social sciences. These are the required attributes allowing for understanding of clients' illnesses in the context of their experience, personalities and culture.

Nonetheless, knowledge or rapid access to the best available evidence by forensic nurses on its own is not sufficient to enable them to give optimal care for CSDE needs of the client. What forensic nurses must know is whether the evidence at hand would make a difference to the client in question, and, when it would, what the possible consequences of applying that evidence would be for the client. This is where the ethical and legal challenges for the forensic nurse reside with reference to the skills and judgement required in applying and interpreting evidence to impact on care and treatment (Guyat and Rennie 2002).

Indeed, it could be argued that the good forensic nurse uses the ever-growing body of evidence that constitutes the science of forensic nursing, and delivers it in a sensible, genuine and compassionate manner. It is perhaps, the art of forensic nursing (Watkins 2001, Addo 2006b, Barker

2009). Ignoring the science and art of harmonising the elements of CSDE and basing decisions alone on "expert" knowledge without involving the client in decision-making is likely to harm clients in more ways than can be imagined (Department of Health 1991, Blofeld 2003, Mental Welfare Commission of Scotland 2007).

Where decisions are made, and unproven expensive care and treatment interventions to clients are implemented, without consideration of their CSDE needs, and which provide no benefits and contribute no positive difference to their quality of life, then negligence and malpractice charges emerge due to breach of contract and duty of care (Baillie and Strachan 2008). Furthermore NHS Scotland (2008) found that philosophical and religious beliefs emerge as the most significant influence on conceptualisations of mental well-being, even for younger people who have received a Western education. It was also highlighted in the report that people may hold more than one frame of reference for conceptualising mental well-being. Cortis (2004) found inadequate understanding of culture and spirituality by staff led to limited implementation of "holistic" care with Pakistani clients in hospital.

Service providers and staff

Clinical governance requires corporate accountability of all stakeholders in the provision of forensic services to demonstrate continuous improvement of the quality of their services and safeguarding of high standards of care, by creating an environment in which clinical excellence will flourish (Baillie and Strachan 2008).

When forensic services focus on safety alone, this can result in professionals acting on beneficent obligations towards clients, which often lead to paternalistic assessments of clients' best interests. Legal issues relating to the provision of CSDE in forensic nursing practice relate to (a) incorrect diagnosis of the client, leading to inappropriate care and treatment provided, (b) improper and or poor supervision and failure to monitor the overall well-being of the client, alongside the prevention of unwarranted adverse events with psychotropic medications and iatrogenic incidents with clients. Issues of organisational structure, culture, ethos and commitment to engage with CSDE are needed (Blofeld 2003). Alongside this are resource developments to enable staff to acquire the relevant expertise to practise ethically and legally with respect to CSDE issues and the clarification of roles and responsibilities that need to be addressed, before any amount of training or education of forensic nurses can be effective (Drake et al 2001).

An ethical code violation exists when there is lack of enactment of policies in the work environment to enable staff to work with CSDE with forensic clients that shows adherence to legislative requirements and ethical practice to prevent abuse and/or exploitation of the client (Human Rights Act 1998, Millan 2001, HM Government Equality Acts 2006, 2010, Scottish Executive 2006, NMC 2008). One of the key recommendations following investigations of the care and treatment of Mr G by the Mental Welfare Commission of Scotland (2007) stated that the Health Boards must ensure staff are appropriately trained "as to the ethical and legal issues involved, and how to properly address issues of consent". This illustrates the legal and ethical responsibility and accountability enshrined in clinical governance placed on providers to account for their actions (Baillie and Strachan 2008).

The recruitment and selection of staff is another important area that can breach legal and ethical notions of good forensic nursing practice. Where staff do not have the requisite knowledge and skills to work with CSDE issues in forensic nursing, this can lead to negligence in their actions (Department of Health 2004, Baillie and Strachan 2008). The level of job satisfaction that nurses feel towards their work impacts positively on the quality of care offered to clients (Cavanagh 1992, McNeese-Smith 1999). It is clear that the outcome and effectiveness of what clients might gain from nurses' therapeutic use of self rests on the quality of the human relationship established and how the nurse in that context feels about his or her work. The NMC (2008) expects nurses to have the right knowledge, skills, and attitudes to engage with clients in the course of their professional practice. However, Franks (2004) reminds us that, in the provision of nursing care to clients, it is essential to address the particular needs of those who provide the care. Therefore the issues of CSDE are the business of not service providers alone but all stakeholders with an interest in the welfare and treatment of clients in forensic care settings.

Conclusion

This chapter has suggested ways in which service providers, clients and forensic nurses can work together to address ethical and legal issues with CSDE in forensic nursing practice. There is no place for cultural insularity, myopia or tunnel vision, since CSDE is at the heart of person-centred care. The responsibilities for all stakeholders, including clients and their families, are noted with the need to base care and treatment on sound evidence in a mutually respectful fashion. As forensic nursing takes a more holistic approach, which gives attention to the client's CSDE, we should expect that the ethical and legal issues being debated now will become even greater in everyday clinical settings. For it is only when we reach an agreement and have a meaningful dialogue, that we will realise that we share a common humanity, and that no matter what diversity exists between us all, we will have an easier time relating to and showing compassion to each other with a calmness of mind. There are several implications for practice which include the need to ensure the use of appropriate validated cultural assessment tools in the assessment and diagnostic phase of the client's admission. It is argued that this can be achieved through effective communication and negotiation utilising the cultural brokerage model to gain mutual understanding of both parties. The need for requisite knowledge and an understanding of the complexity and multidimensional elements of diversity are important. Nonetheless possessing this knowledge is not enough until all individual nurses have undertaken a reflection of their own values and how that impacts on their ability and willingness to work with compassion in their heart, to know how to engage with the "other" to make a positive difference.

The key points raised in this chapter include:

- Respect for client autonomy is fundamental to person-centred care in forensic mental health nursing.
- Diversity is a multidimensional concept which forensic nurses must know and understand.
- Giving clear and sufficient information to clients to aid facilitating their participation in the decision-making process about their care and treatment are important elements of the informed consent process and client autonomy.
- It is not possible to respect clients' autonomy if there is disregard for their rights to information and informed consent; and a lack of appreciation of the meaning of privacy in clients' cultural contexts.
- Forensic nurses need to clarify their own values to help make decisions and champion the respect for the client's personhood.
- Appropriately validated cultural assessment tools should be used in the diagnostic phase and the client should be involved in the decision-making process.
- Effective communication is essential to achieve collaboration with treatment and care interventions.

References

Addo M (2000) The Role of the Forensic Nurse in Clinical Supervision. In Robinson D, Kettles AM (eds) *Forensic Nursing and Multidisciplinary Care of the Mentally Disordered Offender* Jessica Kingsley, London

Addo M (2001) I am mental illness. *Interdisciplinary Journal of Pastoral Studies. Disabling Society Enabling Love* 136: 3–4

Addo M (2006a) Culture, spirituality and ethical issues in caring for clients with a personality disorder. In: National Forensic Nurses' Research and Development Group: Woods P, Kettles AM, Byrt R (eds) *Forensic Mental Health Nursing: Interventions with people with 'personality disorder* (pp. 60–80) Quay Books, London

Addo M (2006b) *The unseen abyss: Registered Nurses' experience in working with sex offenders – a Hermeneutic Phenomenological Study*. Unpublished PhD Thesis University of Aberdeen

Addo MA, McKie A, Kettles AM, Gibb J, Gass J, Yule M (2010) Are nurses empowered to make decisions about levels of patient observation in mental health? *Nursing Times* 106(9): 26–8

Addo M, Smith I (2008) Equality and diversity: Respecting the person with a learning disability. In: *Forensic Mental Health Nursing: Capabilities Roles and Responsibilities*. Quay Books, London

Arnold E, Boggs KU (2003) *Interpersonal Relationships: Professional Communication Skills for Nurses*. WB Saunders, Philadelphia

Austin W (2001) Relational ethics in forensic psychiatric settings. *Journal of Psychosocial Nursing* 39(9): 12–17

Baillie D, Strachan V (2008) *An Essential Guide to Legal Issues in Scotland for Health Professionals* (4th edn) NHS Grampian, Grampian

Barker P (2001) The Tidal Model: Developing a person-centred approach to psychiatric and mental health nursing. *Perspectives in Psychiatric Care* 37: 2

Barker P (2003) Person centred care: The need for diversity. In: Barker P (ed) *Psychiatric and Mental Health Nursing: The craft of caring*. Arnold, London

Barker P (2009) *Psychiatric and Mental Health Nursing: The craft of caring*. Arnold, London

Beauchamp T, Childress J (1994) *Principles of biomedical ethics* (5th edn). Oxford University Press, New York

Bjarnason D, Mick J, Thompson JA, Cloyd E (2009) *Nursing Clinics of North America*. 44(4): 495–503

Blofeld J (2003) *Independent Inquiry into the Death of David Bennett*. An Independent Inquiry set up under HSG (94) 27. Department of Health, London

Boyd MA (1998) Communication and therapeutic relationship. In: MA. Boyd, Nihart (eds) *Psychiatric Nursing: Contemporary Practice* (pp 247–8) Lippincott, Philadelphia

Byrt R, Aiyegbusi A, Hardie T, Addo M (2007) Cultural and diversity issues: In: *Forensic Mental Health Nursing: Forensic Aspects of Care* (pp 219–35) Quay Books, London

Cameron ME (2003) Legal and ethical issues – Our best ethical and spiritual values. *Journal of Professional Nursing* 19(3): 117–18

Cavanagh SJ (1992) Job satisfaction of nursing staff working in hospitals. *Journal of Advanced Nursing* 17: 704–11

Chalanda M (1995) Brokerage in multicultural nursing. *International Nursing Review* 42(1): 19–26

Cortis J (2004) Meeting the needs of minority ethnic patients. *Journal of Advanced Nursing* 48(1): 51–8

Department of Health (1991) *Review of Health and Social Care Services for Mentally Disordered Offenders and Others Requiring Similar Services*. HMSO, London

Department of Health and Home Office (1992) *Review of Health and Social Services for Mentally Disordered Offenders and Others Requiring Similar Services*. Final Summary Report Cm 2088. HMSO, London

Department of Health (1999) *The Report of the Committee of Inquiry into the Personality Disorder Unit – Ashworth Inquiry*: Stationery Office, London,

Department of Health (2000) *The NHS Plan: A Plan for Investment: A Plan for Reform*. HMSO, London

Department of Health (2001a) *Valuing People: A New Strategy for Learning Disability for the 21st Century*. HMSO, London

Department of Health (2001b) *Building Capacity and Partnership in Care: An agreement between the statutory and the independent social care, health care and housing sectors*. HMSO, London

Department of Health (2004) *Agenda for Change. Knowledge Skills Framework*. Scottish Executive, Edinburgh

Department of Health (2005a) *Delivering Race Equality and the Government's Response to the Inquiry into the Death of David Bennett*. Department of Health, London

Department of Health (2005b) *New Blueprint to Tackle and Eradicate Discrimination in Mental Health Services Over the Next Five Years*. Department of Health, London

Downie RS, Calman KC (1994) *Healthy Respect: Ethics in Health Care* (2nd edn) Oxford Publications, Oxford

Drake RE, Goldman HH, Leff S, Lehman AF, Dixon L, Mueser KT, Torrey WC (2001) Implementing evidence-based practices in routine mental health service settings. *Psychiatric Services* 52: 179–82

Draper H (1998) Sterilisation abuse. Women and consent to treatment. In: Brazier M, Lobjoit M (eds) *Protecting the Vulnerable. Autonomy and consent in healthcare*. Routledge, London

Fernando S (2002) *Mental Health Race and Culture* (2nd edn). Palgrave, Basingstoke

Franks V (2004) Evidence-based uncertainty in mental health nursing. *Journal of Psychiatric and Mental Health Nursing* 11: 99–105

Gallop R (1998) Abuse of power in the nurse–client relationship. *Nursing Standard* 12(37): 43–7

Gillon R (1986) Autonomy and the principle of respect for autonomy. *British Medical Journal* 290: 18068

Guyat G, Rennie D (2002) *User's Guide to the Medical Literature. A Manual for Evidence-Based Clinical Practice*. (1st edn) AMA Press, Chicago

Hammer R (2000) Caring in forensic nursing. *Journal of Psychosocial Nursing* 38(11): 18–24

HM Government (1992) *Report of the Committee on Inquiry into Complaints at Ashworth Hospital*. (The Blom-Cooper Report) HMSO, London

HM Government (1998) *Human Rights Act 1998*. The Stationery Office, London

HM Government (2006) *Equality Act*. The Stationery Office, London

HM Government (2010) *Equality Act, 2010*. The Stationery Office, London

Hodge J, Renwick S (2002) Motivating mentally disordered offenders. In MacMurran M (ed) *Motivating Offenders to Change*. Wiley, Chichester

International Councils of Nurses (2006) *Code of Ethics*. International Councils of Nurses, Geneva

Jezewezki M (1990) Culture brokering in migrant farm worker health care. *Western Journal of Nursing Research*.12(4): 497–513

Jezewezki M (1993) Cultural brokering as a model for advocacy. *Nursing and Health Care* 14(2): 78–85

Johnstone M.J, Olga K. (2009) Ethics and advance care planning in a culturally diverse society. *Journal of Transcultural Nursing* 20(4): 405–16

Lama Dalai (2002) *The Essence of Wisdom*. Abacus, London

Laschinger HKS (2004) Hospital nurses' perception of respect and organisational justice. *Journal of Nursing Administration* 34(7/8): 354–64

Liaschenko J (1994) Making a bridge: The moral work with patients we do not like. *Journal of Palliative Care* 10(3): 83–9

Marsella A (1980) Depressive experience and disorder across cultures. In: Triandis H, Draons J (eds) *A Handbook of Cross-Cultural Psychology* (vol 6). Allyn & Bacon, Boston

McNeese-Smith D (1999) A content analysis of staff nurse descriptions of job satisfaction and dissatisfaction. *Journal of Advanced Nursing* 29(6): 1332–41

Mental Welfare Commission for Scotland (2007) *Not my problem. Summary report from investigation into deficiencies in the care and treatment of Mr G*. MWC, Edinburgh

Mental Welfare Commission (2009) *Too Close to See: Summary of our investigation into deficiencies in the care and treatment of Mr F.* Mental Welfare Commission, Edinburgh

Millan B (2001) *New Directions: Report on the Review of the Mental Health (Scotland) Act, 1984*. Scottish Executive, Edinburgh

Mohr WK (2006) Spiritual issues in psychiatric care. *Perspectives in Psychiatric Care* 42(3): 174–83

NHS Health Scotland (2008) *Research Report – Scoping exercise with Black and minority ethnic groups on perceptions of mental wellbeing in Scotland*, NHS Health Scotland, Edinburgh

NHS Health Scotland (2010) *Dimensions of Diversity: Population differences and health improvement opportunities*. NHS Health Scotland, Edinburgh

NHS Education for Scotland (2009) *Spiritual Care Matters. An introductory resource for all NHS Scotland staff*. NES, Edinburgh

Nursing and Midwifery Council (2008) *Code of Professional Conduct: Standards for conduct, performance and ethics*. NMC, London

Pargament KI (1997) *The Psychology of Religion and Coping: Theory Research, and Practice*. Guilford Press, New York

Peplau HE (1991) *Interpersonal Relations in Nursing: A Conceptual Frame of Reference for Psychodynamic Nursing*. Springer, New York

Post SG, Puchalski CM, Larson B (2000) Physicians' and patients' spirituality: Professional boundaries, competency, and ethics. *Annals of Internal Medicine*.132(7): 578–83

Rawlinson JW (1990) Self-Awareness: Conceptual influences, contributions to nursing, and approaches to attainment. *Nurse Education* 10: 111–17

Registered Nurses' Association of Ontario (2007) *Professionalism in Nursing*. Registered Nurses' Association of Ontario, Canada

Ross L (1994) Spiritual aspects of nursing. *Journal of Advanced Nursing* 19(3): 439–47

Royal College of Nursing (2010) Spirituality: Survey aims to shape RCN position on complex area. *RCN bulletin* 245: 2

Sackett DL (1996) Evidence based medicine: What it is and what it is not. *British Medical Journal* 312, 71–2

Schachter D, Kleinman I, Prendergast P, Remington G, Schertzer S (1994) The effect of psychopathology on the ability of schizophrenic patients to give informed consent. *Journal of Nervous Mental Disorder* 182(6): 360–2

Scott PA (1998) Morally autonomous practice. *Advanced Nursing Sciences* 21(20): 70–80

Scott PA, Valimaki M, Leino-Kilpi Dassen T, Gasull M, Lemonidou C, Arndt M (2003) Autonomy, privacy and informed consent 1: Concepts and definitions. *British Journal of Nursing* 12(1): 43–7

Scottish Executive (2003a) *Mental Health (Care and Treatment) (Scotland) Act 2003*. Scottish Executive, Edinburgh

Scottish Executive (2003b) *An introduction to the Mental Health (Care and Treatment) Act 2003,* Edinburgh, Scottish Executive

Scottish Executive (2006a) *Rights Relationship and Recovery: The Report of the National Review of Mental Health Nursing in Scotland*. Scottish Government, Edinburgh

Scottish Executive (2006b) *The 10 Essential Shared Capabilities for Mental Health Practice: Learning Material (Scotland)*. NHS Education for Scotland, Edinburgh

Swinton J (2000) Reclaiming the soul: A spiritual perspective on forensic nursing. In: Robinson D, Kettles A (eds) *Forensic Nursing and Multidisciplinary Care of the Mentally Disordered Offender*. Jessica Kingsley, London

Swinton J (2001) *Spirituality and Mental Health Care: Rediscovering a 'Forgotten' Dimension*. Jessica Kingsley, London

Swinton J, Boyd J (2002) Autonomy and personhood: The forensic nurse as a moral agent. In: Robinson D, Kettles A (eds) *Forensic Nursing and Multidisciplinary Care of the Mentally Disordered Offender* (p 113) Jessica Kingsley, London

Wallace B (2000) Nurses and consent. *Professional Nurse* 15(11): 72–3

Watkins P (2001) *Mental Health Nursing: The Art of Compassionate Care*. Butterworth–Heinemann, Oxford

Woods P, Collins M, Kettles AM (2002) Forensic nursing interventions and future directions for forensic mental health practice. In: *Therapeutic Interventions for Forensic Mental Health Nurses*. Jessica Kingsley, London

CHAPTER 8

Ethical issues in forensic community work

Michael Coffey and Jeanette Hewitt

Introduction

Contemporary community mental healthcare of people discharged from forensic services continues to present practitioners and service users with a range of challenging problems. The tension between espoused values of involvement, partnership and autonomy and those of risk management and public protection are ones which have to be addressed in routine practice. For practitioners to deliver ethically aware services that are fair and equitable they must endeavour to tease out the range of issues that are likely to arise in their day-to-day practice. In this chapter we focus our attention on the delivery of care to people discharged on Section 41 conditions, hereafter referred to as "conditional discharge". First we outline the context of contemporary community mental healthcare for those on conditional discharge. We then move on to discuss the goals of community mental healthcare and examine how these are set in tension with the demands of public protection. We observe that the goal of treatment may be primarily seen as advancing the public protection agenda at the expense of purely therapeutic outcomes. We then provide a discussion of the balance to be struck between safety and autonomy in the provision of community care. Within this context we explore issues of reciprocity related to the limitation of liberty for the purposes of providing treatment. Lastly we address the issues of risk and note a renewed discussion about confinement within mental health that may place disproportionate limits on the mentally ill when compared with other members of society.

The legal context of care

The principal legislation governing detention and treatment of people with mental illness in England and Wales is the Mental Health Act 1983 and the later amendments in the Mental Health Act 2007. The Crown Courts have at their disposal a range of provision within the Mental Health Act which they may use when convicting people of serious criminal offences against the person in the context of a diagnosable and treatable mental illness. Section 37 of the Mental Health Act allows the Crown Court to detain a person, on conviction of a serious offence, in hospital, for treatment, and this section is often used in conjunction with Section 41, which prevents and restricts discharge unless granted by the Home Office or a Mental Health Review Tribunal. In the majority of instances where discharge is granted it is on a conditional basis subject to supervision and monitoring arrangements which may include attendance for treatment, permitting the care team access to living arrangements, attendance at organised day-time activities and restrictions on travel or contacting particular individuals. Other requirements can include conditions of residence, curfews and unannounced urine and breath tests to detect drug and alcohol use. In all cases the Home Office retains the right to recall individuals to hospital and it may do so on the advice of the supervising care team, or, more unusually, independently of this advice.

Conditional discharge is an important strategy for the rehabilitation and eventual discharge of individuals from the forensic mental health system. It provides opportunities for both service users and workers to gauge the level of preparedness for eventual independent living which implies the possibility of less monitoring and surveillance of mental health and risk behaviours. It has been suggested that powers such as conditional discharge offer the means of shifting, in a titrated way, "the locus of responsibility from the system to the patient" (Skipworth and Humberstone, 2002: 48).

In the year 2008, 407 people were discharged from hospital to the community on conditions (Ministry of Justice 2010). It has previously been estimated that 25% of people conditionally discharged are likely to be recalled to hospital at some point due to concerns about their risk or their mental health (Street 1998) and most recent figures indicate that approximately 3% of those discharged between 1999 and 2006 committed serious offences following discharge (Minisstry of Justice 2010). Mental health workers engaged in the support and supervision of people on conditional discharge are charged with monitoring the mental health, risk status and social circumstances of service users. This involves multiple and regular visits by workers as well as the use of more covert and discreet methods of monitoring by proxy agents such as workers employed by voluntary agencies. In interactions with service users, and in worker accounts of aftercare, these more discreet forms of monitoring may be glossed as extra forms of support. However there remains a clear expectation that non-statutory organisations providing services such as housing and daytime activities should pass on relevant information about behaviours to the aftercare team. This additional layer of monitoring enables decisions in relation to movement of people towards great autonomy or safety (Heyman et al 2004). The degree to which service users are or should be informed of these arrangements is difficult to determine.

The focus on community care

Community mental healthcare, since its contemporary conception in the mid-1950s, has sought to advance the deinstitutionalisation of people with mental ill health and provide services in more everyday community settings. The occupancy of inpatient beds fell from its peak of 350 per 100 000 population in 1954 to 151 per 100 000 population in 1982 (Boardman 2005). The closure of old mental hospitals and the move towards community provision has gathered pace in the last 20 years (Bell and Lindley 2005). Goodwin (1997) has summarised the variety of factors driving forward community care which included the development of new medications; the appearance of more enlightened professional attitudes; imperatives to reduce the cost of expensive hospital services; increased lobbying from organised groups of carers and service users; the influence of anti-institutional critiques; and the emergence of anti-psychiatry ideas. These factors have combined to raise questions about bio-medically-dominated, hospital-centred mental health services (Goodwin 1997). Taken together these developments have led to a greater emphasis on the provision of care and treatment outside of the large institutions that had themselves become synonymous with enquiries into failures in care (Martin 1984). Community mental healthcare has been seen to offer distinct advantages for the treatment of mental illness (Leff et al 1994), and has helped deliver an improved quality of life for many users of services (Anderson et al 1993) although cautions about uncritical adoption of the policy have been voiced (Pattison and Armitage 1986).

Although there is no one coherent description of the values and goals of community mental healthcare, workers do appear to share an interest in promoting independence, supporting recovery and ensuring prompt responses to mental health crises. Woodbridge and Fulford (2004) have outlined a clear values-based process in the provision of mental health services that many workers in any setting would find appealing (see *Box 8.1*). These notions of involvement and partnership suggest collaborative relationships built on trust and honesty with the ultimate aims of ensuring the delivery of user-focused healthcare and independence. Collaborative relationships with a therapeutic focus have been shown to be a necessary but not sufficient condition for better outcomes in mental healthcare (Hewitt and Coffey 2005). Much work is expended on achieving collaborative relationships within forensic mental health settings and some evidence exists to suggest that supportive relationships more generally may have protective effects leading to reduced episodes of violent behaviour (Estroff et al 1994).

Box 8.1. Ten pointers to good process in values-based practice

Practice skills

1. *Awareness*: of the values present in a given situation. Careful attention to language is one way of raising awareness of values
2. *Reasoning*: using a clear reasoning process to explore the values present when making decisions
3. *Knowledge*: of the values and facts relevant to the specific situation
4. *Communication*: combined with the previous three skills, this is central to the resolution of conflicts and the decision making process

Models of service delivery

5. *User-centred*: The first source for information on values in any situation is the perspective of the service user concerned
6. *Multidisciplinary*: Conflicts of values are resolved in values-based practice (VBP) not by applying a "pre-prescribed rule" but by working towards a balance of different perspectives (e.g. multidisciplinary team working)

Values-based practice and evidence-based practice (VBP and EBP)

7. *The "two feet" principle*: All decisions are based on facts and values (EBP and VBP thus work together)
8. *The "squeaky wheel" principle*: We only notice values when there is a problem
9. *Science and values*: Increasing scientific knowledge creates choices in healthcare, which introduces wide differences in values

Partnership

10. *Partnership*: In VBP decisions are taken by service users and the providers of care working in partnership

Woodbridge and Fulford (2004)

An ongoing focus of community mental health services has been to secure and extend the tenure of community living for service users (Stein and Test 1980). This has been promoted through the use of intensive case management, assertive outreach and crisis resolution and home treatment services which aim to preserve community status and prevent or limit hospital admission (Hoult 1986, Muijen et al 1994, Burns and Firn 2002). Forensic services have been directed towards similar approaches (Shepherd 1993) and some evidence exists that many adopt them (Judge et al 2004) although evidence for effectiveness remains limited (Mohan et al 2004). There are however some distinct problems with forensic services using these approaches, which does not appear to have been addressed in the literature and which we now turn to in our discussion.

Balancing care with compulsion

One of the prime requirements of forensic mental health services has been the safe management of risk behaviours. The development of "risk thinking" has been pervasive in all mental health services to the extent that decisions on care and treatment are influenced by considerations of risk, despite the term itself being poorly defined and understood (Pfohl 1978, Rose 1998). While services may ostensibly operate in ways that provide transition towards eventual discharge and greater liberty it is also the case that movement may occur in the opposite direction too. Heyman et al (2004) have applied the concept of a risk escalator to forensic services. A risk escalator is defined as

> *...a system, designed or emergent, which is oriented towards managing a defined health risk, and which is made up of a set of sub-systems, ordered in terms of different trade-offs between autonomy and safety, through which service users may move.*
>
> (Heyman, 2005: 44)

To operate as a risk escalator a system must be able to differentiate between steps in treatment relative to assessed risk, attempt congruence between the safety/autonomy balance in relation to assessed risk and have the potential to move people towards greater autonomy or safety dependent upon these assessments (Heyman et al 2004: 310). Traditionally the assessment and management of risk behaviours has been conducted behind the walls of large institutions but contemporary moves towards community care have introduced new challenges of providing assessment, support and treatment in an arena that is open to much more public and professional scrutiny.

Much of the care offered by forensic community mental health services appears to be based on the notion that comprehensive evidence-based services will deliver better mental health outcomes which in turn will reduce risk and help protect the public from dangerous risk behaviours of the mentally-ill (Skipworth and Humberstone 2002). However, this view is essentially advancing a public protection agenda or in other words public protection is being seen as a useful outcome of treatment. The degree to which forensic community services can be safely assumed to achieve the delivery of evidence-based services must however remain open to question (Judge et al 2004). Notions of evidence-based practice may be a pervasive rhetoric in health and social care work but the reality of day-to-day practice can deviate significantly from this ideal.

There appears to us to be a number of problems that can occur in the provision of community forensic services. We identity three such problems here and provide an outline discussion of these to demonstrate the complexities of ethical and moral judgements in the provision of community services to this group.

First, workers must achieve a balance between the safety of the individual/community and provide opportunities for greater autonomy and independence from services.

Second, there are also problems to be resolved in relation to reciprocity. This relates to the deprivation of usual everyday liberties for the purposes of receiving treatments which may not be evidenced, to help improve the condition.

A third problem arises when the individual follows treatment diligently and events peripheral to their mental health but central to their assessed level of risk intervene to prompt recall to hospital. This challenges notions of supported recovery and movement towards greater liberty from continued surveillance.

Safety and autonomy

Autonomy is held as an important good for people, associated with ideas of individual liberty, self-determination, freedom of choice and the right to make independent decisions for the self, and the acceptance of responsibility for one's moral positions (Fairbairn 1995). The individual has the ability to choose to think and act in a certain way, based on internal influences where intentions are under personal control and not the result of un-reflected social manipulation or coercion (Varelius 2003). Autonomy is sometimes seen as a potentially variable state, since what a person thinks and does cannot be explained without reference to his or her own activity of mind (Dearden 1972). Therefore, any temporary or enduring phenomenon that interferes with cognitive capacity might restrict the level of autonomy a person is able to possess. This seems to be a relatively clear-cut position when regarding certain categories of brain insult or injury (e.g. cerebral hypoxia, post-ictal states, encephalopathy, etc), or where toxicity, disease or drugs have induced fluctuating levels of consciousness. Arguably, it is more ambiguous when considering mental disorder, such as schizophrenia or the spectrum of learning difficulties, where there is a tendency to presume diminished autonomy due to the "controlling influences" of illness or reduced mental capacity.

The moral principle of respect for autonomy includes obligations to "acknowledge a person's right to hold views, to make choices, and to take actions based on personal values and beliefs" (Beauchamp and Childress 2001: 63). It also requires more than non-interference in others' personal affairs; it includes obligations to build up or maintain others' capacities for autonomous choice (Hewitt and Edwards 2006). Respecting this moral principle involves more than simply acknowledging that people are entitled to their opinions. It entails, in some circumstances, enhancing a person's capacity to make autonomous choices. Respecting autonomy also entails respecting a person's choices, "so long as their thoughts and actions do not seriously harm other persons" (Beauchamp and Childress 2001: 64).

Action taken that denies another the possibility of exercising autonomy over his or her life is seen as paternalistic (Fairbairn 1995). Within the principle-based approach to biomedical ethics advocated by Beauchamp and Childress (2001), respect for autonomy has only a prima facie standing and can be overridden by competing moral considerations:

> *Our obligations to respect autonomy do not extend to persons who cannot act in a sufficiently autonomous manner (and cannot be rendered autonomous) because they are immature, incapacitated, ignorant, coerced, or exploited. Infants, irrationally suicidal individuals, and drug-dependent persons are examples.*
>
> (Beauchamp and Childress 2001: 65)

People with mental illness are often conceptualised by psychiatric approaches to ethics as being non-autonomous due to the controlling forces of their condition. This means that respect for autonomy is not considered to be the trumping principle in treating people with mental illness, since their capacity to be autonomous is seen to be impaired. Within this paradigm, compulsory treatment and/or detention and ongoing supervision would not be considered to be a violation of a person's autonomy as there is no conflict between autonomy and paternalism in preventing the "non-autonomous acts" of people with mental illness (Beauchamp and Childress 2001). Instead, obligations of non-maleficence and beneficence can be deployed in the justification of paternalism to ensure the well-being of others and that no harm befalls persons, which is due to action or inaction by moral agents.

Paternalism is conceptualised by Beauchamp and Childress (2001) in either weak or strong terms. Weak paternalism allows an agent to intervene "on grounds of beneficence or non-maleficence only to prevent substantially non-voluntary conduct" (p.181). Weak paternalism can therefore only be used where the person is considered to be incapable of autonomous, rational action. Strong paternalism involves beneficent intervention, by virtue of the need to protect the person, despite the fact that the intervention is contrary to the person's wishes and that risky choices and actions are informed. This applies to persons who are considered to be autonomous and rational, but where moral considerations are seen to outweigh respect for the principle of autonomy.

In psychiatry, the paternalism employed is seen to be of a weak nature, since the status label of mental illness implies a condition of non-autonomy and irrationality. The term mental illness implies that persons with such a diagnosis are more likely to be dangerous to themselves or others than are persons without such illnesses (Szasz 2003), and acts of paternalism are therefore seen as necessary to govern people who, because of mental illness, cannot govern themselves (Roberts 2004). Therefore, paternalism is seen here as being justified if the person is at risk of a significant, preventable harm, which intervention will probably prevent; the projected benefits outweigh risks to the patient and the least autonomy-restrictive alternative is chosen (Beauchamp and Childress 2001: 186). Paternalism, which overrides a non-autonomous person's wishes, choices or actions, does not involve a conflict between beneficence and autonomy, since capacity to be autonomous is impaired (Veatch 1989). Acts of paternalism are justified by invoking the concept of mental illness and by suggesting that mental illness, particularly hallucinations and delusions, diminish a person's capacity to act in an autonomous manner (Beauchamp and Childress 2001).

Determinations of the suitability of supported placements appear to hinge on achieving a balance between safety and autonomy. The prominence of concerns about risk can mean that the person's autonomy is relegated in decisions of discharge. This is understandable to a degree, especially in circumstances where there is a history of serious risk behaviours. On purely clinical grounds it may be justified but there is evidence that it is considerations of risk and the wish to limit risk behaviours that hold sway in determinations of discharge (Cardiff Local Health Board 2004).

Leaving hospital and returning to live in the community is a critical juncture in the treatment trajectory of any condition. Discharge from forensic settings may be a time of increased anxiety for both the individual service user and for those charged with monitoring their aftercare. Conditional discharge provides the means for graduated, planned and controlled departure from hospital. Workers have to weigh up the potential for risk behaviour towards others or the person him or herself, with the needs of the person for rehabilitation and recovery. Discharge to a supported placement may allow continued surveillance and monitoring that would not otherwise be available to workers if the person had returned home or to another independent setting.

Decisions on the use of supported placements may be made purely on the recovery and rehabilitation needs of the individual. For instance, in the absence of particular independent living skills, supported accommodation can provide opportunities to socialise and learn new skills, such as managing household budgets or cooking. In such circumstances the longer-term goal of autonomy is suspended for a more limited form to enable the individual to build the necessary skills to move on to more independent living.

However, decisions on supported placements may be in part dictated by concerns to maintain high levels of monitoring and supervision, particularly in cases where there is a history of failed supervision. In such a scenario the person may be required to live in a 24-hour supported placement; to take prescribed psychotropic medication; provide access to the aftercare monitoring team; be subject to curfews; be required to provide random samples of urine or hair for analysis to detect drug use; be required to attend particular daytime activities; and have other limits placed on his or her movements and contacts. This range of conditions can severely limit the movements and autonomy of the person. Opportunities to socialise, develop new relationships and social supports, achieve inclusion through employment or mainstream community activities may all be limited or prevented by such close control and monitoring.

The very nature of aftercare monitoring itself may militate safety and diminish autonomy. Opportunities to integrate with communities, achieve social bonding and pursue non-illness identity careers may be prevented by what can be the persistent and intrusive nature of community support and aftercare. People discharged on Section 41 may have visits from nurses, social workers, doctors, support workers, housing officers and the police. In a very real sense these visits serve to highlight the person to the rest of the community as someone in need of extensive support services, perhaps even as someone who needs close supervision. In such circumstances there is a real likelihood that rather than providing the means to recovery, aftercare supervision and monitoring may perpetuate stigmatised identities and increase the social isolation of the person.

Reciprocity

The trade-off between autonomy and safety may be a transaction that is worthwhile on the basis that limited autonomy is a reasonable short-term price to pay for comprehensive evidence-based treatment. Withdrawal or limits on certain everyday civil liberties, such as restrictions on travel or congregation, or social activities, such as visiting the local public house, may be seen as acceptable conditions when agreeing to discharge plans, especially when set against continuing detention. Ostensibly these restrictions are placed upon the person not only to reduce risk behaviours but also to allow the delivery of treatment for mental illness. The evidence for efficacy of many treatments for mental illness is however limited. For example some medications, such as neuroleptics, do not reduce symptoms for approximately 30% of people (Kane and Leiberman 1987). In some, symptoms may be reduced but unpleasant symptoms are not completely removed. Many people taking these medications experience persistent, unpleasant and potentially fatal side effects. Similarly the availability, fidelity and efficacy of non-pharmaceutical treatments is variable. This prompts a question about the continuing limits on liberty for the purposes of providing treatments that are known not to work for some and which may prove unavailable or even dangerous to others.

Riskiness

Risk management is concerned with preventing future harms, which are perceived as being predictable and manageable. There is an increased awareness of risks in society and a perception that this increased knowledge can lead to more effective prevention strategies (Ryan 1999). Mental health policy development in the UK has become increasingly dominated by the need to prevent violence and alleviate public concerns about the presumed dangers of the mentally ill living in the community. Moon (2000) has suggested that the failures in supervision of the mentally ill living in the community have now given rise to a renewed discourse of confinement within mental health policy targeted at people seen to be the most unpredictable and dangerous. Risk management has become the expected focus of contemporary mental health services, and responsibility has increasingly been devolved to individual workers when systems fail to prevent violence. Links between violence, dangerousness and mental illness have become embedded in cultural consciousness over the course of hundreds of years (Moran 1985). The media's reporting of violence attributed to mentally disordered individuals in the last decade has fuelled beliefs that dangerousness is an inevitable consequence of mental illness and that this behaviour is predictable, measurable and controllable (Hewitt 2008).

Mental healthcare provision for people discharged from forensic services therefore occurs against a backdrop of growing concern about the perceived risk of violence posed to the general public by people with mental illness (Wright and Stockford 1999). Public concern has inspired policy responses and considerable research in the fields of criminal justice and mental health in attempting to devise methods of predicting dangerousness, and, at the micro level of service delivery, risk assessment and management, is the expected focus of contemporary mental health services (Hewitt 2008).

A central question arises as to whether a just society can legitimately curtail the autonomy of a section of that society, because the status label of mental illness is seen to confer increased riskiness. Edwards (1999) argues that:

> *…the level of risk for which a risk assessment is considered appropriate must be above that to which all humans are exposed, otherwise people with mental health problems might properly claim they are being unfairly singled out for "special" attention or scrutiny of their lifestyle.*
>
> Edwards (1999: 141)

Therefore, the principle of justice would seem to demand that there be robust evidence to support the notion of riskiness and mental illness, if the paternalistic intervention of ongoing surveillance is to be employed.

Such evidence is however far from conclusive and policies formulated on a concept of dangerousness have been heavily criticised by mental health professionals who have argued that violent patients form a very small sub-section, and efforts would be better directed at improving care for all (Hewitt 2008).

Psychiatry is distinguished from most other medical disciplines in its extensive powers to apply coercive treatments and its central role in the custody and control of the mentally ill (Dreβing 2004), but is not without its critics (e.g. Szasz 1970, 2003). The power relationships in psychiatry have a marked asymmetry between clinicians and patients. This is not present to the same extent in general medicine and would seem at odds with the partnership values usually advocated in mental health nursing and the promotion of independence and recovery. Roberts (2004) argues that, simply being identified as a patient is enough to disempower somebody:

> *As a "patient", a person is required to submit to medical authority, to learn to listen and accept medical instruction and also to respond with gratitude for any attention given. This experience may be compounded in psychiatry where a person may have a history of being a "patient" and of experiencing negative consequences following attempts to exercise power and autonomy. Threats of being "sectioned", treatment without consent and generally having others decide what is in one's best interests may all be factors in the development of a state of disempowerment and learned helplessness.*
>
> Roberts (2004: 586)

The person's sense of personal identity is threatened by his or her reduced moral and legal status as a "mental patient". Notions of "riskiness" are also likely to diminish respect for the patient's autonomy, where management of public concerns converge with professional obligations to reduce the risks, which are seen to be conferred by a label of mental illness. Risk management concerns are likely to have an even greater weight where patients have the additional label of "forensic" attached. Paternalism in this context may have an equal remit of control as it does beneficent intervention.

The rights-based justification for user involvement in mental health services relates to the acquisition of equal rights of citizenship for people with mental illness (Hird and Cash 1999). Hird and Cash (1999) observe that

> *...taking risks with life and health is accepted to be part of normal life for non-service users. For example, two individuals, say a rock climber and a smoker, may each look at the other and argue for control of the other's activities while defending their own freedoms.*
>
> Hird and Cash (1999: 152)

In other words, while society at large may indulge in risky behaviour, which constitutes a potential harm to self and/or others, such behaviour is rarely curtailed by the sort of paternalistic intervention to which a person with mental illness might be subject. Therefore equal rights of citizenship are not extended to people with mental illness in terms of respecting their right to full self-determination. The challenge for mental health nurses is therefore to balance the paternalistic remit of psychiatry and professional obligation with espoused values of partnership and person-centredness, which underpin contemporary mental health practice.

Conclusion

Contemporary forensic community mental healthcare is a site of complexity. This complexity is the result of an interweaving of health and social care needs, concerns about public protection, respect for libertarian ideals and the challenging nature of social responses to mental ill-health. Mental health nurses must develop greater awareness of the tensions in providing forensic mental health services within the community so that they can meaningfully engage in dialogue with service users, other professions and the general public. It is in day-to-day interaction with users of services that mental health nurses must achieve a balance between the supposed dichotomies of care and control.

Therapeutic interaction requires more openness and honesty with users of services about the limitations and expectations of community provision. To do otherwise is likely to lead to more alienation and disenchantment with health and social care provision. There is a delicate balance to be struck here, between on the one hand providing a realistic picture of life post-discharge, and aftercare requirements, and on the other hand meeting the information needs of providers to enable them to make judgements about risk behaviours.

Although the provision of community forensic services has been evident for many years, there still remains relatively little research in this field. This is slowly starting to change and new knowledge about the make-up and provision of services is beginning to emerge. However there are significant gaps in relation to evidence of how people experience services and how community return is negotiated by them. New research approaches might focus on face-to-face negotiations between workers and service users in relation to aspects of aftercare monitoring and delivery of community services. In doing so it is likely that issues of safety, autonomy, reciprocity and risk will be further elucidated, thus offering us greater insights into how these tensions are resolved in everyday community practice.

References

Anderson J, Dayson D, Wills W, Gooch C, Margolius O, O'Driscoll C, Leff J (1993) The TAPS Project. 13: Clinical and social outcomes of long-stay psychiatric patients after one year in the community. *British Journal of Psychiatry* Suppl **19**: 45–56

Beachamp T, Childress J (2001) *Principles of Biomedical Ethics*. New York: Oxford University Press

Bell A, Lindley P (Eds.) (2005) *Beyond the Water Towers: The Unfinished Revolution in Mental Health Services 1985–2005,* Sainsbury Centre for Mental Health, London

Boardman J (2005) New services for old: An overview of mental health policy. In Bell A, Lindley P (eds) *Beyond the Water Towers: The Unfinished Revolution in Mental Health Services 1985–2005*. Sainsbury Centre for Mental Health, London

Burns T, Firn M (2002) *Assertive Outreach in Mental Health - A manual for practitioners* Oxford University Press, Oxford

Cardiff Local Health Board (2004) *Independent External Review into a Homicide at Prestatyn Wales on 25th March 2003*. ECRI, Hertfordshire

Dearden RF (1972) Autonomy and education. In: Dearden RF (ed) *Education and the Development of Reason (*p. 453) Routledge and Kegan Paul, London,

Dreβing H (2004) Compulsory admission and compulsory treatment in psychiatry. In: Schramme T, Thome J (eds) *Philosophy and Psychiatry* (pp.352–6) Walter de Gruyter, Berlin

Edwards S (1999) Risk assessment in the context of mental health care: Some moral considerations In: Ryan T (ed) *Managing Crisis and Risk in Mental Health Nursing,* (pp.141–8) Stanley Thornes, Cheltenham

Estroff SE, Zimmer C, Lachicotte WS, Benoit J (1994) The influence of social networks and social support on violence by persons with serious mental illness. *Hospital and Community Psychiatry* **45**(7): 669–79

Fairbairn G (1995) *Contemplating Suicide: The Language and Ethics of Self-Harm*. Routledge, London

Goodwin S (1997) *Comparative Mental Health Policy: From institutional to community care*. Sage, London

Heyman B (2005) Health risk escalators. In: Bibace R, Laird J, Valsiner J. (eds) *Science and Medicine in Dialogue: Thinking Through Particulars and Universals* (pp. 43–62) Greenwood Publishing Group, Westport CT

Heyman B, Shaw MP, Davies JP, Godin P, Reynolds L (2004) Forensic mental health services as a risk escalator: A case study of ideals and practice. *Health Risk and Society* **6**(4): 307–25

Hewitt J (2008) Dangerousness and mental health policy. *Journal of Psychiatric and Mental Health Nursing* **15**(3): 186–94

Hewitt J, Coffey M (2005) Therapeutic working relationships with people with schizophrenia: Literature review. *Journal of Advanced Nursing* **52**(5): 561–70

Hewitt J, Edwards SD (2006) Moral perspectives on the prevention of suicide in mental health settings. *Journal of Psychiatric and Mental Health Nursing* **13**(6): 665–72

Hird M, Cash K (1999) Mental health service-users and risk. In: Ryan T (ed) *Managing Crisis and Risk in Mental Health Nursing* (pp. 149–61) Stanley Thornes, Cheltenham,

Hoult J (1986) Community care of the acutely mentally ill. *British Journal of Psychiatry* **149**: 137–44

Judge J, Harty MA, Fahy T (2004) Survey of community forensic psychiatry services in England and Wales. *Journal of Forensic Psychiatry and Psychology* **15**(2): 244–53

Kane JM, Leiberman J (1987) Maintenance pharmacotherapy in schizophrenia. In Meltzer HY (ed) *Psychopharmacology: The third generation of progress*. Raven Press, New York

Leff J, Thornicroft G, Coxhead N, Crawford C (1994) The TAPS Project. 22: A five-year follow-up of long-stay psychiatric patients discharged to the community. *British Journal of Psychiatry* Suppl **25**: 13–17

Martin JP (1984) *Hospitals in Trouble*. Blackwell, Oxford

Ministry of Justice (2010) *Statistics of Mentally Disorder Offenders 2008 England and Wales*. Ministry of Justice, London

Mohan R, Slade M, Fahy TA (2004) Clinical characteristics of community forensic mental health services. *Psychiatric Services* **55**(11): 1294–8

Moon G (2000) Risk and protection: The discourse of confinement in contemporary mental health policy. *Health and Place* **6**: 239–50

Moran R (1985) The origin of insanity as a special verdict: The trial for treason of James Hadfield (1800). *Law & Society Review* **19**(3): 487–519

Muijen M, Cooney M, Strathdee G, Bell R, Hudson A (1994) Community psychiatric nurse teams: intensive support versus generic care. *British Journal of Psychiatry* **165**(2), 211–17

Pattison S, Armitage P (1986) An ethical analysis of the policies of British community and hospital care for mentally ill people. *Journal of Medical Ethics* **12**(3): 136–42

Pfohl SJ (1978) *Predicting Dangerousness*. Lexington Books, Lexington Mass

Roberts M (2004) Psychiatric ethics; a critical introduction for mental health nurses. *Journal of Psychiatric and Mental Health Nursing* **11**: 583–8

Rose N (1998) Living dangerously: Risk thinking and risk management. *Mental Health Care* **1**(8): 263–6

Ryan T (1999) Risk knowledge and mental health nursing. In: Ryan T (ed) *Managing Crisis and Risk in Mental Health Nursing* (pp 3–13) Stanley Thornes, Cheltenham,

Shepherd G (1993) Case Management. In: Watson W, Grounds A (eds) *The Mentally Disordered Offender in an Era of Community Care: New Directions in Provision*. Cambridge University Press, Cambridge

Skipworth J, Humberstone V (2002) Community forensic psychiatry: Restoring some sanity to forensic psychiatric rehabilitation. *Acta Psychiatr Scand Suppl* 106(412 suppl.): 47–53

Stein LI, Test MA (1980) Alternative to mental hospital treatment. I. Conceptual model, treatment program, and clinical evaluation. *Archives of General Psychiatry* **37**: 392–7

Street R (1998) *The Restricted Hospital Order: From court to the community*. Home Office Research Study 186. Home Office, London

Szasz T (1970) *Ideology and Insanity*. Penguin Books, Middlesex

Szasz T (2003) Psychiatry and the control of dangerousness: On the apotropaic function of the term "mental illness". *Journal of Medical Ethics* **29**: 227–30

Varelius J (2003) Autonomy Subject-Relativity, and Subjective and Objective Theories of

Well-Being in Bioethics. *Theoretical Medicine* **24**: 363–79

Veatch RM (1989) *Medical Ethics*. Jones & Bartlett, Boston

Woodbridge K, Fulford B (2004) *Whose Values? A workbook for values-based practice in mental health care*. Sainsbury Centre for Mental Health, London

Wright P, Stockford A (1999) Risk management of mentally disordered offenders in the community. In: Ryan T (ed) *Managing Crisis and Risk in Mental Health Nursing* (pp. 105–23) Stanley Thornes, Cheltenham,

CHAPTER 9

Women's enhanced medium secure care: A personal account

Wendy Ifill

For the past 29 years, I have been a seasoned traveller of the mental health services, and have come across all sorts of people and situations. My first contact with the services was when I was 14, and now, in my 40s, I am still doing the rounds. I've been on acute wards, high-dependency wards, hostels, low secure units; and, when I was younger, I also spent a while in a women's prison on the mental health wing.

Not only am I still battling with my problems, but it has left me with a string of offences, and a long criminal record, which will probably affect my future progress, once back in the community.

However, my current placement is different, and for once, I hold more faith and confidence in its working for me. WEMS, meaning women's enhanced medium secure service, has only about three units in the country, and is a pilot scheme, which has been running about three years.

What was an advantage to me in the first place, was that it was an all-women's ward, which I prefer; although there are some male staff, which is good because I think it's important to keep up some male contact.

One of the first things that is different about a WEMS unit compared to other women's units, is that it has a higher ratio of staff. This enables people to be treated at different levels and so it is able to accommodate individual needs at the varying stages people are at. This works most of the time in theory, although not always in practice.

The WEMS unit I currently reside in is run by Nottinghamshire Healthcare NHS Mental Health Trust, although it's not in Nottingham. The unit seems to me to be progressive in its forms of treatment, offering different types, including arson treatment, mindfulness, substance misuse, and a wide range of occupational therapy, leisure therapy, education, sports and leisure and other activities. This for me means a healthy balance between structured groups and more leisurely pursuits.

This unit, like many others I have been on, has its share of violence and aggression, in which I have played a minor part. Other units I have been in have used seclusion in varying amounts. I vary in my views about the use of seclusion, and still do. On units I have been on that don't use it, individuals have been restrained for long periods or extensive medication has been used. My current WEMS unit does use seclusion and I have been in it on a few occasions, and felt I needed it then. Restraint or large doses of medication would have probably been the only alternatives.

One of the most important features for me of the WEMS unit is that, as I have mentioned before, it is just for women. I have found on mixed wards in the past that the men can be very domineering and take over. Also, mixing men with women can be very inappropriate, especially if many of the men have committed offences against women. Saying this, there are still some groups where the women mix with the men, but this is very much by choice, whereas years ago when there were mixed wards, women had no choice.

One of the things that I feel works well on the ward that I am on is that each woman is treated individually. What's appropriate for one may not be for another, depending on their needs.

So far, few women have moved on from the WEMS service, so it's hard to establish if it's successful or not. However, in the time in which I have been there, I have felt some benefit.

I'm less aggressive and impulsive and for once, feel more settled. It will, however, be interesting to see if the WEMS service works, or if it's just another flash in the pan.

CHAPTER 10

"Enhanced" women's secure services: Reflections and strategies for treatment design

Rebecca Lawday

Introduction

This chapter provides background to the development of specialist services for women in secure healthcare. It was originally submitted as part of a collection of works entitled *Managing Self-Harm: Psychological Perspectives* (Motz 2009). The chapter considers what is meant by "enhanced" medium secure care, and presents the overarching "treatment stage" model that is applied within the women's service at Arnold Lodge medium secure service in Leicester. It presents considerations as to specific treatment needs, multi-professional working and integrating approaches as well as discussing responsivity factors such as engagement, the importance of therapeutic relationships and the process of change, all especially in relation to self-injury.

Women in secure services

Women who access secure mental health services have been the subject of increased interest and funding following many years of campaigning by organisations such as WISH (Women in Secure Hospitals). Following publication of documents such as *Making a Difference* (Department of Health 2000), *Into the Mainstream* (Department of Health 2002a, b, 2003), the National Institute for Mental Health in England (NIMHE) briefing paper on women's mental health services (Department of Health and NIMHE 2003), and recommendations in the Tilt report (Tilt et al 2000) guidance has been provided on modernising our mental health services. The Tilt report, a review of security at high secure hospitals, made a number of recommendations relevant to the physical and procedural security needs in high security care, as well as recommending a further review of medium secure provision. An objective was for patients to be cared for in conditions/environments commensurate with their level of risk and need. Specifically, recommendations supported the accelerated discharge of women patients not thought to require high secure care. This included the importance of accommodating gender-specific needs, and papers outline factors considered most important in the design of such services. Understanding and managing self-injury has become central to the design of services, both in the physical design of new services and in the development of treatment strategies, policies and care pathways.

Whereas the overall prevalence of mental disorder in men and women is not thought to differ significantly there have been differences observed in the presentation of mental disorder, and social and offending profiles between women and men in secure care. The difficulties particularly relevant to women who present to mental health services or who are detained in prison in the UK are anxiety, depression, eating disorders, borderline personality disorder and symptoms of post-traumatic stress disorder as well as postnatal depression and psychosis. Behaviours that cause concern include fire-setting and criminal damage as well as parasuicidal behaviours.

In prison women were found relatively to be more likely than men to have a history of self-harm. Estimates of a history of childhood abuse and self-harm are reported as 70% and 90% respectively for women in high secure hospitals (Coid et al 2000). Self-injury has complex functions, but is reported by patients to be utilised as a means of managing problematic relationships, strong emotions and difficult memories. When detained in secure services the likelihood is that both strong emotions and difficult memories will be triggered, and relationships can be a source of tension.

"Re-traumatisation" can occur within organisational and therapeutic processes that are viewed by the individual to be oppressive. Survivors of complex trauma can be reminded of, and continue to interact in ways reminiscent of, previous abusive experiences. The reciprocity of interpersonal dynamics on the ward can lead to confirmatory statements and actions by others that serve to support trauma-related beliefs. Examples of some institutional practices that some patients have identified as having the potential to re-confirm traumatic experiences have included organisational processes (e.g. restraint procedures and the use of seclusion and observations), therapeutic processes (e.g. enforced medication, physical examination, "interrogative" interviewing), and systemic processes (lack of choice, control and power). These factors may contribute to self-injury. A task for developing and established services is to effectively manage the tension created by both understanding, and setting limits on, self-injury and other extreme responses.

Importantly, concern has been expressed that women in secure services often experience longer lengths of stay and transfers between facilities resulting from the risk they are deemed to pose to themselves as well as incidents of assaults against members of staff and fellow patients. One of my own clinical observations has been that the risks associated with an individual's potential for harm towards others in such services often appear inflated by an "urge" to self-harm: This is especially when the act itself is not an easily-achievable option (planning is required), when it is accompanied by intrusive experiences (hallucinations, images, thoughts) and when there is (as yet) a lack of well-rehearsed alternatives to coping with distress. An "expressive" assault on another then becomes part of a "re-victimisation" pattern that ultimately leads to the individual being punished, contained or transferred, historically up levels of security. Alternatively, the act is followed by self-punishment, often through self-injury, and so the cycle continues.

Women's enhanced medium secure care

The current objective to reduce the numbers of women inappropriately detained in high secure hospitals has led to the development of a number of women-only services in both the public and private sector. Arnold Lodge women's service provides one of the three current NHS pilot Women's Enhanced Medium Secure (WEMS) services, designed for women who require enhanced levels of care and treatment within a medium secure setting. The national programme has identified a group of women who do not require Category B, high secure care, but are neither considered to be effectively managed in conditions of standard medium secure care. Recommendations were for services to provide an enhanced level of "procedural" and "relational" security beyond that available in standard medium secure care.

The physical design of the service at Arnold Lodge considered the need to minimise the risks associated with self-injury (i.e. likelihood, frequency, intensity and lethality) as the distinction between self-injury with and without suicidal intent is a complex one, both for patients and staff. Following on from advice regarding the physical design of units and the enhancement of relational security, the unit has been built being mindful to a preference for open spaces, separate/separable intensive care areas, quiet areas, family visiting areas and limited beds (10 in each ward).

"Procedural security", important to the development of WEMS services, refers to organisational policies and processes for maintaining safety, preventing absconding, preventing entry/possession of contraband, and, in the case of WEMS services, in managing access to articles used to harm selves or others.

"Relational security", an organic process based on attachment theory, is defined as the nature and quality of therapeutic relationships, reflected in patient/staff ratios, interaction processes, training, and interventions provided by staff. In the case of WEMS services, patients talk not just about the need for additional staff but also that they hope that staff will convey an understanding of self-injury above and beyond that experienced previously in other services.

The general principles identified in section 8 of *Into the Mainstream* (Department of Health 2002) highlights the need for a workforce to utilise therapeutic relationships to create security. Skills such as listening; being non-judgemental, empathic and respectful; understanding and managing complex problems; consistency and continuity of care; and staff as role models are encouraged.

Developing a model of care and treatment

A review of the literature (Lart et al 1999) suggests a lack of systematic information on current service models and therapeutic interventions in women's services with published research being descriptive. Specific examples of positive practice were highlighted by the Department of Health at Northgate Hospital, Newton Lodge and St Andrews Hospital. The lack of published research comparing different models of care may have been a reflection of the requirements of academic journals for control groups that cannot always be achieved in smaller forensic services, who tend to adopt a more "eclectic" approach. Individualised packages of treatment are recommended and provided from a variety of professional approaches. Where this is the case (as in Arnold Lodge), describing overarching treatment models of care becomes apparently complicated.

In addition to this, an approach needs to consider the application of the "what works" core principles of risk, need and responsivity (see Andrews and Bonta 2003) and to ensure that the responsivity principle is gender-informed. A service that can provide a number of therapeutic opportunities, from a range of theoretical backgrounds, combined with a patient group presenting a complex array of psychological, interpersonal and biological needs is not likely to fit neatly into a treatment model restricted to a single approach. There are a number of key issues to consider:

- The need to pay attention to the literature on the validity and utility of specific approaches to treating personality disorder.
- The need to prepare for specific criminogenic needs associated with women in secure services.
- The need to consider issues of treatment integrity with the above.
- The need to acknowledge the significant role of trauma.

- The need to accept complex presentations (post-traumatic stress disorder, psychoses and personality disorder).
- The need to value the contribution of different professionals and patients, working towards a common goal using an integrative approach (reflective of New Ways of Working).
- The need to build in a process that supports a philosophy of empowerment, values the role of the therapeutic relationship, provides containment through consistency, and promotes sustainable change.

Specific approaches

When planning the design of psychological input to a WEMS service, considering the empirical support for specific interventions that have used episodes of self-injury as outcomes is a reasonable first step. Hawton et al's (1998) systematic review of randomised control trials highlighted problem solving therapy and dialectical behaviour therapy as having support for helping reduce incidents of self-injury. Given what we know about the patient population, services should also employ psycho-social interventions aimed at reducing the impact of stress, and should make attempts to address specific areas of need such as arson and substance misuse.

Complex trauma: The need for consistent therapeutic relationships

A characteristic that is often referred to in the interface between patients and staff in secure services is the potential for "splitting". Although sometimes now used as a pejorative term, when working closely with individuals for whom relationships can be dangerous, and their own identity and self-esteem is fragile, one needs to be careful to manage expectations. It is difficult for some patients with complex type-II traumatic experiences to manage their relationships with those in the role of care-provider/authority. From an analytical perspective, in multi-disciplinary teams, co-workers can become "split" into those who represent to the patient the punitive figure the patient/"inner child" is angry at, those that represent the abusive carer that the patient feels vulnerable around, and those that represent the longed for connection, acceptance, nurturing and something different.

Jeff Young (2005) describes how individuals with borderline personality disorder are observed to flip between these modes/self states so rapidly that it can feel like different team members are talking about different people. In applying this thinking to self-injury in secure settings, the motive of the patient in deciding to injure herself might immediately appear different to different people. In the case of the punitive figure he/she may think that the patient acted to express the intense anger she experienced in their interaction, or to punish herself; in the case of the abusive figure he/she may consider the act to be one done to alert attention to her vulnerabilities; in the case of the idealised figure, he/she might consider the act to be a pattern of coping that we have come to understand, but that the patient has difficulty replacing with something less damaging. Ensuring adequate time and systems for communication and team reflection on such processes is recommended, alongside developing a shared narrative and accepted use of language.

Multi-disciplinary teams (MDT)

With the risk of "splits" in the team, the complexity of psychological disturbance in this patient group, and the different professional/theoretical backgrounds and experiences from which members of an MDT originate, it should not be assumed that there would automatically be a consistent approach to the care of each patient. Procedures for the management of decisions, discussion of approaches and interactions, and the shared understanding of treatment stages should reflect this need. Procedures for effective communication and reflection currently include computerised clinical notes, a simplified access/observation procedure, nursing handover by nurse-in-charge, feedback by visiting professionals, ward communications books, daily management meetings, daily patient ward/business meetings, weekly MDT business meetings, fortnightly ward rounds, care programme approach process, monthly women's service meetings as well as individual professional and group staff supervision arrangements. There are many opportunities for communication and integration, but such systems each require careful implementation and review. We call this approach "integrative eclecticism".

Empowerment

The development of a transparent treatment model highlighting needs and expectations emerged from an understanding of women's needs being linked to the issue of disempowerment as reflected in historical economic, social, political and cultural attributes and opportunities (i.e. access to resources, opportunities and decision making). In forensic settings it is difficult not to replicate such experiences given the lack of control patients often have over decision making in their care. Patients are observed to make attempts to empower themselves, sometimes in "dangerous" ways, such as interpersonal conflicts as well as self-injury.

According to WISH (Stafford 1999) women surveyed in high secure hospitals were mostly from large working class families, had experienced early abandonment or loss of a carer, had problematic attachment to foster families and over one-third were looked after in children's homes. In terms of attainment, 23% were sent to special schools, 75% had no educational qualifications and over 25% were never employed. As an adult 76% were solely dependent on social security payments prior to admission, over 80% had not experienced a stable partnership as an adult, but 40% had children – mostly as lone parents.

It is also the case that women in secure care may have regularly received messages that they are not to talk, not to share – to keep secrets. Anna Motz (2004) writes

> *...women use their bodies to articulate what cannot be spoken or thought about... their bodies become quite literally the sites of battles and modes of communication.*

Guidance from the *Into the Mainstream* document is that,

> *Psychological therapies adhere to the principles of empowerment, partnership and giving women a sense of control over the pace and movement of the therapeutic process.*

Overcoming such protection becomes a *readiness* consideration.

Readiness for treatment

In their recent overview of Australasian work on *treatment readiness* Andrew Day and colleagues (2007) sought to articulate and further develop the construct. They describe how, whereas the term responsivity has been concerned with adjusting treatment delivery in a way that maximises learning, "treatment readiness" is an overarching term which encompasses both the internal components of responsivity (e.g. offender motivation, problem awareness, emotional capacity to engage with psychological treatment, goals and personal identity), and external components that may be specific to the custodial environment in which treatment is commonly offered (e.g. availability of programmes, institutional social climates, legal pressure to attend; see Ward et al 2004).

When developing a new service, it is not only the patients who are asked to commit to a treatment model, but the service and staff have needs in respect of commitment, training and co-ordination to enhance the readiness of the establishment to provide effective treatment. This will continue to develop after a service opens its doors to patients, no matter how long the preparation period.

Jeffcote and Travers (2004) highlighted the need to consider issues of engagement carefully in designing psychological services for women in secure settings:

> *Apparent engagement may be misleading, reflecting the woman's expertise at being "a good girl" and leading the professional into collusion. Lack of engagement can be misconstrued as a lack of motivation rather than reflecting a deep sense of worthlessness or fear of being known by another... Women often experience a strong pressure to "prove" they always fail.*

Issues of treatment readiness have historically meant that patients with complex presentations that include personality disorder have found themselves excluded from services, or have themselves had difficulty engaging with or remaining in treatment. Patterns of behaviour, coping and inter-relating are entrenched and have become self-fulfilling, leading very often to an assumption that the path to change is a hopeless one. Particularly in medium security there is a sense of hope (and combined fear in some cases) that the next step could be living more independently. Without the pace and process towards this objective being carefully staged the anxieties associated with rejection can become overwhelming; without the building of therapeutic relationships, the establishment of safety, and further therapeutic stages/phases, the likelihood of therapeutic success is limited.

The question of change

Reflecting the issue of change in our treatment models is essential. Services designed to provide enhanced relational security should understand that positive change is often slow, with many setbacks. When facing crises it is common for professionals to consider patients to have lost all of the progress they have made; this has sometimes been termed "sabotage". Feelings of hopelessness, betrayal, disappointment and anger in staff are common given the cyclical nature of patient pathology. For patients themselves, fear and anxiety prevent personal development, growth and exploration, and for many women this fear and anxiety is associated with the therapeutic relationships they are asked to make in forensic settings. Being explicit about the language of change can help to manage expectations and alleviate anxieties around what should be provided from the inception of new services. As mentioned, readiness is a measure of the service as well as for the patient. One approach that has been utilised for understanding the sequence through which behaviour changes is Prochaska and DiClemente's (1992) naturalistic descriptions of changes in addictive behaviours. The six-stage process that they describe (pre-contemplation, contemplation, preparation, action, maintenance, termination) is combined by John Livesley to reflect four core stages:

- *Problem recognition involves recognising and accepting problems and developing a commitment to change.*
- *Exploration, whereby a collaborative description is used to develop an understanding of a given problem, its associated feelings and thoughts.*
- *Acquisition of alternatives suggests new ways of responding to situations and handling feelings and impulses: a problem-solving stage that seeks to find new solutions to old problems.*
- *Consolidation and generalisation, where steps are taken to ensure that new learning is strengthened and applied to everyday situations.*

(Livesley 2003: 91)

Such an approach is used to organise the management of specific problems, ranging from self-harming behaviour to maladaptive interpersonal patterns. Although these core strategies are described by Livesley in relation to individual therapy, they can be applied to an overarching model of treatment approach. He writes,

> *...evidence suggests that the non-specific component makes the greatest contribution to change; an approach based on generic mechanisms promises to provide the most effective way to manage and treat core pathology.*
>
> (Livesley, 2003: 115)

Therapeutic strategies are suggested by Livesley that complement the approach supported by Marsha Linehan and colleagues in the application of dialectical behaviour therapy (see *Table 10.1*). These can be amalgamated as:

- The importance of building and maintaining a therapeutic relationship.
- Establishing and maintaining a consistent treatment process (adhering to the treatment frame).
- Utilising validation ("communicating to the patient that her responses make sense and are understandable within her current life context or situation", Linehan 1993: 223).
- Building and maintaining motivation.

The application of validation to the treatment of self-injury is through:

- Recognising and accepting behaviour and experience.
- Acknowledging areas of competence.
- Facilitating a search for meaning.
- Managing validation ruptures.
- Avoiding invalidating interventions.
- Counteracting self-invalidation and reducing self-derogation.

Table 10.1: Psychological "treatment-stages" model for the Women's Services at Arnold Lodge

Structured day (on ward) and therapy services	*Individual work focus*	*Group work focus*
Therapeutic stage: Change management		
Daily business/feedback meetings Social, recreational and leisure activities – stabilising structure Physical health promotion and exercise	MD assessments Timelines and formulation Therapeutic, collaborative relationship building	
Therapeutic stage: Safety. Pre-treatment – Orientation and commitment		
Daily business/feedback meetings Social, recreational and leisure activities Physical health promotion and exercise and motor skills Motivational work Pattern of occupation Use of intensive care unit in crisis periods Tiers of response to incidents of self-harm	Timelines and formulation Pharmacology and concordance Review of physical health Psychoeducation and dialectical treatment orientation Coping strategy enhancement Grounding/mindfulness Named nurse session	Psychoeducation groups (mental health awareness) Pre-therapy groups: Lifestyles programme
Therapeutic stage: Containment. Stage 1 – Attaining basic capacities		
Daily business meetings Vocational placement exploration Distress signature work	Individual SPS/DBT sessions MDT support sessions Named nurse session	DBT-informed skills groups – mindfulness
Therapeutic Stage: Control and Regulation. Stage 2 – Reducing post-traumatic stress		
Daily business/feedback meetings Soothing and expressive activities (e.g. gardening group, creative opportunities – art, music and drama) Staged leave opportunities	Cognitive behavioural strategy intro: • Trauma-focused CBT • CBT for psychosis • Schema/mode work Individual body-centred/ somatosensory approaches Individual SPS/DBT sessions MDT support sessions Named nurse session	Social problem solving DBT-informed skills groups – mindfulness (Cognitive analytic music therapy pilot)

Table 10.1. cont/

Table 10.1. cont/		
Therapeutic Stage: Exploration and Change. Stage 3 – Increasing self-respect		
Daily business/feedback meetings Education and daily living skills Further leave opportunities Linking somatosensory work to meaningful therapeutic activities	Individual sessions (CBT approaches continue) MDT support sessions Named nurse session	Social skills/communication/esteem Mental health awareness Substance misuse programme Arson treatment programme
Therapeutic Stage: Integration and Synthesis. Stage 4 – Achieving individual goals		
Daily business/feedback meetings Daily living skills continue Family work and parenting skills	MDT support sessions Named nurse sessions (on leave where appropriate)	Daily business/feedback meetings Systemic approaches (e.g. family work) Pre-discharge group
MD = multidisciplinary, SPS = social problem solving, DBT = dialectical behaviour therapy, CBT = cognitive behavioural therapy		

Evidence from behavioural literature indicates that in order to change a behaviour one needs to be exposed to a different, novel experience and to both suppress the desire to act in one way and learn to associate another behaviour with the experience. This can only be achieved through learning (reinforcement processes). This needs time and patience. Those who have come to utilise any model of staged change will understand that a new experience will require consideration, action and maintenance. Our treatment stages model acknowledges the same phenomena, and therefore allows for and understands occasional "lapses" into old ways of relating/acting – this includes self-injury. It is understood by all parts of the multi-disciplinary team that the women will harm themselves, but it is clearly expressed that this is something that we (and they in the most part) would like to be different.

Treatment stage model

The over-arching psychological "treatment-stages" model for the women's services at Arnold Lodge is based on recognition of the need to provide opportunities for meaningful change, at a pace that is individualised, but which tends to follow a predictable sequence. This sequence gives an overall structure to treatment and provides a framework for integrating different kinds of specific, change-focused interventions.

Treatments are offered across professional groups and support each other through recognition of treatment stages. These stages were proposed by John Livesley (2003) and broadly are described by the terms change management; safety and containment; control and regulation; exploration and change; and integration and synthesis. The multi-modal approaches within these stages are summarised in *Table 10.1*. The opportunity for change is provided through therapeutic relationships, increased self-knowledge, the provision of new experiences and the acquisition of new behaviours. The methods of communicating treatment stages to patients are important. Patients can receive a written overview of the stages and how this relates to their care.

The provision of a ward-based daily programme provides support to all of the treatment stages by creating a holding and facilitating environment, by promoting engagement and familiarity essential to safety and containment, by offering new experiences to support exploration and change, and by allowing the opportunity for structured interpersonal activities, allowing learning to be applied and integrated into daily life.

Summary

There has been some support for the use of a stages of change/"treatment stages" model across services designed for treating individuals with complex needs. The Transtheoretical Model of Change (Prochaska and DiClemente 1984) has been influential in considering motivation, engagement and readiness in forensic settings and is integral to some programmes currently delivered in Dangerous People with Severe Personality Disorder (DSPD) sites in the UK for men as well as other women's enhanced services. For the women's service at Arnold Lodge, the treatment model/process described here allows for the co-ordination of a number of complementary approaches through a series of treatment phases and through balancing the principles of validation and change. This has promise in terms of simplicity, integrity, transparency and alliance with existing approaches. Individual treatment evaluation will inform the overall picture of effectiveness but so too will a description of the process of the stages themselves, alongside an anticipated reduction in problematic behaviours or symptoms.

Acknowledgement

The Editors would like to thank Routledge, Taylor and Francis Group and Rebecca Lawday for kind permission to reproduce in this chapter most of: Lawday R (2009) Self-harm in women's secure services: Reflections and strategies for treatment design. In: Motz A (ed) *Managing Self-Harm. Psychological Perspectives* (Chapter 8, pp 157–79). Routledge, Taylor and Francis Group: Hove.

References

Andrews DA, Bonta J (2003) *The psychology of criminal conduct* (3rd edn). Anderson, Cincinnati OH

Coid J, Kanton N, Gault S, Jarman B (2000) Women admitted to secure forensic services: Comparison of women and men. *Journal of Forensic Psychiatry* **11**(2): 275–95. Cited in Department of Health (2002) *Women's Mental Health: Into the Mainstream. Strategic Development of Mental Healthcare for Women*. HMSO, London

Day A, Howells K, Casey S, Ward T, Birgden A (2007) Treatment readiness: An overview of Australasian work. *Issues in Forensic Psychology* **7**: 21–5

Department of Health (1999) *Secure Futures for Women: Making a Difference*. NHS Executive Department of Health, London

Department of Health (2000) *Making a Difference*. Department of Health, London

Department of Health (2002a) *Women's Mental Health: Into the Mainstream. Strategic Development of Mental Healthcare for Women*. Department of Health, London

Department of Health (2002b) *Into the Mainstream: Analysis of Responses to the Consultation* Document accessed 10th June 2010 and available from: http://www.dh.gov.uk/prod_consum_dh/groups/dh_digitalassets/@dh/@en/documents/digitalasset/dh_4062101.pdf

Department of Health (2003) *Mainstreaming Gender and Women's Mental Health: Implementation Guidance*. Department of Health, London

Department of Health and NIMHE (2003) *Women only and Women-Sensitive Mental Health Services* (Expert Briefing). Department of Health and NIMHE, Leeds

Hawton K, Avensman E, Townsend E, Bremner S, et al (1998) Deliberate self-harm: Systematic review of efficacy of psychosocial and pharmacological treatments in presenting repetition. *British Medical Journal* **317**: 441–47. Cited in Department of Health (2002) *Women's Mental Health: Into the Mainstream. Strategic Development of Mental Healthcare for Women*. Department of Health, London

Jeffcote N, Travers R (2004)Thinking about the needs of women in secure settings. In Jeffcote N, Watson T (eds) *Working Therapeutically with Women in Secure Mental Health Settings* Jessica Kingsley. London, Philadelphia

Lart R, Payne S, Beaumont, et al (1999) *Women and Secure Psychiatric Services: A literature review*. Bristol: Bristol University. Cited in Department of Health (2002) *Women's Mental Health: Into the Mainstream. Strategic Development of Mental Healthcare for Women*. Department of Health, London

Lawday R (2009) Self harm in women's services-reflections and strategies for treatment design. In Motz A (ed) *Managing Self Harm: Psychological Perspectives* Routledge, Hove

Linehan MM (1993) *Cognitive Behavioral Treatment of Borderline Personality Disorder*. Guilford Press, NY, London

Livesley WJ (2003) *Practical Management of Personality Disorder*. Guilford Press, NY,

London

Motz A (2004) Hiding and being lost: The experience of female patients and staff on a mixed sex ward. In Jeffcote N, Watson T (eds) *Working Therapeutically with Women in Secure Mental Health Settings*. Jessica Kingsley, London, Philadelphia

Motz A (ed) (2009) *Managing Self Harm: Psychological Perspectives* Routledge, Hove

Prochaska JO, DiClemente CC (1984) *The Transtheoretical Approach: Crossing traditional boundaries of therapy*. Dow Jones-Irwin, Homewood IL

Stafford P (1999) *Defining Gender Issues: Redefining Women's Services*. WISH, London. Cited in Jeffcote N, Watson T (eds) (2004) *Working Therapeutically with Women in Secure Mental Health Settings*. Jessica Kingsley, London, Philadelphia

Tilt R, Perry B, Martin C, et al (2000) *Report of the Review of Security at the High Security Hospitals*. Department of Health, London

Ward T, Day A, Howells K, Birgden A (2004) The multifactor offender readiness model. *Aggression and Violent Behaviour* **9**: 645–73

Young J (2005) Schema therapy workshops. Cambridge

CHAPTER 11

The emotional labour of prison nursing

Elizabeth Walsh

Introduction

This chapter considers the emotional labour of prison nurses as narrated by them through interviews and clinical supervision undertaken as part of a doctoral study (Walsh 2007). It is well documented that nursing patients can be emotionally demanding for nurses and can result in stress and burnout (Landa et al 2008, McVicar 2003). Putting aside one's own feelings and troubles to care for another is, at times, difficult for the most professional of nurses, however, by considering the concept of emotional labour, this chapter considers how nurses working in prison, caring for some of the most socially excluded and despised individuals, experience and manage the emotional labour of caring for them.

The literature surrounding prison nursing often regards the challenges facing nurses as centred on the competing philosophies of caring and custody (Gulotta 1986, Droes 1994, Doyle 1999, Dale and Woods 2001); however, this chapter considers emotional labour as central to the challenges facing nurses working in prison. Clearly the secure environment within which prison nurses work has an impact on their practice, but so does the nature of the prisoner patient, and indeed, the culture of the prison world.

The context of prison nursing in England and Wales

The current prison population is 84 115 in England and Wales, both male and female (HM Prison Service 2008). It is estimated that over 1 million people per year are affected by imprisonment, be they in prison themselves or have a family member in prison. The healthcare needs of this population are similar to those in the community. However, it is suggested that 90% of the prison population have a diagnosable mental health problem (including personality disorder), a substance misuse problem, or both, and 80% of prisoners smoke (Department of Health and HM Prison Service 2001). In addition to the possible pre-existing health needs of prisoner patients, there are health needs created as a consequence of imprisonment. Examples of these include the lack of direct access to over-the-counter medications, restriction on family networks/support, overcrowding, and limited opportunities for self-care. Overcrowding in prisons is currently high on both the political and media agendas as the prison population in England and Wales reaches capacity and police cells are commandeered to house prisoners. In addition to overcrowding affecting the care needs of prisoners, Vere-Jones (2007: 5) highlights it as a problem for nurses working in prison:

> *...overstretched prison nurses cannot provide the therapeutic intervention that inmates require because of overcrowding.*

A multidisciplinary team comprising doctors, nurses, physiotherapists, chiropodists, dentists, radiographers, specialist nurses, opticians, and drug workers, for example, provide healthcare and health-related services to prisoners. Interestingly, the multidisciplinary team in a prison comprises a far wider spectrum of professionals than in a primary care team outside prison. For example, the nurse in the prison setting may also liaise with probation officers, discipline (prison) officers, psychologists, physical education staff and educational staff in caring for a prisoner.

The role of the nurse in a prison is varied and complex. Prisoners present a range of health problems, often spanning the spectrum of traditional nursing specialities. Hence, nurses working in prison need skills in mental health nursing, general nursing (both medical and surgical), primary care/practice nursing, learning disability nursing and children's nursing (for those nurses working with young offenders and juveniles). This presents a professional challenge to practitioners, educationalists and researchers alike. Not only are nurses working in prison providing nursing care to the prison population but they also have a role similar to that of the prison officer in maintaining security and order. This demands skills and competencies in both nursing care and security.

On a practical level, prison nursing staff can expect to deal with a wide range of illness and disease including chronic illness, mental health problems, drug and alcohol misuse, acute medical conditions and trauma. In addition, nurses provide health screening services for all prisoners entering the prison system and inpatient services for medical, surgical and psychiatric care. Nurses in prison also provide well man clinics, chronic disease management clinics and primary healthcare/practice nursing similar to that provided at a local GP surgery. Prison nurses practise in a prison community, away from the world outside. This inevitably requires them to engage with prisoners, sometimes on a daily basis over long periods of time, in a setting which is often emotionally highly charged. It is no wonder that prison nursing practice entails high levels of emotion work.

Caring in custody

It has been well documented that the culture within which prison nurses work impacts on their practice (Norman and Parrish 2002, Wilcox 2002, Schafer 1997). In an anecdotal article, Stevens (1993) highlights the collision of cultures that nurses experience when practising in the prison environment. *Table 11.1*, adapted from Stevens (1993), illustrates the two main cultures prevalent in a prison where healthcare and security are competing priorities.

The impact on the nurse of working with these competing priorities can be significant and it is suggested that it is the resultant emotional labour with which they engage in attempting to meet the caring and custodial elements of their role, that can cause difficulties. Mann (2004: 211) cites Festinger's theory of cognitive dissonance, which maintains that:

> *...whenever an individual simultaneously holds two cognitions that are psychologically inconsistent, they experience a negative drive state called dissonance, which is a state of discomfort or tension.*

The impact of this state of discomfort and tension will vary from individual to individual, however, it is suggested that the long-term

Table 11.1. Conflicting cultures

Element	*Healthcare*	*Prison*
Values	Basic goodness All individuals are essentially the same	Evil is present Criminal traits exist
Beliefs	Individuals who say they are sick should receive attention People obey the rules	Individuals who say they are sick are trying to get out of something People break the rules
Norms	Respect the patient Anger and hostility are acceptable behaviours when a person is ill. Assistance is offered, anger is redirected Resisting treatment calls for counselling with restraints being the last resort Assumption of danger to self is minimal	Distrust the inmate Anger and hostility are not acceptable. Hostile inmates necessitate higher security Resisting arrest is not tolerated and restraints are the first resort (handcuffs) Assumption of danger to self is ever present

impact of sustained cognitive dissonance will impact negatively on the nurse working in prison.

Emotional labour

Emotional labour has been described by Hochschild (1983: 7) as

> *The management of feeling to create a publicly observable facial and bodily display.*

She elaborates on this by suggesting that

> *...this labour requires one to induce or suppress feeling in order to sustain the outward countenance that produces a proper state of mind in others...this kind of labour calls for co-ordination of mind and feeling, and it sometimes draws on a source of self that we honour as deep and integral to our individuality.*

Hochschild (1983:147) suggests that jobs that have an element of emotional labour share three common characteristics: they require face-to-face/voice-to-voice contact with the public; they require the worker to produce an emotional state in another person and they allow the employer, through training and supervision, to exercise a degree of control over the emotional activities of employees.

Other authors have applied the concept of emotional labour to a broad spectrum of occupations such as counselling (Mann 2004), call centre work (Mulholland 2002), police work (Rutter and Fielding 1988, Stenross and Kleinman 1989), prison work (Tracy 2005), and fast food work (Leidner 1993). However, within the arena of nursing and healthcare, Pam Smith is regarded as a seminal writer (see Smith 1992). Emotional labour has been highlighted in a wide range of nursing specialties such as gynaecology (Bolton 2000), palliative care (James 1992, Frogatt 1998), midwifery (Hunter 2004), general nursing (Henderson 2001), intensive and critical care (Beeby 2000), elderly care (Gattuso and Bevan 2000), and paediatric and neonatal intensive care (Greenall 2001, Way 2003). The concept has also been considered from the perspective of the student nurse (Pfund et al 2004).

The emotional labour of prison nurses

Mann (2004: 208) identifies three components of emotional labours:

- The faking of emotion that is not felt.
- The hiding of emotion that is felt.

- The performance of emotion management in order to meet expectations within a work environment.

In considering emotional labour, it is clear that it relates to nurses working in any setting. In prison, the emotional labour experienced by the nurse is thought to be underpinned by relationships with three main areas: the prisoner, fellow colleagues and the institution within which the work takes place, for example, the prison/health service.

These are external relationships; however, there is also an internal relationship which is what is suggested here to be at the heart of the emotional labour of the prison nurse, and the one relationship that is difficult to uncover: the relationship the nurse has with him or herself. This "intranurse" relationship provides the nurse with two internal perspectives on practice: the professional, "What I should do", which is often in conflict with the more emotional "What I want to do". In terms of nursing in prison, consider the more emotional "What I want to do" in light of caring for prisoners who are particularly difficult to manage or who may provoke negative feelings in the nurse. These negative feelings are rarely acknowledged as they can sometimes feel inappropriate and unprofessional. However, the dissonance and resultant strain caused by these conflicting feelings is significant. Glasberg et al (2007: 392) note the impact of moral strain on stress levels and burnout amongst nurses and suggests that

> *...healthcare professionals experience a troubled conscience when they feel that they cannot provide the good care that they wish – and believe it is their duty – to give.*

This is also highly relevant for the prison nurse working within a system where healthcare is a competing priority with security.

Figure 11.1 illustrates the sources of emotional labour impacting on the prison nurse and demonstrates where the resultant dissonance and conflict is placed as a result.

It can be seen from *Figure 11.1* that there are three external relationships with which nurses engage that impact on the internal relationship they have with themselves: the intranurse relationship. In discussing each of these relationships, a picture is built detailing the areas of prison nursing practice which, when experienced on a daily basis, will, over time, entail significant levels of emotional labour. There is a clear link between high levels of emotional labour and high levels of stress, and Mann (2004: 212) notes that "research has shown links between emotional labour and burnout". She asserts that emotional exhaustion, depersonalisation and diminished personal accomplishment are common components of burnout. In

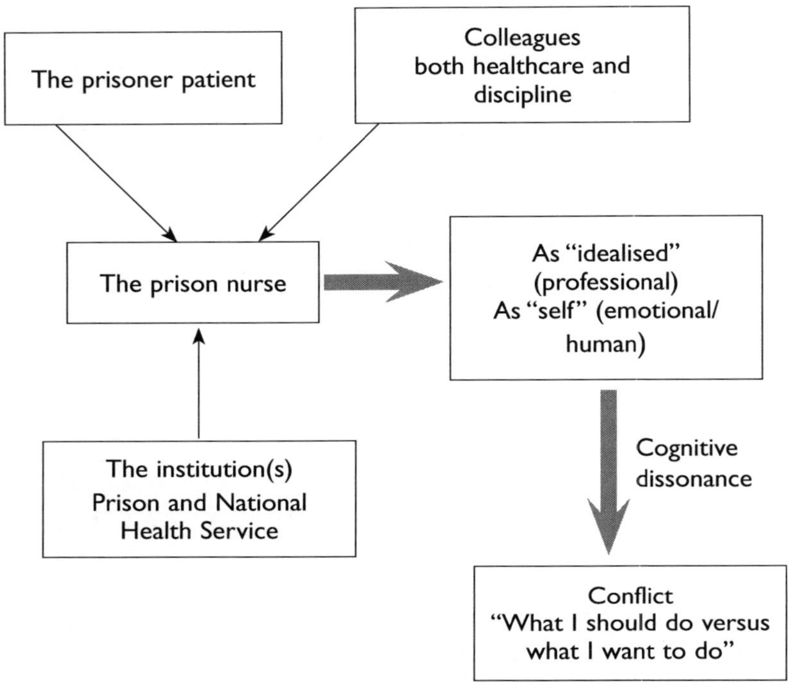

Figure 11.1. The sources of emotional labour impacting on the prison nurse.

addition, McVicar (2003) notes that the impact on the individual of sustained distress can include sadness, depression, pessimism, negative attitudes, fatigue, increased smoking/alcohol consumption, elevated arterial blood pressure, indigestion, and constipation/diarrhoea. It is suggested that sustained high levels of poorly managed emotional labour for the prison nurse will result in high levels of stress with negative consequences, both physical and psychological. This in turn can affect staff recruitment and retention, morale, sickness levels and ultimately impact on patient care.

The nurse–prisoner patient relationship

The nature of the nurse–patient relationship in prison is very different to that outside prison. In considering the relationship between nurse and prisoner patient, there are three main areas that are felt to be challenging for the prison nurse: prisoner aggression and manipulation; the effect of the prisoner's offence on care; and challenges to developing a nurse–patient relationship (Walsh 2007).

Through interviewing prison nurses and asking them to reflect on their practice, incidents of aggression and manipulation have a clear effect on care:

> *You see, one way or another, prisoners will always try to con you. One way or another, and it's how they do it that's annoying. If a prisoner comes up and is very, very angry or aggressive, my attitude is I just don't want to know him. It's like, "You come back and speak to me when you're calmer. I won't put up with it." Then my instant reaction is, "I don't want to know. I'm not going to help you." If they come back and they've calmed down, then of course, I will do whatever needs to be done.*
>
> (Prison nurse in Walsh 2007)

This nurse highlights the impact of aggression and manipulation on care provision insomuch as care is sometimes denied within rigid boundaries set in the face of aggression. However, in terms of emotional labour, it is the impact of having to adopt this approach to caring for a prisoner patient that is of interest. Nurses spoke of feeling worn down and tired of dealing with aggressive prisoner patients (Walsh 2007).

The impact of a prisoner's offence on care is an area which many people who do not work in prison feel would be the most difficult to manage. In terms of emotional labour, it has serious implications which are often not explored, as to do so would entail reflecting deeply on practice and may encourage difficult feelings to be confronted. Droes (1994) suggests that nurses in her study looked beyond the prisoner's past behaviour which, although taking perseverance and patience, enabled them to accept prisoners as human beings, which, in turn, made it easier for them to care. However, Holmes and Federman (2003) report that nurses working with prisoners modify their own representation of inmate patients in order to care, since modifying their own representation of the patient is easier than modifying their own behaviour. Walsh (2007) found that nurses working with prisoners whose offences they knew about, actually modified their own behaviour insofar as they became more detached:

> *It does affect you….I mean, yes, I wouldn't sometimes like to give them the steam off my tea, that's how I feel, and then they go, "Oh, I've got a headache, have you a couple of paracetamol?" or whatever and I think to myself, "Why don't you go and rot somewhere?" I don't want to help them and I think that's human. I don't punish myself for that because I would only think it; I wouldn't say it. Much as I might like. I wouldn't. I'd just be like, "Yep – there you go"…It does, it kind of affects the way you behave towards them. Definitely does. Yes it's hard. You know what though, I'm a smiley kind of person, it's just the way I am, and I try not to when I'm dealing with one particular inmate…I wouldn't, I just couldn't bring myself to smile at him. I just used to mumble. I was never*

> *rude, because he was on medication, I would say, "Do you want this today – do you want this now or tonight?"; that was how I would say it when normally I would say to them, "Do you want this now, or later, or do you want to take it away with you?", something like that – a bit more chatty. It did, it wears you down. It wore me down because I'm not like that you know.*
>
> (Prison nurse in Walsh 2007)

There are many prison nurses who deny that the prisoner's offence has any impact on the care they provide. In many instances this will be true, however, although care will still be provided regardless, it is the manner in which that care is provided which, it is suggested, will have implications for the emotional labour of these nurses. As the nurse above notes, it is not that care is not provided, but that it is provided in a way that is more detached. It is this detachment that affects the intranurse relationship and the subsequent feelings that this detachment promotes within the prison nurse which is at the centre of emotional labour.

The nurse–discipline officer relationship

The relationship between prison nurses and discipline officers can be difficult primarily due to the underpinning philosophies within which both operate. Discipline officers are by their very role, working within a custodial philosophy whereas nurses are working within a caring discourse. Both are competing priorities within a prison setting and consequently, there is conflict. Glasberg et al (2007) note that interpersonal conflicts impact significantly on stress and burnout in nurses. In Walsh (2007) the issues of communication, understanding, responsibility and a professional divide were highlighted as issues which often bring this conflict to the fore. This is not to say that nurses and discipline officers are always in conflict. On the contrary, there are often times when both officers and nurses work well together. However, when the custodial and caring philosophies clash, nurses can experience high levels of emotional labour as they attempt to "perform emotion management in order to meet expectations within a work environment" (Mann 2004: 208).

The expectations placed upon nurses by discipline officers often relate to the need to maintain security, both psychological and physical. For example, nurses may want to unlock a prisoner in order to attend to a physical health need, or they may want to engage with the prisoner as they would a patient in the community by sharing information about themselves in order to foster a trusting relationship. Both courses of action could be viewed by discipline staff as threats to security. As a consequence, nurses have to adjust their behaviour to meet the expectations of the prison and its culture, thereby engaging in emotional labour to do so successfully.

In her study concerning the experience of caring for inmate patients in the USA, Weiskopf (2005: 339) suggests that nurses experienced caring as "an attempt to negotiate the boundaries between the cultures of caring and custody". She refers to complex challenges, numerous frustrations, and substantial limitations placed on the nurse–patient relationship. In addition, it was not only the nurse–patient relationship that was difficult, but also the relationship with correctional officers. Weiskopf suggests that it is these boundaries, that are so central to the environment, which caused the greatest frustration for the nurses in trying to develop a professional relationship with inmates.

The prison routine, which is rigidly imposed on nurses, can limit access to prisoner patients and has been highlighted as having a marked impact on care provision and possibilities, thus causing cognitive dissonance for prison nurses:

> *It's difficult really. You are trying to ensure that they get the healthcare they need, but sometimes it's difficult in the environment to provide it. It's like sometimes the person only needs a cup of tea and a chat, but finding the time when you can actually do that is very difficult.*
>
> (Prison nurse in Walsh 2007)

Another nurse noted how stressful it is to administer medication within a specified time frame:

> *Like for example, when you are working in a treatment room and it's busy. Depending on the wing and how busy it is – on the busiest wing you'd see around 60 to 80 prisoners in the course of an hour, hour and a half. It's like a conveyor belt system. It's really stressful.*
>
> (Prison nurse in Walsh, 2007)

Given that nurses working in prison are experiencing high levels of emotional labour, it is important to consider the ways in which this emotional labour can be managed more effectively in order to reduce stress and promote well-being.

Managing emotional labour

As has already been noted, extended exposure to the cognitive dissonance caused as a result of engaging in emotional labour causes stress. One way in which people often manage this dissonance is through what Menzies

Lyth (1988) refers to as defences against anxiety. These defences manifest themselves in a variety of ways, such as depersonalisation and categorisation of the patient, the elimination of decisions by ritual task performance, performance of checks and counter checks, and avoidance of change. In Walsh (2009a) nurses described such defences against anxiety through their discussion of routines and practice:

> *I like the fact that you can hand your keys in at the end of the day and go home and you don't necessarily have to think about things. For me, the handing in of the keys is the cut off point. Whereas when I worked on a ward, I was like, "How's that little old lady in bed 2? Is she OK tonight?", so I find that my cut off point, actually doing that, makes me feel like, no, I'm at home now. I think to myself when I went home they were all alive and happy – tomorrow's another day.*
>
> (Prison nurse in Walsh 2007 and Walsh 2009a: 146f)

Depersonalisation of the patient can be seen in prison through the way in which nurses, particularly when dealing with more difficult prisoners, prefer to connect with them on a purely functional, needs-approach basis rather than engaging in the development of a traditional nurse–patient relationship, based on mutual trust (Johns 1996).

Another theoretical perspective to consider in managing emotional labour is that of emotional intelligence. Emotional intelligence has gained a great deal of interest of late, promoted primarily in popular culture by Daniel Goleman (see Goleman, 1996); however, the concept was introduced by Salovey and Mayer (1990). However, further development of the concept led them to redefine it as:

> *...the ability to perceive accurately, appraise and express emotion; the ability to access and/or generate feelings when they facilitate thought; the ability to understand emotion and emotional knowledge; and the ability to regulate emotions to promote emotional and intellectual growth.*
>
> (Mayer and Salovey 1997: 10).

In relation to nurses working in prison, this concept is important on a number of levels that match with the relationships described earlier, such as with the prisoner, colleagues and institution. For example, it is important for the prison nurse to be able to perceive accurately, and appraise and express appropriate emotion when dealing with prisoners. Those with low levels of emotional intelligence may encounter hostility if their reactions to emotionally charged situations are inappropriate. Therefore, the nurse with high levels of emotional intelligence will be able to manage relationships with prisoners, colleagues and the institution far more effectively, which will ultimately impact on the overall emotional labour and its subsequent consequences on the internal intranurse relationship.

Given that it tends to be the effect of the cognitive dissonance in the intranurse relationship which can have adverse effects on the prison nurse, it is important that the emotional intelligence of prison nurses is developed to its maximum potential in managing emotional labour. One way in which it is suggested emotional labour can be developed is through the mechanisms of reflection and clinical supervision.

Clinical supervision

According to Davey et al (2006: 239) "there is [no] one definition of clinical supervision". Bond and Holland (1998) suggest that definitions proposed by authors tend to highlight the elements of clinical supervision that they themselves feel are most important. In her concept analysis of clinical supervision, Lyth (2000) asserts that

> *Clinical supervision is a support mechanism for practising professionals within which they can share clinical, organisational, developmental and emotional experiences with another professional in a secure, confidential environment in order to enhance knowledge and skills. This process will lead to an increased awareness of other concepts including accountability and reflective practice.*
>
> (Lyth 2000: 728)

In Walsh (2007), clinical supervision was utilised as a way of supporting prison nurses to develop their emotional intelligence whilst providing a safe space to enable them to manage their emotional labour. Through regular monthly clinical supervision sessions over six months, key themes emerged which the nurses felt contributed to their emotional labour: conflict with colleagues, both healthcare and discipline; their position within the prison hierarchy; professional safety; nursing practice; self-confidence; empowerment; and accountability.

These issues were discussed through supervision in terms of the way in which they impacted on the intranurse relationship. In evaluating and reflecting on these supervision sessions, these nurses noted a positive change in their levels of confidence, and an ability to come to terms more effectively with the stresses and challenges of their practice. They reported an increased awareness of the need for reflection both on and in practice, which they felt led them to an altered perspective. One nurse remarked that she felt more positive about her practice and more able to cope with the challenges she had previously felt unable to manage. Engaging with clinical supervision had enabled these nurses to utilise the time and space for clinical supervision to think more deeply about their practice, and the supportive element of it had led to one of the nurses remaining at the prison rather than seeking alternative employment elsewhere. It was also noted to be important that, although having clinical supervision was useful for these nurses, the fact that the supervisor had experience of prison nursing, and thus understood the context of the supervisees' practice, was vital to its success. Given the nature of clinical supervision as focused on the needs of the supervisee (the nurse) this is unsurprising.

More detailed discussion of these concepts and the way in which they were perceived by these nurses can be found in Walsh (2007, 2009b). Support for the development of clinical supervision in prison healthcare settings can be found in Walsh et al (2007) and Freshwater et al (2002a, b, 2007), .

Conclusion

Emotional labour is often felt, but not fully understood, by many nurses working in prison. Prolonged exposure to it manifests itself in many ways, such as through stress, which leads to staff sickness, low morale and frustration, all of which can impact on patient care. Drawing on the work of Walsh (2007), this chapter suggests that many of the challenges facing prison nurses in their daily practice are rooted in three key relationships: with the prisoner, with colleagues and with the institution. The challenges inherent within these relationships have a significant impact on the intranurse relationship, which is the internal relationship that nurses have with themselves. This internal relationship often appears to be in a state of discomfort or tension, due to the cognitive dissonance experienced between the professional self and the emotional self; the "What I want to do versus what I should do". This tension can be effectively uncovered and worked out through reflection on practice and clinical supervision. Given that the emotional intelligence of prison nurses is paramount in managing effective relationships between themselves and prisoners/colleagues/institutions; clinical supervision can also serve to develop the emotional intelligence of the prison nurse, thus reducing the impact of emotional labour on the intranurse relationship.

All nurses need to be engaged in some form of reflection on and in practice. Formal clinical supervision serves as a way for nurses to structure their reflection and be supported through uncovering what can often turn out to be uncomfortable and sometimes distressing emotions. As one prison nurse reported:

I think there are certain crimes, you know, we are all human and sometimes. It gets me. There was one…erm, a child abuser. I read about it in his medical notes, he was in healthcare. You know, that time, it really gets me really; it was a baby, a baby. I went into the toilets and cried, you know..I cried that night.

(Prison nurse in Walsh 2007)

This is an extreme emotional reaction and fortunately, in the day-to-day practice of prison nurses, is not common. However, it could be suggested that negative emotions are commonly felt by prison nurses, but not confronted or indeed, managed appropriately. After all, in some prison environments, showing certain emotions is inappropriate and not in keeping with the expectations of the institution; such behaviour is a departure from traditional prison culture (Crawley 2004). However, this experience is a very real possibility for nurses working in prison and indeed, many of them will have experienced similar high levels of emotion such as anger, frustration or disgust which can impact on their mental well-being, due to dissonance in the intranurse relationship. The first stage in managing these emotions is to admit feeling them, with the second stage being to engage in regular clinical supervision in order to receive support.

References

Beeby JP (2000) Intensive care nurses' experiences of caring: Part 2: Research findings *Intensive and Critical Care Nursing* **16**(3): 151–63

Bolton S (2000) Who cares? Offering emotion work as a 'gift' in the nursing labour process *Journal of Advanced Nursing* **32**(3): 580–6

Bond M, Holland S (1998) *Skills of Clinical Supervision for Nurses: A Practical Guide*. Open University Press, Buckingham

Crawley E (2004) Emotion and performance. Prison officers and the presentation of self in prisons. *Punishment, Society* **6**(4): 411–27

Dale C, Woods P (2001) *Caring For Prisoners*. RCN, London

Davey B, Desousa C, Robinson S, Murrells T (2006) The policy and practice divide. Who has clinical supervision in nursing? *Journal of Research in Nursing* **11**(3): 237–48

Department of Health and HM Prison Service (2001) *Changing the Outlook: A Strategy for Developing Mental Health Services in Prison*. Department of Health, London

Doyle J (1999) A qualitative study of factors influencing psychiatric nursing practice in Australian prisons. *Perspectives in Psychiatric Care* **35**(1): 29–35

Droes N (1994) Correctional nursing practice. *Journal of Community Health Nursing* **11**(4): 201–10

Freshwater D, Walsh L, Storey L (2002a) Prison health care: Developing leadership through clinical supervision. *Nursing Management* **8**(8): 10–13

Freshwater D, Walsh L, Storey L (2002b) Prison health care. Part two: Developing leadership through clinical supervision. *Nursing Management* **8**(9): 16–20

Freshwater D, Walsh E, Esterhuizen P (2007) Models of effective and reflective teaching and learning for best practice in clinical supervision. In Bishop V (ed) Clinical Supervision in Practice(2nd edn). Palgrave Macmillan, Basingstoke

Froggatt K (1998) The place of metaphor and language in exploring nurses' emotional work. *Journal of Advanced Nursing* **28**(2): 332–8

Gattuso S, Bevan C (2000) Mother, daughter, patient, nurse: Women's emotion work in aged care. *Journal of Advanced Nursing* **31**(4): 892–9

Glasberg AL, Eriksson S, Norberg A (2007) Burnout and 'stress of conscience' among healthcare professionals. *Journal of Advanced Nursing* **57**(4): 392–403

Goleman D (1996) *Emotional Intelligence*. Bloomsbury, London

Greenall FM (2001) Doctor–nurse communication in the neonatal intensive care unit: An anthropological analysis. *Journal of Neonatal Nursing* **7**(4): 110–4

Gulotta K (1986) Factors affecting nursing practice in a correctional healthcare setting. *Journal of Prison and Jail Health* **6**(1): 3–22

Henderson A (2001) Emotional labour and nursing: An underappreciated aspect of caring work. *Nursing Inquiry* **8**(2): 130–8

HM Prison Service (2008) Available from: www.hmprisonservice.gov.uk/resourcecentre/publicationsdocuments/index.asp?cat=85 [last accessed 22 September 2008]

Hochschild A (1983) *The Managed Heart*. University of California Press, London

Holmes D, Federman C (2003) Constructing monsters: Correctional discourse and nursing practice. *International Journal of Psychiatric Nursing Research* **8**(3): 942–62

Hunter B (2004) Conflicting ideologies as a source of emotion work in midwifery. *Midwifery* **20**: 261–72

James N (1992) Care = organisation + physical labour + emotional labour. *Sociology of Health and Illness* **14**(4): 488–509

Johns JL (1996) A concept analysis of trust. *Journal of Advanced Nursing* **24**: 76–83

Landa JMA, Lopez-Zafra E, Martos MPB, Aguilar-Luzon MC (2008) The relationship between emotional intelligence, occupational stress and health in nurses: A questionnaire survey. *International Journal of Nursing Studies* **45**: 888–901

Leidner R (1993) Fast Food Fast Talk: Service Work and the Routinization of Everyday Life. University of California Press, Berkley

Lyth GM (2000) Clinical supervision: A concept analysis. *Journal of Advanced Nursing* **31**(3): 722–9

McVicar A (2003) Workplace stress in nursing: A literature review. *Journal of Advanced Nursing* **44**(6): 633–42

Mann S (2004) 'People–work': Emotion management, stress and coping. *British Journal of Guidance, Counselling* **32**(2): 205–21

Mayer JD, Salovey P (1997) What is emotional intelligence? In Salovey P, Sluyter DJ (eds) *Emotional Development and Emotional Intelligence: Implications for educators*. New York: Basic Books

Menzies Lyth I (1988) *Containing Anxiety in Institutions Selected Essays*. (Vol 1) Free Association Books, London

Mulholland K (2002) Gender emotional labour and teamworking in a call centre. *Personnel*

Review **31**(3): 283–303

Norman A, Parrish A (2002) *Prison Nursing*. Blackwell, Oxford

Pfund R, Dawson P, Francis R, Rees B (2004) Learning how to handle emotionally challenging situations: The context of effective reflection. *Nurse Education in Practice* **4**: 107–13

Rutter DR, Fielding PJ (1988) Sources of occupational stress: An examination of British police officers. *Work and Stress* **2**: 291–9

Salovey P, Mayer JD (1990) Emotional intelligence. *Imagination Cognition and Personality* **9**: 185–211

Schafer P (1997) When a client develops an attraction: Successful resolution versus boundary violation. *Journal of Psychiatric and Mental Health Nursing* **4**: 203–11

Smith P (1992) *The Emotional Labour of Nursing*. Basingstoke: Macmillan

Stenross B, Kleinman S (1989) The highs and lows of emotional labor: Detectives encounters with criminals and victims. *Journal of Contemporary Ethnography* **17**: 435–52

Stevens R (1993) When your clients are in jail. *Nursing Forum* **28**(4): 4–5

Tracy SJ (2005) Locking up emotion: Moving beyond dissonance for understanding emotion labor discomfort. *Communication Monographs* **72**(3): 261–83

Vere-Jones E (2007) Prison pressures endanger care. *Nursing Times* **103**(6): 5

Walsh E (2007) *An Examination of the Emotional Labour of Nurses Working in Prison*. PhD Thesis, Bournemouth University

Walsh E (2009a) The emotional labour of prison nurses working in Her Majesty's (HM) Prison Service. *Journal of Forensic Nursing* **5**(3): 143–52

Walsh E (2009b) The emotional labour of nurses who work in Her Majesty's (HM) Prison Service. *Journal of Forensic Nursing* **5**(3): 143–52

Walsh E, Dilworth S, Freshwater D (2007) Establishing Clinical Supervision in Prison Health Care Settings: Phase three. A report for Offender Health. Department of Health Bournemouth University, Bournemouth

Way C (2003) In their own words: Paediatric intensive care nurses' experiences of withdrawal of treatment. *Paediatric Intensive Care Nursing* **4**(1): 17–31

Weiskopf C (2005) Nurses experience of caring for inmate patients. *Journal of Advanced Nursing* **49**(4): 336–43

Willcox A (2002) Nursing in prisons: Understanding educational needs through a case study approach. *Learning in Health and Social Care* **1**(4): 180–90

CHAPTER 12

An experience as a prison in-reach mental health nurse

Glynnis Vann and Richard Byrt

Working in the prison

Glynnis Vann

Approaching the prison, you see a huge concrete and high walled building with barbed wire around it. Large metal gates and signs warn the public, and entrance boxes, for occasional security upgrades, add to the general atmosphere, which is scary and daunting. Once inside, this does not change unless you work there regularly, and then you become desensitised. What is an everyday occurrence for staff, makes others gasp and say they are fascinated or frightened. Ethically, the impact of such environments on prisoners, including the many individuals with mental health problems or learning disabilities, can be questioned (Stern 2006, Blom-Cooper 2008).

No chairs, toilets or water

The corridors are long and cold winds blow through them all the year round, especially in winter. It can be cold on the warmest days, due to the concrete and shade. The corridors are not heated and prisoners are discouraged from wandering and hanging around there as impulsive and violent threats and bullying attacks are a regular occurrence. The healthcare department is off one of these corridors. The prisoners are allowed to attend the healthcare department from the wings for medication, before 8 am, at lunchtime and at 4 pm. They also attend for appointments with doctors and nurses. However, soon after 8 am, there is a roll call, and the prisoners are held in the caged healthcare area until this is completed, often for up to two hours, with no chairs, no access to toilets and no water. Whilst prisoners wait for medication, there are arguments, and bullying occurs on a regular basis. Individuals are supposedly not allowed to smoke at this time, but many do so, and those who do not are subjected to passive smoking. All the prisoners are subjected to the cold and many to verbal abuse, which is often from staff when the prisoners complain. The way in which these people are treated shows a lack of "respect for persons" (Kant 1969): a concept which was considered in *Chapter 2*.

Walking through this waiting area is frightening, but unavoidable, as it is the main thoroughfare to the Healthcare Department. A good coping mechanism is to be assertive and respectful, to stop and discuss general issues with prisoners, pass the time of day or just smile to acknowledge they are there.

I observed the Healthcare Manager take cups of coffee to prisoners in the waiting area on one occasion, but he was told there was a security issue with hot fluids and a risk of harm to himself and others. In relation to "respect for persons" and establishing therapeutic communication, it was frowned upon by prison officers and other staff when any perceived signs of what was seen as "weakness", in the form of compassion, were observed. Often, as healthcare staff, we were subjected to verbal abuse, touching, comments about our age and appearance, and complaints about the system, even if this was unconnected with the role we carried out.

"Anyone for Hep B?"

Nursing staff sometimes failed to show respect for patients. They were often rude and abusive in return for the abuse they received, and regularly closed the medication hatch in response to prisoners voicing their frustration. Nursing and healthcare staff were in a superior position, and were not dealing with complaints in an appropriate manner.

The Nursing and Midwifery Council (2008, 2010) emphasises the registered nurse's duty of care to maintain confidentiality. However, during the holding time, when up to 30 prisoners waited for the hepatitis clinic, the nurse used to call loudly into the area: "Anyone for Hep B?". Often prisoners missed appointments because they were unwilling to admit to needing this service. This also happened when the infection control nurse visited. When challenged, the nurse involved said it did not matter.

There were many other breaches of confidentiality. HIV results and follow up appointments were left on the desk for entry onto the system. The office was cleaned by prisoners who were felt to be reliable and trustworthy, but I observed one reading an HIV positive result which showed the prisoner's name, number and location. This prisoner had yet to be informed of the result. I reported this immediately to management, and was treated differently afterwards. Following this, I was moved to a small and inappropriate office space.

Lack of communication about individuals' risk

In one large prison where I worked, many of the prisoners were serving long sentences for a variety of crimes. However, the extent and nature of individuals' risk was unknown. This lack of risk assessment meant that individuals were faced with an increased threat of attack.

Transfers between prisons regularly occurred, and ordinarily a letter would arrive, stating that a prisoner transferred to the establishment had previously received care from a mental health professional. As with many prisons (Durcan 2008), there was no primary mental health team, so members of the in-reach team, including myself, dealt with these individuals. However, we were not always informed that they had been transferred to the prison, and were never sent any care programme approach documentation or risk assessment and management paperwork. Often, colleagues in other institutions were unwilling to share this, or the relevant documentation was inappropriate, inadequate or simply not completed. Related computerised information was not always available. These inadequacies are clearly not in accordance with the Nursing and Midwifery Council (2009) guidance on record keeping.

In one incidence, "Mr X" was transferred from another prison. I checked his documentation and did not notice any flagged initial risks or untoward issues. I was unaware of any particular risks, and perhaps desensitised. As with other prisoners, and for reasons I found difficult to understand, Mr X's security file, indicating potential risks, arrived after his transfer. After I had introduced myself, I gave Mr X an appointment slip, which he scrunched up and threw into my face, and swore, informing me he did not want it, and asking me to go.

A related ethical question concerns how nurses manage to maintain Carl Rogers' (1967, 1990) core principles of congruence, empathy and unconditional positive regard in the face of such hostility (Aiyegbusi and Clarke–Moore 2009, Bowers 2002). This question was considered in *Chapter 11*.

I looked in Mr X's inmate medical record, and found that a high secure hospital would be admitting him from prison when a "bed was available". I then communicated with the consultant who initially assessed this client, and he visited him in prison. I found that Mr X had a history of serious violent offending. The consultant decided to section him for further assessment. However, unfortunately, the prisoner was due for release two days after he was due to be transferred. I spoke to the Governor about the risks, and we decided a plan of action, which involved moving the prisoner to the segregation unit until he was told that he was to be sectioned. This would hopefully mean that he would be in a safe environment, as his reaction was expected to be violent and aggressive. I also felt I would possibly be a target of his reactive anger, as the consultant had not informed him of his transfer plans.

However, prison staff apparently informed Mr X of the plan for high secure hospital admission. Subsequently, I was told by prison officers that he had said that he would slash my throat if he saw me. I informed my manager, who did not appreciate the gravity of this risk, or see it as important. Prison governors and my own managers did not give me the opportunity to reflect or give feedback on this action, although I did consider the scenario in supervision.

Because of the potential risks to me, I was even more determined to avoid Mr X. The plan agreed by the Governor was that, over the weekend, Mr X would be moved to the segregation unit; and three days following this, be transferred to the hospital, escorted by four prison officers and a healthcare nurse, as per protocol. The staff involved were hand picked for their size and experience. I felt I had managed the risks as best I could.

On Monday morning, to my surprise, I passed Mr X in the corridor. He looked at me with such venom, the hairs stood up on the back of my neck. What had gone wrong? As far as I was aware, I had managed the risks and communicated with prison management. I asked the segregation unit staff what had happened. They informed me that the wing manager had decided that, since the prisoner was "only a risk to me", he would be managed on the wing until he was to be informed of his move, on the day of his transfer.

Implications for the safety of other prisoners and staff

Richard Byrt

This scenario has implications for risk assessment and risk management, and the safety of both prisoners and staff, in relation to sound ethical nursing and multidisciplinary practice, and Health and Safety at Work legislation (Dimond 2005).

The Nursing and Midwifery Council (2010) Code makes it clear that both staff and managers who are registered nurses would have responsibilities to manage risk in this situation:

- *You must act without delay if you believe that you, a colleague or anyone else may be putting someone at risk.*
- *You must inform someone in authority if you experience problems that prevent you working within this Code or other nationally agreed standards.*
- *You must report your concerns in writing if problems in the environment of care are putting people at risk.*

Nursing and Midwifery Council (2010: 6) quoted in Ford et al (2010: 48)

In Glynnis's account, the safety of other prisoners and staff appears to have been compromised because, despite the decision made by Glynnis and the Governor, some officers decided to give Mr X prior information about his transfer, and to avoid transferring him to the segregation unit. This appears to have affected the duty of care to make a decision which was beneficent (promoted the best outcome for most people) and non-maleficent (avoided serious harm: Adshead 2010). It has been argued that individuals with mental illness are likely to be harmed by long periods of segregation from other people (King et al 2008); and that, therefore, delays in transferring Mr X to the high secure hospital meant that it was in his interests to remain on the prison wing until his transfer. Related absolutist ethical positions (see *Chapter 2*) are that Mr X's needs and interests must take precedence over those of other people; or that service recipients should always be told the truth (Chodoff 2006). Either of these absolutist perspectives may have informed the prison officers' decision. However, from a utilitarian perspective (Chodoff 2006, Adshead 2010: see *Chapter 2*), it could be argued that detrimental effects to others from Mr X's possible assaults outweighed the harms to him from segregation; and that nurses could take steps to reduce any adverse consequences of this isolation from others. Furthermore, Maden (2007) has argued that trauma results not only from being assaulted (*Chapters 5 and 6*), but also to mental health clients if they are not prevented from perpetuating assaults. Maden (2007) argues that this is an additional reason why mental health professionals have a duty of care to prevent clients with mental health problems from engaging in violent acts. However, stigmatisation of these individuals should be avoided (Morris 2006). Maden (2007) points out that only a minority of those of us with mental health problems engage in violent behaviours.

Glynnis's account also indicates the importance of clear communication between staff of different disciplines, and understanding and appreciation of each other's complementary and/or conflicting perspectives. Various authors have described how the aims and goals of nurses and other healthcare staff may conflict with those of prison officers and their managers (Maeve and Vaughan 2001, Durcan 2008). The experiences described by Glynnis in this chapter, and by some other nurses (Maeve and Vaughan 2001, Walsh 2009), indicate the difficulties that some may experience in delivering care of a high ethical standard. In part, these may relate to conflicting expectations, within wider society and the prison itself, that prisoners are both punished and have their healthcare needs met ("custody versus therapy": Maeve and Vaughn 2001, Seddon 2007).

Finally, Glynnis's account relates to literature on the importance of both managerial support and clinical supervision in relation to nurses' experiences of patients' violence and aggression (McKenna and Paterson 2006, Ford et al 2010); and the importance of "a strategic organisational response" to this (McKenna and Paterson 2006: 231).

References

Adshead G. (2010) Principles of ethical reasoning in forensic psychiatry. In Bartlett A, McGauley G (eds) *Forensic Mental Health. Concepts Systems and Practice*. Oxford University Press, Oxford

Aiyegbusi A, Clarke-Moore J (Eds) (2009) *Therapeutic Relationships with Offenders. An Introduction to the Psychodynamics of Forensic Mental Health Nursing*. Jessica Kingsley, London

Blom-Vann L (2008) *The Penalty of Imprisonment. Why 60% of the Prison Population Shouldn't Be There*. Continuum, London

Bowers L (2002) *Dangerous and Severe Personality Disorder: Response and Role of the Psychiatric Team*. Routledge, London

Chodoff P (2006) Involuntary hospitalization of the mentally ill as a moral issue. In Green SA, Bloch S (eds) *An Anthology of Psychiatric Ethics*. Oxford University Press, Oxford

Dimond B (2005) *Legal Aspects of Health and Safety*. Quay Books, Dinton Salisbury.

Durcan G (2008) Prison Mental Health Nursing. In National Forensic Nurses' Research and Development Group: Kettles AM, Woods P, Byrt R (eds) *Forensic Mental Health Nursing: Capabilities Roles and Responsibilities*. Quay Books, MA Healthcare, London

Ford K, Byrt R, Dooher J (2010) *Preventing and Reducing Aggression and Violence and Aggression in Health and Social Care: A Holistic Approach*. MK Publishing, Keswick

King K, Steiner B, Breach SR (2008) Violence in the supermax: A self-fulfilling prophecy. *The Prison Journal* **88**(1): 144–68

Kant I (1969) The Moral Law: Kant's Groundwork of the Metaphysics of Morals. London. Hutchinson. (Translated by Paton HJ) Cited in: Thompson IE, Melia KM, Boyd KM, Horsburgh D (eds) (5th edn) *Nursing Ethics*. Churchill Livingstone/Elsevier, Edinburgh

McKenna KJ, Paterson B (2006) Locating training within a strategic organizational response to aggression and violence. In Richter D, Whittington R (eds) *Violence in Mental Health Settings. Causes Consequences Management*. Springer, New York

Maden T (2007) *Treating Violence: A Guide to Risk Management in Mental Health*. Oxford University Press, Oxford

Maeve MK, Vaughn MS (2001) Nursing with prisoners: The practice of caring, forensic nursing or penal harm nursing? *Advances in Nursing Science* **24**(2): 47–64.

Morris G (2006) *Mental Health Issues and the Media: An Introduction for Mental Health Professionals*. Routledge Taylor and Francis Group, London

Nursing and Midwifery Council (2008) *Confidentiality Advice*. Nursing and Midwifery Council London. Available via www.nmc-uk.org/

Nursing and Midwifery Council (2009) *Record Keeping. Guidance for Nurses and Midwives*. Nursing and Midwifery Council, London. Available via www.nmc-uk.org/

Nursing and Midwifery Council (2010) *The Code. Standards of Conduct Performance and Ethics for Nurses and Midwives*. (Revised) Nursing and Midwifery Council, London. Available via www.nmc-uk.org/

Rogers C (1967) *On Becoming a Person: A Therapist's View of Psychotherapy*. Constable, London

Rogers C (1990) A client-centred/person-centred ppproach to therapy. In: Kirschbaum H, Henderson VL (eds) *The Carl Rogers Reader*. Constable, London

Seddon T (2007) *Punishment and Madness. Governing Prisoners with Mental Health Problems*. Routledge Cavendish Taylor and Francis Group,Abingdon

Stern V (2006) *Creating Criminals. Prisons and People in a Market Society*. Fernwood Books, Halifax Nova Scotia..

Walsh E (2009) The emotional labour of nurses who work in Her Majesty's (HM) Prison Service. *Journal of Forensic Nursing* **5**(3): 143–52

CHAPTER 13

Ethics of involving service users in forensic nursing education

Julia Terry

Introduction

Mental health service users have a unique insight into the very nature of mental illness and healthcare, putting them in a position of expertise. However, this expertise, although readily available, has been largely ignored and untapped by mental health professionals, and has not been valued to make a difference by those in power (Campbell 1998). During the last 20 years this has started to change with greater evidence of service user involvement in healthcare provision, although geographically this remains variable. This chapter explores mental health service user involvement in education programmes, particularly in relation to the ethics of the changing relationship between nurses and service users. Whilst there have been examples of user involvement in professional education programmes, in the main the literature has focused on user involvement in research, and how service users are increasingly becoming equal partners in this process. How mental health service users are best involved in nurse education programmes, particularly forensic courses, requires considered thought. This chapter briefly highlights mental health service user involvement in nurse education, debating the ethics of participation and true inclusion, and exploring issues that relate to forensic nurses and service users themselves. Demographic changes in society confirm that mental health nurses are increasingly working with a growing population of forensic service users (Whyte 1997), meaning the value of user involvement in nurse education is all the more significant.

Development of the mental health service user movement

The involvement of service users in the planning and development of mental health services is essential if professionals are to understand the experience of mental illness and ensure relevant care provision, since user involvement can shape the research and education agenda (Spiers et al 2005). Whilst there is an increasing awareness of the contribution that users can make to the development of future practitioners, in both service and educational settings, there are many geographical areas where progress has been slow (Basset et al 2006).

The concepts of user involvement are complex and have been debated and contested over many years, with no comprehensive definition that encapsulates involvement activities yet available (Welsh Assembly Government 2004). Whilst user involvement may include the giving of information and consultation at one end of the spectrum, it can progress to the formal establishment of partnerships between users and professionals at the other end (Welsh Assembly Government 2004). National Service Frameworks and recent policy guidance (Department of Health 1999; Welsh Assembly Government 2005) stress the importance of user involvement. Standards require services to develop arrangements to ensure service users and carers constructively participate in the design, planning, delivery, monitoring and evaluation of mental health services generally (Department of Health 1999). There is recognition that choice is an important factor, as users may wish to be involved in ways that range from simply being listened to, through to structured service user involvement in all levels of decision-making (Department of Health 2009), with many users wishing to see more people with personal experience of mental health problems employed in mental health services.

Despite notions of growing empowerment, people with mental health problems experience a dilemma. Whilst they are welfare consumers, this may mean they are viewed as inferior and in the role of care recipient, since the power remains with the provider (Campbell 1998). Developments in user involvement have seen users invited into positions of influence, but with service providers often controlling the nature of that relationship, user status appears elevated, but may be restricted regarding actual involvement (Campbell 1998). In order to promote a true culture of inclusion, service users will often require support and training to enable full participation and to minimise harm (Royal College of Nursing 2007). Likewise staff working in statutory and higher education sectors would benefit from training on user involvement, particularly around the aims and objectives, so they have had an opportunity to explore the possibilities and to openly discuss effective working strategies. User involvement needs to be approached at a systems level to ensure organisational and consumer issues are considered at the outset (Repper and Breeze 2007). Any omission in this area can be deemed unethical, as service users should be fully informed and clear about what to expect from their involvement. A lack of information may deny people the opportunity to exercise their autonomy. Discrimination may still be a real possibility. Ethical issues relating to access, diversity, consent and confidentiality are all highly pertinent with regard to user involvement. If such issues are not planned for and addressed, a culture of true inclusion will be impossible, thus making a mockery of user involvement at the expense of service users themselves. Genuine user involvement can best be demonstrated when service users and carers believe and perceive they are being involved (Welsh Assembly Government 2004). In terms of improving the status of mental health service users, one key difference would be to enable change in their relationships with the world around them, including relationships with mental health services, care providers and staff (Campbell 1998).

People with a mental illness diagnosis will have had experiences specific to them, yet it has been highlighted that there is a view that users may lack objectivity regarding the quality of care they have experienced, which may have led to reluctance to seek their views (Coffey 2006). Yet we can no longer treat users as passive recipients of healthcare, because if services are to be effective, users need to play an active role (Birmingham 1997); and their involvement provides a valuable and insightful perspective.

The National Service Frameworks for Mental Health (Department of Health 1999; Welsh Assembly Government 2005) state that a skilled workforce should have the time and skills to work in partnership and prepare care plans with full user involvement. Genuine involvement requires building users' confidence, providing relevant and timely information about services, and providing suitable space for users to express their views (Welsh Assembly Government 2008). In addition to engaging with users in meetings, providers need to consider other ways of obtaining views such as through letters and email, and providing feedback regarding how users' views have been acted upon. The offender population has often been excluded from the patient and public involvement agenda, which denies the contribution of insight and experience from those who have been through the system, and it is vital that this group has its voice heard (Bradley 2009).

Service users can not only offer fresh ideas for service provision, but can also offer advantages when involved in the education of professionals delivering care. Involving service users in nurse education can help improve its quality and relevance. It is vital that the ethics of user involvement in professional programmes are considered at the outset. Issues such as ensuring information for participants is accessible and making sure views are properly respected can inform an understanding of the ethics of user involvement. Principles of good practice for user involvement in service provision (Welsh Assembly Government 2005) and in research are highlighted (Staley and Minogue 2006), whilst in relation to user involvement in education guidance is less obvious, although it can be suggested that the same principles apply.

In professional mental health training programmes patients have traditionally held a passive role, often with limited awareness or choice that their experiences have been exploited to further the education of health professionals. This is slowly changing as service users are becoming active educators, benefiting both themselves and students (Livingston and Cooper 2004), as they usefully contribute to professional programmes in a more active role. The service user expertise is defined by experience, and this distinctive first-hand perspective gives them a unique role in teaching.

Involvement of users in education programmes

Traditionally healthcare professionals undertake an undergraduate or postgraduate qualification, comprising registration by a professional body, such as the Nursing and Midwifery Council in a university setting. Programmes include a taught academic element, balanced with direct practice experience; and standards are to be achieved in both areas in order to achieve qualification.

The National Service Framework for Mental Health (Department of Health 1999) proposed that service users be involved in planning, providing and evaluating professional training programmes, signifying a cultural shift. Professional education has been steeped in a culture of practitioners as experts, imposing their frames of reference upon service users (Tew et al 2004). Now we are seeing principles of partnership emerging, with a more holistic understanding of mental distress and a greater recognition of contributions from the wider community, which promote the model of recovery. The ethos of partnership values the expertise of service users and carers, and this partnership must form the foundation of mental health education (Tew et al 2004). In order to shape the attitudes, values and skills of the future mental health workforce, it is not only the content, but also the process of education that is important. The Ten Essential Shared Capabilities set out by the National Institute for Mental Health in England, is the underpinning framework for the entire mental health workforce (Hope 2004), with working in partnership given top priority. The Chief Nursing Officer recommends all training programmes reflect these principles (Department of Health 2006).

The concept of involving service users and carers in all aspects of curricula is far from new. However, practice examples remain sparse (Masters et al 2002). Service users, through their experience of living with mental distress, and increasing involvement in research, are developing a knowledge base of immediate relevance to mental health practice. This may be complementary to currently taught programmes, and at times may challenge professional orthodoxies and the power bases that hold fast to them (Tew et al 2004). Users may wish to promote alternative models of recovery that they have found beneficial, which may be at odds with other views in the classroom and it is essential that these discussions are managed sensitively and inclusively.

Benefits of service user involvement in education programmes include students stating positive impacts upon their personal world views and practice (Khoo et al 2004). Students felt face-to-face contact with a user educator was more beneficial than a lecture, as this confirmed the reality of users' stories, and initiated positive feedback as users encouraged students to identify improvements they could make in practice (Rush 2008). This has been highlighted as a process of transformative learning, whereby students undergo a process of realising their emotions, making sense of the experience and resolving to take future action. Much of this appears to result from the role reversal with students as the people who are "helped" and the user educator as the "helper" (Rush 2008).

In the UK the Mental Health in Higher Education (MHHE) project was established in 2003, aiming to increase discussion about learning and teaching on mental health across disciplines, with service user involvement emerging as a central tenet of its work (Basset et al 2006). The MHHE project has introduced national workshops, network building, such as the Developers of User and Carer Involvement (DUCIE) group, and the production of a good practice guide, *Learning from Experience* (Tew et al 2004). Further guidance can be sought via the National Continuous Quality Improvement Tool for Mental Health Education which facilitates an assessment of post-qualification mental health education programmes, measuring meaningful user involvement (Centre for Clinical and Academic Workforce Innovation 2005). The tool facilitates an evaluation of programme relevance to the NHS and Social Care modernisation agenda, and is intended for use with users and carers to weigh their involvement in the planning, design, delivery and evaluation of programmes. Whilst a number of assessment tools and practice guides exist that aim to promote user involvement, without national evaluation it is difficult to know the utilisation of such tools.

Ethical issues arise from user involvement in education programmes, such as attention paid to dignity, welfare and the rights of participating individuals (Staley and Minogue 2006). Users should not be distressed by taking part, although it must be noted this is a real possibility as they may be reliving painful issues by talking about illness experiences with students. Users need to know what they are actually consenting to when they agree to participate in programme delivery. This highlights the main ethical principles that require consideration when involving users in education, which include non-maleficence, confidentiality and justice (Keogh and Daly 2009). The beneficence to the user educators, which may be in terms of an opportunity to share their story or to be remunerated for their participation, need to be transparent. A user's autonomy should not be compromised, and aims and expectations from both the higher education institution and user need to be clear at the start. Fundamentally, a steering group and a user involvement policy setting out rights and responsibilities on either side are worthwhile (UK Mental Health Research Network 2005).

In terms of involving forensic service users in education, they may not only revisit their experiences of mental distress, but also reflect on negative experiences of detention, including forced treatment, in the classroom. In terms of dilemma, negative experiences of coercion reported by service users have often referred to a restriction of freedom (Gilburt et al 2008); yet nurses are aware there is virtually no public support for this client group, as public views focus on containment as a priority. While forensic nurses are dealt the task of integrating competing conflicts of therapeutic and security roles, their mission is to establish an ethos of a health-orientated and person-valuing culture (Burrow 1998). This may be assisted by hearing forensic users' experiences in the classroom, however nurses may continue to struggle with the dual aspects of their role, and be less than sympathetic to the user voice.

Research into user involvement in education programmes has not just focused on classroom delivery, but also on true involvement across the curriculum, including process evaluation (Masters et al 2002). One user educator stated:

> *It represents a fundamental philosophy about user/carer involvement and about respect for people who use the services. It isn't an add-on extra – it is something essential to the way the course is delivered. In its own way it changes the focus and balance of power completely – and this is how it should be.*
>
> (Masters et al 2002: 314)

Users who have more comprehensive involvement, such as being included in curriculum planning, classroom delivery and evaluation aspects of courses would obviously have greater programme knowledge. However, an unprepared and inexperienced external speaker may have little idea what to expect without adequate discussion and preparation. Recommendations for service user involvement frequently recommend training for both users, students and academics to ensure there are systems of support and preparation available (RCN 2007, Rush 2008), with some higher education institutions running preparatory courses aimed at empowering service users, developing presentation skills, and increasing confidence and support, with good effect (Hanson and Mitchell 2001). It is worth noting that a number of useful guides on user involvement in education programmes have been developed (Tew et al 2004, Miller and Waters 2006, Lloyd et al 2007).

The use of service user educators also raises the issue of appropriate standards, as all training in universities must meet an appropriate level. There is a dearth of literature on what is necessary to ensure that users conform to an appropriate standard of objectivity and communication skill (Livingston and Cooper 2004) but this may be equally true of all external speakers on courses. Aspects of quality assurance and control are vital in all professional programmes, and whilst one would expect that service users would give a subjective view; content, style and delivery of all teaching sessions require a monitoring and evaluation process to ensure relevance. This usually occurs through peer review and module or programme evaluation. Indeed it can be difficult to control for quality for all speakers on nursing programmes, and effective evaluation processes can certainly help with this. Preparation, prior to user delivery in the classroom, with students themselves, is a worthwhile activity, as this helps them appreciate that delivery by service users may be different to other experiences. Students may need to exercise tolerance, as users are not usually teachers, nor are they necessarily used to speaking to groups about their experiences. Students would benefit from considering user involvement issues before they experience directly taught sessions, and this may best be done in a supportive environment, with education staff and users themselves, in a way that promotes exploration of existing attitudes and values.

Involving users in mental health programmes

The education of forensic nurses is based on formal and informal rules (Goffman 1961), with formal education relating to teaching the academic rules of "the book", and informal education relating to learning the ropes, or rules of the institution. This has been viewed as the difference between the ideal, versus actual realities in practice, creating a theory–practice divide. There have been moves to examine the true nature of forensic nursing, with suggestions for a progressive model of education that empowers students, equipping them with critical thinking skills to guide service development (Carton 1998). Research and literature focusing on user involvement has only begun to emerge in the last two decades; now a progressive educational model would surely include user involvement.

Studies that centre on the role of the forensic mental health nurse have identified a focus on task-orientated competencies, knowledge, skills, values and attitudes (Bowring-Lossock 2006). While managers identify self-awareness, and effective decision-making as essential nursing qualities (Wilson 1998), in contrast service users seek to engender human qualities such as good interpersonal skills in mental health nurses (Repper and Breeze 2007). It has been shown that service user involvement in the classroom can lead to nurses connecting better with clients' experiences and understanding the impact of these, with more individualised interventions likely to follow (Wood and Wilson-Barnett 1999). This would suggest that forensic mental health service users do have a role in the education of nurses, in order to promote the human qualities they wish to experience in care settings. However, continued allegiance to the medical model of mental health, may have led to discriminatory attitudes with perceptions that those who experience mental distress are ill all the time; and educational institutions may continue to demonstrate stigmatising attitudes, viewing service users as unreliable or even dangerous (Tew et al 2004). Identifying staff who wish to engender a more inclusive approach, and develop supports to change such cultures can be achieved successfully by developing effective working relationships with service users and carers.

Conversely, attitudes may only in part be related to following the medical model, as the notion of stigma arises from the process of labelling, which is not specific to mental illness. Whilst more positive social attitudes may now be perceived towards those with mental illness, negative associations persist for mentally disordered offenders (Chaloner 2000). Forensic service users are liable to experience both the mental illness label and the criminal offender label, which are not easily eroded. Frequently staff attitudes can be judgemental about the trustworthiness, reliability and permanence of mental illness in users (Short et al 2009), attributing negative aspects of users as inherent to the personal make-up of the individual rather than recognition that illness behaviours can be episodic, and offending behaviour may have been entirely illness-related.

Maintaining a resolute user-centred approach needs to underpin any educational programme that focuses on preparing nurses for legislative roles which may result in power and coercion, with an ethical and lawful educative framework as the essential goal (Hurley and Linsley 2007). As mentioned previously, key processes, such as transparent policies that address the nature and aims of user involvement, remuneration, safety issues, and the preparedness of users, require consideration at the outset. However, whilst the ethics of forensic service user involvement in education may be noble in theory, it may be difficult in practice (Chaloner 2000).

Forensic mental health nurses have usually undertaken three-year mental health nurse training to diploma or degree level, and obtained employment in a forensic setting, in many cases with prior employment in generic mental health provision. Opportunities for continuing professional development may be in the form of in-house training days, or academic courses, such as a university module or higher degree in working with mentally disordered offenders. Service user involvement in postgraduate mental health education is currently sparse, which could be a missed opportunity. If user involvement promotes positive change, postgraduate students are experienced practitioners, and in a prime position to advocate change in practice settings (Khoo et al 2004). At the time of writing, a brief trawl of all the Higher Education Institutions' websites in the UK offering an MSc programme in Forensic Mental Health was conducted. Educational programmes included on these sites, which are usually open to all disciplines, made no mention of service user involvement in their courses.

In a review of mental health services and prisoners, Brooker et al (2003) states that prisoners who have experienced mental health problems need to be recruited, trained and provided with appropriate support to enable them to contribute, as they are a disenfranchised group. The same approach may be beneficial in user involvement in educative settings.

The provision of support is vital to user educators, as individuals may perceive their vulnerability as increased by sharing personal stories to a room of strangers; and it is difficult to predict which individuals would be more at risk of distress (Livingston and Cooper 2004). User researchers have highlighted that, ethically, it is vital that user educators are offered feedback about their involvement, that self-disclosure of mental distress is valued, that there is discussion about power relationships, and that relevant information is accessible and available (Lindow 2002). Whilst the importance of preparation and a transparent process has been reflected upon, there is a lack of national standards for involving users and carers in nursing programmes, which differs from social work education (Welsh Assembly Government 2005). A buddying system has been adopted in other areas of user involvement, for example in research where a user partners with a more experienced researcher for support. The same model can be utilised in educative settings, whereby an educator who understands the principles of user involvement and is supportive, can assist a user to grow in confidence, initially engage in some joint teaching, and provide reflective and support time as required.

Views of forensic mental health service users have seldom been sought in relation to nurse education. However, one consultation with a range of service users explored how users could be involved in an integral way in mental health nurse training, and included users in a medium secure unit in South Wales (Miller and Waters 2006). Forensic service users' comments focused on nurses' attitudes, and a wish not to see nurses who were "power mad". The users consulted were keen to be involved in the training of mental health nurses, and felt they may be able to give a particular insight into the extra discrimination and stigma experienced by them in forensic settings (Miller and Waters 2006).

Involvement of forensic service users has developed in the area of research, for example the National Forensic Mental Health Research and Development Programme, where forensic service users are included as expert reviewers for research proposals and help identify research priorities (Spiers et al 2005) Whilst user involvement in forensic research has been limited to small-scale involvement, much can be learned from good practice (Faulkner and Morris 2002).

Considering the challenges that may be inherent when involving users in the actual delivery of nurse education, such as security and confidentiality (Faulkner and Morris 2002), it is worth considering alternatives to users being in the actual classroom. For example, teaching staff may choose to present forensic service users' views using presentations and journal papers which focus on this client group. Nonetheless, the ethics of these alternatives need to be weighed, as one systematic literature review of forensic mental health service users' views highlighted, out of 22 studies, none had discussed ethical issues, and only six had sought ethical approval (Coffey 2006). Forensic service users can be seen as a disempowered group, as there are issues of control, privacy and power, as they are literally a captive audience (Coffey 2006), and vulnerable to exploitation.

The users themselves have voiced creative suggestions as to how they could be involved in mental health nurse training, such as nurses attending open days in forensic settings and attending talks by users (Miller and Waters 2006). Users have also suggested they could participate in assessments of student nurses' competencies on placement, which has been proposed in terms of assessing skills around developing therapeutic relationships (Speers 2008). Attending student evaluations post placement, and users sending in questions for student nurse interviews were also put forward as users' suggestions of how they could be involved (Miller and Waters 2006). Another option may be to bring users into the classroom via video or a video link, which again presents ethical dilemmas. A university education intends students to critique the world presented to them and they might well ask about the ethics and process of using clients in this manner.

Whilst empowerment seeks to shift the balance of power between service providers and those who use these services, users themselves can be disempowered by the statutory regulations that detain people for compulsory treatment, under the mantle of protection (Barnes et al 2000). Again the nature of forensic service users means they experience disempowerment, and we do not wish to return to former decades where patients were fetched from the local asylum and paraded as specimens in the classroom. Although, if properly executed, videos and video links certainly have some potential for the inclusion of service users. There has been an increase in the use of digital stories as a way of building capacity for the service user voice in mental health (University of Birmingham 2010), with this medium having the potential to reach wider audiences, and capitalise on service users' time, therefore being a cost-effective method of user involvement in teaching.

There are established examples of forensic service user involvement in prison councils and health service development, including the expert patient programme, which could be built upon (Sainsbury Centre for Menal Health 2008). This implies from an ethical stance that there need be few limits on the potential of forensic service users' involvement in mental health nurse training. However such users are often regarded as inferior, or having less value compared to service providers, which does not engender an effective climate for collaboration (Faulkner and Morris 2002). Breaking down such attitudinal barriers presents a great challenge.

Barriers are frequently cited at the mention of user involvement in a number of contexts. First, there is the issue of representativeness, and whether a user's views will be typical of mental health service users' views in general. Concern has been raised that there is over-use of certain users, or that opportunities for involvement in education provide a platform or soapbox for individuals to talk about negative experiences, with blatant personal agendas. Yet as research points towards the benefits of user involvement in professional programmes, this need not exclude users from leading class discussions (Khoo et al 2004).

Bassett et al (2006) identified further barriers to user involvement in higher education. These included hierarchies that exclude; stigma; disempowering processes, such as the use of jargon and bureaucratic meetings; clever excuses; a value base with knowledge given highest priority; lack of a team approach; lack of support; and rigid and inflexible payment systems. Preparatory work, and time spent nurturing and supporting all people involved in service user involvement processes in higher education can provide solutions to such barriers. Bassett et al (2006) suggest establishing ground rules, challenging all jargon, and encouraging parties to discuss how they are feeling can be helpful to service users, as they may hear university staff feel disempowered and insecure, and consider how to counter opposition from influential colleagues. As creative teaching methods are increasingly encouraged, user educators will often feel comfortable in moving away from "chalk and talk" approaches, so there may be few barriers in terms of teaching and learning methods. Knowledge of community networks and service users' own support strategies are important, as this can nurture relationships between user educators and their supporters or organisations; additionally users working in pairs can be helpful (Bassett et al, 2006).

If we are seeking to develop and promote a climate of empowerment, which is bred from trust, openness, honesty and genuineness, coupled with an acceptance of people as individuals (Hawks 1992), then empowerment is seen as a collaborative process between nurse and service user, whether in practice or the classroom. Nurses should therefore seek out processes that promote empowerment, and be aware of their own powerful position. Service users who have encountered negative institutional experiences are all too aware of the powerful positions that clinical staff hold, and they may well encounter the same in academic institutions. This could be far from empowering if a higher education institution favours a paternalistic model, which characterises attitudes or systems that subsequently reduce individuals' freedoms and responsibilities. In terms of raising awareness in forensic nurses, and perhaps enlightening service users, a discussion of practices where there is presumption of authority of the powerful over the less powerful, whether in practice or education, is a worthy debate.

In a training environment, forensic service users in the role of user educator, may be deemed as having power, as they have the ear of students, which raises the question of whether students would feel intimidated by this relationship. Perhaps only forensic mental health nurses themselves can say if they would be concerned that the service user may wish to ask them searching or personal questions, which might lead to this information being used later in a way that disadvantaged them as individuals.

It is difficult to know the expectations of service users if they embark on involvement as user educators in a higher education setting. Essentially they are likely to experience a hierarchical structure and an institutional feel, where there is a notion of expertise (Bassett et al 2006). Service users may not be greeted with a warm welcome by all, as a culture of inclusiveness may not be apparent; indeed lecturers may perceive user educators as a threat, as some staff may not wish to relinquish their expert role.

There are security and public protection issues when involving forensic service users in education settings (Spiers et al 2005). It is standard practice for teaching staff to be checked by the Criminal Records Bureau, and students need to feel that visiting speakers are safe to be with and will conduct themselves in a professional manner. This is no mean feat if the average forensic service user is subject to conditions of the Mental Health Act 1983 (amended 2007), and would require rigorous risk assessment long before the option of sharing their stories or co-facilitating a classroom session. Examples of developments in user involvement in education, such as the development of funded user educator roles as substantive posts (Simons et al 2007), may be more difficult for a forensic service user to attain if they are confined by restrictions regarding employment, due to the nature of their care.

Ways that user educators are employed may vary, as some are directly employed, with advantages being access to higher education institution resources, continuity and sustained development of skills, although users may not feel like equal team members and may still lack support. Alternatively, contracts may be developed with user organisations or self-employed user educators, which can promote independence and flexibility, although users may feel like outsiders with this less reliable source of income (Tew et al 2004). Payment for user involvement is essential, including for meetings and travel expenses, and suggestions are that users are paid the standard hourly visiting lecturer rate (Tew et al 2004), with smaller payments for preparatory training attendance. Service user involvement must be budgeted for, expenses reimbursed and they should be paid at a level consistent with others in the teaching team (Sainsbury Centre for Mental Health 2008) although the rules on paying people receiving benefits can make payments difficult (Turner and Beresford 2005). This again raises ethical issues about the equity and justice of user involvement in education. Many users have said they are happy to contribute their time, with views that this may promote change in education, and be an opportunity to give something back. However, if users are not treated on an equitable basis, this seems tangibly to undervalue their involvement.

Current nursing practice demands increased sensitivity to the advocacy needs of users and commands thoughtful reflection of complex legal and ethical dilemmas that arise from a system focused on managed care, which can disadvantage those it seeks to protect (Hurley and Linsley 2007). Nurses may require a neutralising view to counter the dominant ideology of control, and user involvement in forensic nurse education may provide this, assisting nurses in thinking about ethical principles, dilemmas, and basic rights, aimed at promoting practice with an increased user focus.

Conclusion

Whilst no singular event will cause a radical overhaul in the culture of nurse education, and whilst power imbalances will continue for a considerable time, there is room for optimism that true inclusion and partnership working with service users will overcome attitudes of fear and mistrust, with user involvement in the classroom becoming more frequent (Hanson and Mitchell 2001). More work needs to be done to establish forensic service users in the process of user involvement, and to develop tools to evaluate outcomes (Spiers et al 2005). If user involvement in the education of forensic mental health nurses is to enhance skills in ways that are prioritised by users themselves, it must be developed in partnership with service providers (Repper and Breeze 2007). The ethical principles of service user involvement in education centre on the unique contribution users can make in influencing the development of the very professionals delivering their care. It is also vital that systems for supporting user educators are in place, monitored and evaluated. Whilst the demands of involving users in education programmes is acknowledged, there is considerable evidence of added value which has been reflected in programme design and evaluation and students' learning outcomes. Whilst forensic mental healthcare continues to seek an ethical basis for practice, service user involvement in forensic mental health nurse education may be a step towards addressing some of the current ethical dilemmas. User educators are not only empowering themselves, they are empowering the mental health nurses of today and tomorrow to ensure services are client-centred.

References

Barnes D, Carpenter J, Bailey D (2000) Partnerships with service users in interprofessional education for community mental health: a case study. *Journal of Interprofessional Care* **14**(2): 189–200

Basset T, Campbell P, Anderson J (2006) Service user/Survivor involvement in mental health training and education: Overcoming the barriers. *Social Work Education* **25**(4): 393–402

Birmingham L (1997) Should prisoners have a say in prison healthcare? *British Medical Journal* **315**(7099): 65–6

Bowring-Lossock E (2006) The forensic mental health nurse – a literature review. *Journal of Psychiatric and Mental Health Nursing* **13**: 780–5

Bradley (2009) Lord Bradley's review of people with mental health problems or learning disabilities in the criminal justice system. Available at: www.dh.gov.uk/prod_consum_dh/groups/dh_digitalassets/documents/digitalasset/dh_098698.pdf [Last accessed 3 March 2010]

Brooker C, Repper J, Beverley C, Ferriter M (2003) Mental Health Services and Prisoners: A Review for the Department of Health. Available from www.dh.gov.uk/uk/assetRoot/04/06/43/78/04064378.pdf

Burrow S (1998) Therapy versus security: Reconciling healing and damnation. In Mason T, Mercer D (eds) *Critical perspectives in forensic care*. Macmillan Press, Hampshire

Campbell P (1998) Listening to clients. In Barker P, Davidson B. *Psychiatric Nursing: Ethical Strife*. Hodder Arnold, London

Care Council for Wales (2005) *Standards for involving service users and carers in the Degree in Social Work in Wales*. Care Council for Wales, Cardiff

Carton G (1998) Nurse education: Scribes and scriptures. In Mason T, Mercer D (eds) *Critical perspectives in forensic care*. Macmillan Press, Hampshire

Centre for Clinical and Academic Workforce Innovation (2005) *National Continuous Quality Improvement Tool for Mental Health Education* (2nd edn). University of Lincoln

Chaloner C (2000) Ethics and morality. In Chaloner C, Coffey M (eds) *Forensic Mental Health Nursing: Current approaches*. Oxford: Blackwell Science

Coffey M (2006) Researching service user views in forensic mental health: A literature review. *Journal of Forensic Psychiatry, Psychology* **17**(1): 73–107

Department of Health (1999) *National Service Framework for Mental Health: Modern standards and service models*. Department of Health, London

Department of Health (2006) *From values to action: The Chief Nursing Officer's review of mental health nursing*. Department of Health, London

Department of Health (2009) *New Horizons: A shared vision for mental health*. Department of Health, London

Faulkner A, Morris B (2002) *User Involvement in Forensic Mental Health Research and Development*. NHS National Programme on Forensic Mental Health Research and Development. University of Liverpool

Gilburt H, Rose D, Slade M (2008) The importance of relationships in mental health care: A qualitative study of service users' experiences of psychiatric hospital admission in the UK. *BMC Health Services Research* **8:** 92

Goffman E (1961) *Asylums: Essays on the social situation of mental patients and other inmates*. Doubleday, New York

Hanson B, Mitchell D (2001) Involving mental health service users in the classroom: A course of preparation. *Nurse Education in Practice* **1**: 120–6

Hawks J (1992) Empowerment in nursing education: Concept analysis and application to philosophy, learning and instruction. *Journal of Advanced Nursing* **17**: 609–18

Hope R (2004) *The Ten Essential Shared Capabilities: A framework for the whole of the mental health workforce*. Department of Health, London

Hurley J, Linsley P (2007) Expanding roles within mental health legislation: An opportunity for professional growth or a missed opportunity? *Journal of Psychiatric and Mental Health Nursing* **14**: 535–41

Keogh B, Daly L (2009) The ethics of conducting research with mental health service users. *British Journal of Nursing* **18**(5): 277–81

Khoo R, McVicar A, Brandon D (2004) Service user involvement in postgraduate mental health education. Does it benefit practice? *Journal of Mental Health* **13**(5): 481–92

Lindow V (2002) Being ethical, having influence. *Openmind* **116**: 18–19

Livingston G, Cooper C (2004) User and carer involvement in mental health training. *Advances in Psychiatric Treatment* **10**: 85–92

Mental Health Act 1983 (amended 2007) Available at: www.iosu.gov.uk/acts/acts2007/pdf/ukpga_20070012_en.pdf [last accessed: 10 February 2010[

Miller L, Waters R (2006) *Redressing the balance: User involvement in the training of mental health nurses in Wales*. Mind Cymru,Cardiff

Lloyd M, Carson A, Bleakley C (2007) Exploring the needs of service users involved in planning and delivering mental health services and education. Available at: www.health.heacademy.ac.uk/projects/miniprojects/mlloyd_reportsummary [Last accessed: 3 March 2010

Masters H, Forrest S, Harley A, Hunter M, Brown N, Risk I (2002) Involving mental health service users and carers in curriculum development: Moving beyond 'classroom' involvement. *Journal of Psychiatric, Mental Health Nursing* **9**: 309–16

Repper J, Breeze J (2007) User and carer involvement in the training and education of health professionals: A review of the literature. *International Journal of Nursing Studies* **44**: 511–19

Royal College of Nursing (2007) *User involvement in research by nurses*. Royal College of Nursing, London

Rush B (2008) Mental health service user involvement in nurse education: A catalyst for transformative learning. *Journal of Mental Health* **17**(5): 531–42

Sainsbury Centre for Mental Health (2008) *A review of service user involvement in prison mental health research*. December 2008. Sainsbury Centre for Mental Health, London

Short V, Cooper J, Shaw J, Kenning C, Abel K, Chew-Graham C (2009) Custody vs care: Attitudes of prison staff to self-harm in women prisoners—a qualitative study *Journal of Forensic Psychiatry, Psychology* **20**: 408–26

Simons L, Tee S, Lathlean J, Burgess A, Herbert L 7 Gibson C (2007) A socially inclusive approach to user participation in higher education. *Journal of Advanced Nursing* **58**(3): 246–55

Speers J (2008) Service user involvement in the assessment of a practice competency in mental health nursing – Stakeholders' views and recommendations. *Nurse Education in Practice* **8**: 112–19

Spiers S, Harney K, Chilvers C (2005) Service user involvement in forensic mental health: Can it work? *Journal of Forensic Psychiatry and Psychology* **16**(2): 211–20

Staley K, Minogue V (2006) User involvement leads to more ethically sound research. *Clinical Ethics* **1**(2): 1–6

Tew J, Gell C, Foster S (2004) Learning from Experience: Involving Service users and carers in mental health education and training. Available at: http://mhhe.ichameleon.com/silo,files/learning-from-experience-whole-guide.pdf [Last accessed: 10 March 2010

Turner M, Beresford P (2005) *Contributing on equal terms: Service user involvement and the benefits system*. Social Care Institute for Excellence. Shaping our Lives. Policy Press, Bristol

UK Mental Health Research Network (2005) Guidance for Good Practice: Service User Involvement in the UK Mental Health Research Network. Available at: www.mhrn.info/index/library/good-practice/mainColumnParagraphs/0/document/SURGE%Guidance%20for%20Good%10Good%20Practice%2006.pdf [Last accessed: 3 March 2010

University of Birmingham (2010) 'Digital stories' Available at: www.ceimh.bham.ac.uk/tv/DigitalStoriesIntro.shtml [Last accessed: 24 March 2010]

Welsh Assembly Government (2004) *Stronger in Partnership: Involving service users and carers in the design, planning, delivery and evaluation of mental health services in Wales*. WAG, Cardiff

Welsh Assembly Government (2005) *Raising the standard: the revised Adult Mental Health National Service Framework and Action Plan for Wales*. WAG, Cardiff

Welsh Assembly Government (2008) *Stronger in Partnership 2: Involving Service Users and Carers in the design, planning, delivery and evaluation of mental health services in Wales*. October 2008. WAG, Cardiff

Wilson S (1998) The Personal Characteristics of Effective Nurses. Unpublished Bachelor's Project: University of York cited in: Hopkins N, Ousley L (2000) Clinical Psychology and the forensic nursing role. In Robinson D, Kettles A (eds) *Forensic Nursing and Multidisciplinary Care of the Mentally Disordered Offender* (pp. 89–101). Jessica Kingsley: London

Whyte LA (1997) Forensic nursing: A review of concepts and definitions. *Nursing Standard* **11**: 46–7

Wood J, Wilson-Barnett J (1999) The influence of user involvement on the learning of mental health nursing students. *Nursing Times Research* **4**(4): 257–70

CHAPTER 14

Ethical issues in forensic nursing education

Alyson Kettles

Introduction

Nursing education as a whole has changed radically from Florence Nightingale's apprenticeship system to what is now becoming Mrs Bedford-Fenwick's all graduate, university-based education system. Since the two most recent reviews of mental health nursing (Department of Health 2006, Scottish Executive 2006) there has been a fundamental shift in the focus of mental health nursing from the past models of giving care, such as hospital-based, to values, rights and principles-based, whole systems, recovery-focused therapeutic relationships and interventions. There is, also, a drive to ensure that all qualified mental health nurses, including forensic mental health nurses, possess the capabilities (Sainsbury Centre for Mental Health 2004) and skills to do the job properly.

Positive practice, respecting diversity and meaningful involvement of service users and carers are lauded as the ways forward. Yet there is no mention of ethical and legal practice, or the problems that dilemmas (ethical conflicts) cause, in these reviews (Department of Health 2006, Scottish Executive 2006). There is mention of "professional" practice but this is not defined and so it is left to qualified nurses and educators to make what they will of ethical and legal issues relating to nursing education. Even in the National Framework for Pre-Registration Mental Health Nursing Programmes in Scotland (2008a: hereafter referred to as the National Framework) ethical issues are listed as part of the Ten Essential Shared Capabilities (Sainsbury Centre for Mental Health 2004) but then are not referred to again within the document. It does relate to legal issues but these are specific, such as "policies and legislation...relating to people requiring support and protection from neglect, danger, harm or abuse..." for safety and risk. The National Framework does mention personal and professional development and yet again concentrates on skills, capabilities, exemplary personal behaviour, accountability and responsibilities, without discussing ethics as being at the heart of professional development.

In all of these modern drivers there is, at best, only an implicit need to address the issues related to ethical practice. At worst it can be seen as missing entirely. For example, there is a need to address the ethical issues and dilemmas that arise when dealing with patients who are actively suicidal. Yet nowhere in the National Framework (2008) is this addressed.

In forensic nursing education there is an even stronger need to ensure that there is ethical practice because of the public interest in the client group. Maybe not surprisingly, ethics has been cut, either completely or in part, from many nursing education curricula. This is due to the increasing content and subject matter that nurses are now considered to require, as well as to the changes to the practice content to enable students to gain adequate clinical experience.

The advent of the School of Forensic Mental Health and the growing interest in ensuring that forensic nurses have access to appropriate nursing education that is specific to their field means that there are and will be more developments. For example, there is now a Development Framework for Forensic Nurses (NHS Education for Scotland 2008b: hereafter referred to as the Forensic Framework) and the "New to Forensic Mental Health" Teaching Package (NHS Education for Scotland 2008c). However, only the Forensic Framework (2008b) includes any specific reference to ethical practice or behaviour. The Forensic Framework clearly states that "Practitioners must apply ethical practice" and provides a section on the key content of what this statement means. Maybe more surprisingly, the term "dilemma" is not mentioned in any of the documents noted to date. The impressions one is left with from reading this document is that mental health nurses, and forensic nurses in particular, do not come across any dilemmas, or have to deal with them in clinical practice, nor do they have to justify their decisions about any dilemmas to the multidisciplinary teams or to the Nursing and Midwifery Council (NMC), inquiries such as Fatal Accident Inquiries (FAIs) or in courts of law. This is clearly not the case.

Current issues in education

Dishonesty seems to be an increasing problem in academic and clinical settings alike, despite the emphasis on "exemplary personal behaviour" referred to above. Reports of plagiarism and academic dishonesty by both nursing staff and nursing students have risen dramatically (Paterson et al 2003) and Harper (2006) points out a concern that academic dishonesty is a predictor of dishonesty in the workplace. Price (2003) indicates that academic dishonesty is not a single entity, rather it is a range of behaviours by students or by staff, including plagiarism, using or sharing unauthorised information in examinations or claiming to have undertaken fieldwork that has in fact not

Box 14.1. Forms of academic dishonesty

- *Plagiarism*: using words or ideas from published or unpublished sources and presenting it as if it was your own, including context change, missing footnotes and false references, use of search engines in cyberspace co-operation (Ryan 1998, Girard 2004)
- *Collusion*: sharing draft or completed summative work with other students (Price 2003)
- *Examination cheating*: from "looking over the shoulder" to using or sharing unauthorised information and material in examinations (Price 2003, Kolanko et al 2005)
- *Fraudulent fieldwork*: claiming to have undertaken fieldwork or other work/ procedures that have either not been done or have been completed by others without authority to do so (Price 2003), faked home visits and documentation (Bailey 2001)
- *False claims:* making false claims about your situation to gain extensions for assignment work or to gain advantage in examination situations (Price 2003)
- *Theft*: such as breaking into offices to steal examination papers (Tanner 2004)
- *Mobile phone cribbing*: electronic crib notes on mobile phone (Tanner 2004).
- *Fraudulent research*: creating or using false data or reporting, copying, in some cases, entire theses (Lock and Wells 1993)
- *Lying*: about care given/medication/missing clinical placement (Bailey 2001)
- *Forged documentation*: signatures (Bailey 2001)

been done or has been completed by another without authority. *Box 14.1* lists some of the behaviours that constitute academic dishonesty.

This kind of dishonesty leads to its own problems in both nursing and forensic nursing education, which in turn raises concerns about dishonesty in clinical practice and other forms of unacceptable and even criminal behaviour by staff. Much of the evidence from a legal perspective relates specifically to fraud and misconduct in medical practice and research (Hodges 1993, Lock and Wells 1993) rather than in nursing practice. There is also the legal definition of fraud and the broad categories within it, such as acts of omission and acts of commission.

However, much of the literature suggests that in nursing very little of the known plagiarism or academic dishonesty ever gets as far as the courts, or legal liability or professional misconduct committees. Recently, however, there have been reports in the nursing press of an increase in complaints against nurses in clinical practice and that 15% of these complaints are specifically about dishonesty, which include theft and false claims to registration with the Nursing and Midwifery Council (NMC) (Ford 2009). This is a major concern because it would appear that educating nurses about ethical and honest practice is not a major concern when it ought to be and at the same time as the apparent decrease in ethics education, dishonest practice appears to be on the increase. Both academic dishonesty and dishonest practice raise concerns about ethical problems and dilemmas in practice.

There are many forms of academic dishonesty (see *Box 14.1*), some of which are often viewed as minor infringements, such as students working together to produce work that should have been done individually or claiming to have attended events (of various sorts) that they did not attend. However, other forms of dishonesty in the academic system are seen as increasing in severity, from falsifying results, references and clinical experience stories; to students being "signed in" at lectures by other students when they did not attend; right up to the form of dishonesty that is perceived as being the worst, plagiarism.

There are examples of dishonest behaviour reported in the news (Ford 2009) sections of professional journals. For example, a case was reported of a nurse who falsified a passport:

> *A Zimbabwean nurse who used a falsified passport to get a job working with substance misusers at Holloway Prison has been jailed for a year. After Definate Tendayi Mukwe's leave to remain in the UK expired in February 2003, she obtained a bursary for a nursing diploma by altering her passport. She was arrested last December before being convicted last Wednesday of possessing a falsified passport with intent, obtaining money transfers by deception and overstaying her visa.*
>
> (Santry 2009)

Clearly, one of the issues is whether or not there were any indications during this nurse's education that she was likely to go on to conduct herself in this way. As there has been a link shown between academic dishonesty and professional misconduct (Harper 2006) this is an area that requires urgent investigation. Carroll and Appleton (2001) discuss academic dishonesty and how to deal with it. They argue that educators need to be trained to spot academic dishonesty in all its forms. The development of a one-day training course which outlines the problems, presents examples and case studies, suggests strategies for detection and for dealing with the problem once it is identified, and that emphasises the positive aspects of honesty would go a long way to helping staff to deal with it effectively. The relationship with honest and ethical practice needs to be addressed early on in nursing and forensic nursing education.

Current ethics education for nurses

Change is inevitable and so education changes to fit with modern policy, politics, educational theory and thought, and the pace of subject development. Current nursing ethics education considers several issues from legal, ethical and philosophical viewpoints, such as the ideas of beneficence and maleficence. Philosophical education related to ethics includes the ideas of consequentialism and non-consequentialism. Consequentialism looks at the consequences of acts and claims that acts are right to the extent that they produce good consequences and wrong to the extent that they produce bad consequences. This position is known as consequentialism or utilitarianism and the key terms are "good" and "bad". Nursing ethics, like medical ethics, is oriented towards the benefit of patients and so the nurse's primary commitment is to the health, well-being and safety of the patient. Ethical questions and dilemmas arise when the nurse's first duty is no longer to the patient alone. So, for example, when the nurse puts his or her own needs above the patient's needs then there is a dilemma about how to act because there is a conflict between personal and professional action.

Non-consequentialism

This form of philosophy attempts to answer the question of what kinds of acts are right or wrong, independent of the consequences. It is whether or not there is rightness or wrongness inherent in the act itself. These positions are known as formalism or deontologism or non-consequentialism.

Justice, in healthcare terms, is taken to mean the sense of fairness in distributing goods and harms and is held by many to be an ethical right-making characteristic, even if the consequences are or turn out not to be the best. These issues and questions are not just philosophical in nature; they have practical application throughout healthcare but probably nowhere more so than in forensic mental healthcare.

Ethics education for forensic nurses

Forensic nurses do not solely need to learn basic ethical issues such as the types of philosophy involved and the different ways in which they can be perceived. Rather forensic nurses are dealing with deeper and more complex problems than other groups of nursing staff generally deal with, such as multiple pathologies of mental illness, personality disorder, criminal justice, other legal issues such as tribunal procedures and restricted patients, personal and social issues, cultural issues and differences, vulnerability and incapacity, and issues related to the media and publicity.

Therefore some of the additional ethical issues that forensic nurses require to address include the following:

- Reflection on ethical issues and dilemmas.
- Rights versus welfare.
- Conscience.
- Honesty – truth telling.
- Rules and boundaries.
- Limits on rights and rules.
- Moral authority.
- Control and security.
- Fidelity – promise-keeping and contracts.
- Confidentiality.
- Justice and the forensic mental health nurse.
- Beneficence and maleficence.
- Autonomy.
- Research ethics, dilemmas, fraud and governance.
- Clinical dilemmas.

How this is currently delivered

The way this is addressed in the "New to Forensic" package (NHS Education for Scotland 2008c) is by mentoring, supervision and enabling all staff working in the forensic arena to work through the package. Interestingly, the package encourages the first item in the list given above – ethical reflection. Continuous reflection is the cornerstone. However, nowhere is ethical behaviour addressed explicitly but rather is addressed implicitly throughout, such as on page 66 of the document where examples of inappropriate attitudes and behaviours are given. These items are merely listed and there is no further explanation given. The learner is expected to discuss the items and the subject with whoever is supervising and mentoring them through the package. So despite ethics being acknowledged in the Development Framework for Forensic Nurses there is little else to take them further forward. For example, one of the items listed on page 66 is "Friendships with the patient, significant in their intensity, as would be very close friends in life". If a forensic nurse is developing such a friendship with a patient then he or she needs to be honest about what is happening and why. Other staff in the clinical area also need to be honest with the nurse in question and with the patient about what is happening and the possible outcomes of the behaviour. These outcomes may include the nurse finishing the relationship and being moved to another clinical area or the nurse might decrease the intensity of the relationship and be able to continue in a professional capacity without further consequence, or the nurse may choose to leave the hospital and to continue the relationship as a private individual no longer involved in care of the patient. There are other outcomes but these are a few examples of the possibilities. However, the Nursing and Midwifery Council (NMC) has clear views on the ethics of this type of situation and these are expressed through the NMC Code of Professional Conduct (2008) when it says:

> *You must establish and actively maintain clear sexual boundaries at all times with people in your care, their families and carers.*

The ethical position is to ensure that the manager in the area knows about it and can support the nurse to make a professional and ethical decision about how such a relationship might be handled bearing in mind that at all times the nurse must consider the welfare of the patient.

Postgraduate courses

At present postgraduate courses are not geared specifically to forensic nurses and there are many different courses that they could undertake, all with different content. So for example, whilst one forensic nurse might undertake the MSc in Nursing Studies at the University of Aberdeen and take a core module in ethics, another forensic nurse might undertake the BSc/BSc(Hons) in Professional Practice (Violence Reduction) at the University of Glamorgan and have ethical practice included implicitly (as there is no mention in the course programme about ethics). This is not meant as a criticism of particular courses but it does show how each university can develop its own content and aim each degree in different directions depending on the department, its focus and the staff who are constructing the courses. At postgraduate level there is to some degree the assumption that nurses have covered ethics as a component of pre-registration education. This applies to forensic nursing as much as to general mental health nursing at this level.

Policy

Policy for the last 15 years has been to integrate forensic care into general and generic education (Walker 2008). This has led to the current situation where, in the UK, there are only a few short courses available in specific subjects and where nursing staff in particular are aware of and feel that the education system is inadequate for their needs and inadequate to serve the needs of their patient. As a direct consequence of this a group of staff have put together their own proposal for a Virtual School of Forensic Mental Health (http://www.forensicnetwork.scot.nhs.uk/). It has the backing of the profession but we await events to see if it has the backing of the establishment, as the proposal has been submitted but, at the time of writing the outcome is unknown. The School currently offers short courses but the plan is to offer postgraduate degrees in specific forensic mental health oriented subjects including ethics and dilemmas as a part of those forensic-specific degrees.

Third party interests

Forensic mental health nursing no longer sits in the relative isolation that used to be the case (Chaloner 2000: 275). There are many agencies that have an interest in how forensic patients are cared for. For example, the Scottish Government expects to have an input to planning in Scotland; the criminal justice system expects to participate as a key stakeholder in any developments in order to provide a whole systems approach to care; groups such as the Scottish Recovery Network expect their principles to be incorporated into the courses that are likely to be developed. There are many stakeholders who will all have something to say about the potential development of the new School of Forensic Mental Health and who would all like an input into the curriculum planning of postgraduate courses. It is therefore imperative that ethical practice is placed at the heart of clinical practice through explicit inclusion in nursing education courses in both general mental health and forensic nursing.

Conclusion

In conclusion then, honesty is the most important aspect to be brought into professional practice from the ethical perspective. Without honesty from forensic mental health nursing staff, any ethical issues and dilemmas that occur or need to be addressed are compounded from the start. In the example of the nurse–patient friendship given above, if the nurse is not honest about her motives for developing the friendship then inappropriate behaviours and actions can result. Other staff need to be honest and to help the nurse to decrease involvement with the patient and it needs to come out into the open to be dealt with appropriately.

Educating staff to deal with these types of problems in the clinical arena is vital in the forensic field for professional clinical practice to happen and good quality clinical care to be given to the patients.

References

Bailey PA (2001) Academic misconduct: Responses from deans and nurse educators. *Journal of Nursing Education* **40**(3): 124–33

Carroll J, Appleton J (2001) *Plagiarism: A Good Practice Guide*. Joint Information Systems Committee Oxford Brookes University Oxford

Chaloner C (2000) Ethics and Morality. In Chaloner C, Coffey M (Eds) *Forensic Mental Health Nursing: Current Approaches* (pp 267–87). Blackwell Science, Oxford

Department of Health (2006) *From Values to Action: The Chief Nursing Officer's Review of Mental Health Nursing*. Department of Health, London

Ford S (2009) NMC receives hike in complaints about nurses. *Nursing Times*. Available from: http: //www.nursingtimes.net/5003646.article [accessed May 2010]

Girard NJ (2004) Plagiarism: An ethical problem in the writing world. *Association of Operating Room Nurses Journal* **80**(1): 13

Harper MG (2006) High tech cheating. Proceedings from the 1st Nurse Education International Conference – Developing collaborative practice in health and social education. *Nurse Education Today* **26**(8): 672–9

Hodges C (1993) Investigating, reporting, and pursuing fraud in clinical research: Legal aspects and options in England and Wales. In Lock S, Wells F (eds) *Fraud and Misconduct in Medical Research*. British Medical Journal Publishing Group, London

Kolanko KM, Clark C, Heinrich KT, Olive D, Sermbus JF, Sifford KS (2005) Academic dishonesty, bullying, incivility and violence: Difficult challenges facing educators. *Nursing Education Perspectives* **27**(1): 34–44

Lock S, Wells F (eds) (1993) *Fraud and Misconduct in Medical Research*. British Medical Journal Publishing Group, London

NHS Education for Scotland (2008a) *The National Framework for Pre-Registration Mental Health Nursing Programmes in Scotland*. NHS Education for Scotland Edinburgh. Available from www.nes.scot.nhs.uk

NHS Education for Scotland (2008b) *Development Framework for Forensic Nurses*. NHS Education for Scotland, Edinburgh.

NHS Education for Scotland (2008c) *New to Forensic Mental Health Teaching Programme*. NHS Education for Scotland, Edinburgh

Nursing and Midwifery Council (2008) *The Code: Standards of conduct, performance and ethics for nurses and midwives*. NMC, London

Paterson B Taylor L and Usick B (2003) The construction of plagiarism in a school of nursing. *Learning in Health and Social Care* **2**(3): 147–158

Price B (2003) Avoiding plagiarism and related cheating. *Nursing Standard* 18(4): 8th October.

Ryan J (1998) Student Plagiarism in an Online World. *ASEE Prism Magazine* December. Available from: www.asee.org/prism/december/html/student_plagiarism in_an_onlin.htm [Last accessed 12th July 2006]

Sainsbury Centre for Mental Health (2004) *Ten Essential Shared Capabilities: A Framework for the Whole Mental Health Workforce*. Sainsbury Centre for Mental Health, London

Santry C (2009) Prison nurses jailed after falsifying documents. *Health Service Journal* Available from: http: //www.hsj.co.uk/5001652.article [Last accessed May 2010]

Scottish Executive (2006) *Rights Relationships and Recovery: The Report of the National Review of Mental Health Nursing in Scotland*. Scottish Executive, Edinburgh

Tanner CA (2004) Moral Decline or Pragmatic Decision Making? Cheating and plagiarism in perspective. *Journal of Nursing Education* **43**(7): 291

Walker H (2008) The Role of Education. In The National Forensic Nurses' Research and Development Group (eds) *Forensic Mental Health Nursing: Capabilities Roles and Responsibilities* (pp17–26). Quay Books, London

Dark light

Stephen Pope

I feel its presence in my mind
Closing the life I once knew
Taking all I was, leaving nothing behind
An empty shell of a person I once knew
Not this thing you see sitting here
Soulless, lifeless, a prisoner from the light
But once a person full of life
Before being consumed by the Dark Light

CHAPTER 15

Legal and ethical aspects of management of self-harm and suicidal behaviour

Jay Sarkar and Trevor Broughton

Introduction

The rate of self-harm and suicide in England and Wales is high. Over a five-year period (2000–2004), there were 23477 suicides in the general population, a rate of 10.2 suicides per 100000. There were 6367 patient deaths, which represented 27% of all suicides. Of these, 14% (856) were in-patients, a rate of 180 in-patient suicides/year. The commonest methods used for in-patient suicides were hanging (65%) and self-strangulation (30%). Of those who committed in-patient suicide, 29% (251) of deaths occurred on-ward while 27% occurred off-ward. Twenty-two percent (188 suicides) of these patients had been under special nursing observations, indicative indirectly of the swiftness with which the incidents had taken place, and the capacity of the patients to evade detection or give clues to their intentions. Only one-third of the completed suicides were committed by women; the highest risk age-bands for the women were, in order of risk, 35–44 years and 45–54 years. The two commonest diagnoses in those who killed themselves were affective disorders (46%) and schizophrenia (19%); a large proportion of patients (29%) had diagnoses of personality disorder, drug and alcohol abuse and anxiety and adjustment disorders (Appleby et al 2006). Those with a past history of self-harm were more than four times likely to commit suicide than those who did not have this history (Odds ration = 4.3). Two major recommendations of the National Confidential Inquiry into Suicide and Homicide were a more rigorous use of observations to manage access to implements to self-harm with, especially ligating material, and removal of all ligature points.

The legal position

To what extent is intervention justified when someone places his/her own life at risk? When ought we to try and persuade someone, and if required, even compel them by law not to do so? When should we allow people to exercise their basic human right of self-determination and not intervene? These questions do not have straightforward answers. Self-harm is a risky course of action, but so are many other behaviours. Being a soldier, a policemen on duty, a fireman, or playing extreme sports are all examples of how one's chosen profession involves engaging in risky courses of actions, which sometimes lead to death of the individual. Society sanctifies risky courses and indeed puts young men and women in "harm's way" in the armed forces for the greater good of society. There is a notion of "greatest benefit to the highest number of people" that society reaps even if it leads to deaths of some individuals. But, as the benefits from a risky course of behaviour decrease, those risks related to personal goals and wishes not societal, with an associated increase of overall risks in parallel, society no longer supports the individual's course of action. Thus, people engaging in extreme sports do not get life insurance, for, whilst their intention is not to kill themselves, society speaks through its tacit discouragement of such behaviours.

At the other extreme are cases where society determines that individuals do not have the right to pursue a risky course of action with regards to their own life for that life is "worth living" (Glover 1990). That determination is done on the basis that any other "reasonable" person from that particular society, with the necessary mental capacity to consider the pros and cons of living and dying, would choose to live. That determination is often not carried out from the perspective of the individual who wants to self-harm. It is possible that people who are depressed, either long-term as in a severe depressive disorder, or transiently as in various personality disorders or after potentially challenging life events (bereavement, assault, physical injury, financial loss or loss of esteem), forget all that they usually get out of life. On the other hand, individuals who fear death, possibly due to the belief that they would go to hell, may wish they had never been born, but still not want to die. If clinicians are to make these judgements for others, they cannot escape appealing to their own independent beliefs about what constitutes a life worth living and therefore worth saving.

Clearly that cannot be a satisfactory course of action and clinicians require a model of decision-making that is simple, flexible and provides relevant "anchors" to determine a range of strategies to manage the risks of self-harm in a legally justifiable and ethically sound manner. Otherwise, there is a spurious categorisation of life-and-death risks, as well as the capacity of the individual to make such judgements satisfactorily, in artificial boxes of "present" or "absent". Clinicians require a dimensional model that allows risks and capacity to be graded according to the variance that intentions and motivations underlying the wish to self-harm or end one's life characteristically involve (Klonsky 2007).

A "slippery slope" model is depicted in *Figure 15.1*, of ascertaining when a patient's autonomy and right to self-determination with regards to self-harm is permitted by society and the law, and determination of a threshold when clinical paternalism and prevention of self-harm must occur and necessary interventions follow. The determining factors related to one or the other position are listed in the relevant boxes in the figure.

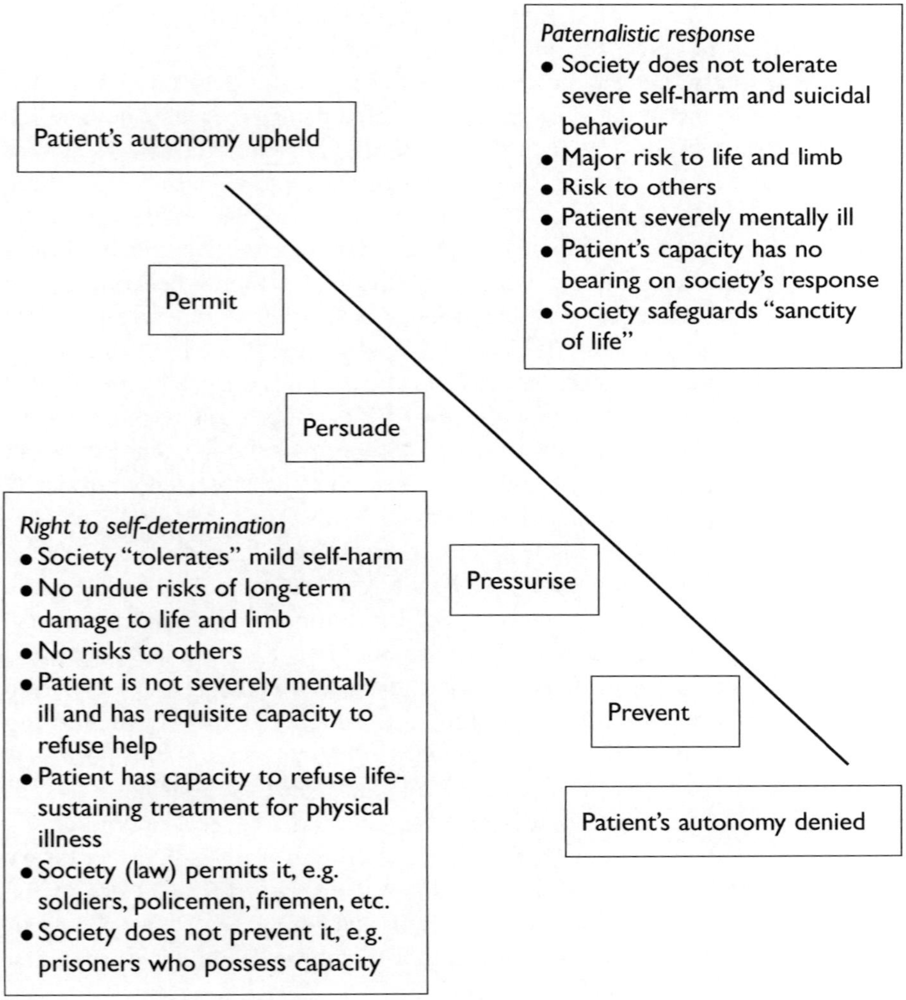

Figure 15.1: 'Slippery slope' model of decision-making.

"Slippery slope" and a staged model of decision-making and responses

There appear to be four "anchors" or thresholds that should trigger certain types of legal determination to justify the necessary interventions to prevent probable significant physical injury and deaths. The first "anchor" obviously is one that places no obligation on any clinician to prevent self-harm. There are many people in the community who self-harm and society does not make it every clinician's duty to prevent them. These would be people who have not come to the notice of statutory services and as such there is no duty of care in law at this stage, beyond being a responsible citizen.

Beyond that particular threshold the clinician has a duty on clinical and ethical grounds and in the "best interests" of the patient, to persuade the self-harmer to desist. This is so when the self-harmer becomes known to statutory services and society expects those services (and individuals within those services) to persuade the person to desist. This may be achieved through using various therapeutic skills of engagement, and problem-solving collaboratively to address the challenges in the patient's life that makes him or her contemplate self-harm. It is necessary to assess the patient's capacity as per criteria established in the Mental Capacity Act 2005, such that if patients are able to rationally consider and express to others the reasons why they wish to self-harm, without any underlying emotional or psychological factors, then their wishes must be respected in law. This is so if the resultant self-harm is mild in nature and is not going to cause serious damage to life and limb. Staff usually cannot physically prevent individuals at this stage from harming themselves.

At the next threshold when gentle persuasion no longer suffices, when risks to self outweigh any perceived benefits of self-harm, even if a person is found to have capacity formally, his or her autonomy is likely to be over-ridden if internationally accepted criteria are used by a suitably qualified and senior psychiatrist to make a mental disorder diagnosis. Consideration must be given to the use of stronger pressure, which may involve monitoring and, if required, informal admission into in-patient care, if the person is mentally disordered. When there are significant risks to serious harm to self, the patient cannot be pressurised into changing the course of action, and is unwilling to be monitored and helped voluntarily, then it becomes necessary to use legislation, i.e. the Mental Health Act (MHA 2007) and detain the patient for reasons of his or her own health and safety. Staff have a duty to ensure the protection of the patient and the patient's autonomy is over-ridden in issues of serious risk of harm to self.

Finally, whilst detained under MHA 2007, for their own safety, some patients may pose high risks of harm to others. There has to be restriction of access to places, everyday objects with which they can self-harm, and liberty and freedom within the institution through high levels of observation, searches, and other forms of monitoring and support. The NMC Code of Practice in relation to ensuring dignity, privacy and respect for patients as well as managing aggression should be followed at all times. When nursing practice has to become unusually restrictive in order to manage high levels of risk, it is judicious to seek a second opinion from the Mental Health Act Commission and legal advice, where appropriate, in order to provide necessary justifications for any future claims for breach of individual human rights by the patient. This approach is summarised in *Figure 15.2*.

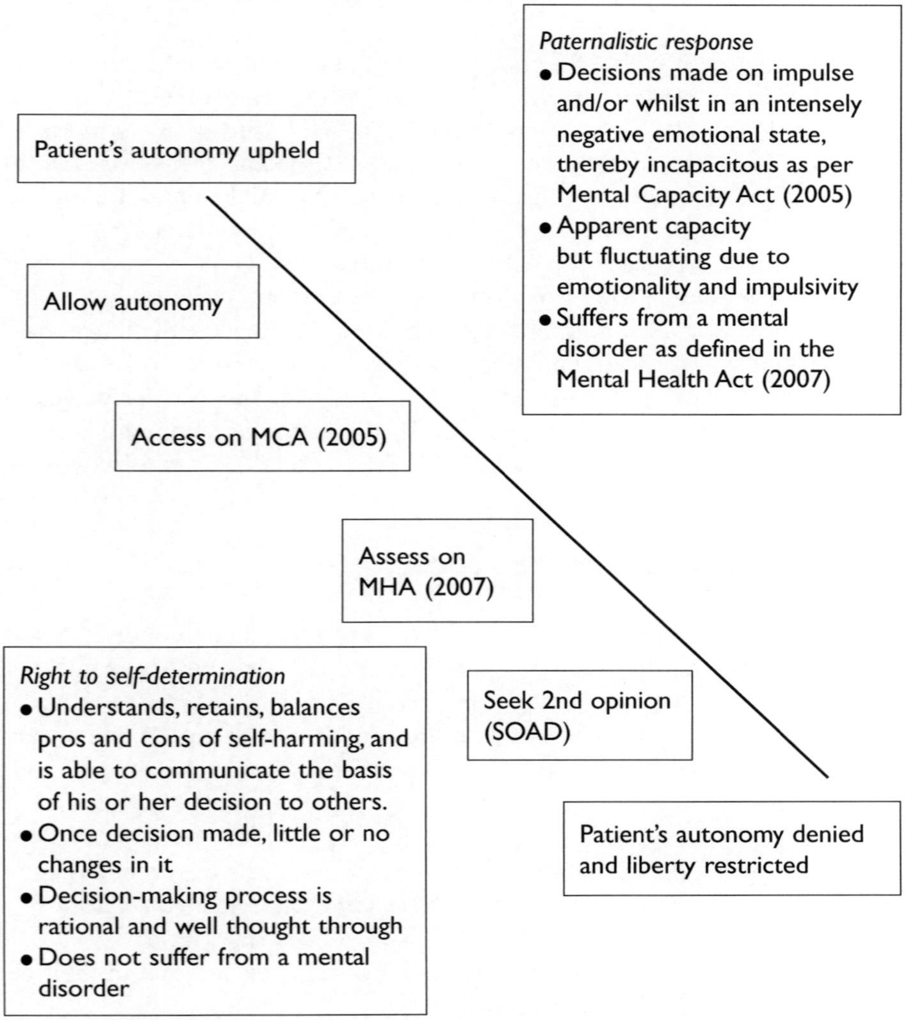

Figure 15.2: 'Slippery slope' model of decision-making. MCA: Mental Capacity Act; MHA: Mental Health Act; SOAD: second opinion appointed doctor.

Mental health legislation

Mental health professionals can use powers enshrined in the Mental Health Act 1983 (amended 2007) and the Mental Capacity Act (2005) in cases where the decision-making capacity of individuals seems impaired. Invariably these legal judgements would be made by senior and experienced health and social care workers responsible for the care of the patient.

The Mental Health Act 1983 (Amended 2007)

The Mental Heath Act 1983 concerns itself specifically with individuals suffering from mental disorder. This is defined at section 1 as "… any disorder or disability of the mind". The Act allows for individuals suffering from such a disorder to be detained for appropriate treatment if it is of a sufficient nature or degree to require hospital treatment. Detention in hospital is necessary as a result of the mental disorder, which poses significant risks to the patient's health and safety, for protection of others, or for prevention or exploitation of a vulnerable individual.

The Act allows treatment against the patient's will, if deemed "appropriate" and treatments for self-harm and prevention of suicide is included within this category, if (and only if) the self-harm was a manifestation of a mental disorder. As the definition of "mental disorder" is very broad, this would include personality disorder if the risks were sufficiently grave.

The Mental Capacity Act 2005

The Mental Capacity Act (MCA) 2005 on the other hand concerns itself with safeguarding individuals who lack decision-making capacity or who foresee themselves losing capacity in the near future (i.e. people in the early stages of dementia who are preparing for a time when they will no longer be *compos mentis*). The MCA is based on several core principles:

- that people are assumed to have capacity unless proven otherwise,
- that everything is done to help people arrive at a decision before declaring them incapable,
- that whatever is done for people lacking capacity be done in their best interest, and
- consideration needs to be given to the least restrictive intervention.

Lack of capacity has to result from a diagnosable mental disorder, much like the MHA 1983, whether this disturbance is permanent or temporary. The MCA includes several assessments that need to be completed where capacity is questioned. Of course in emergency situations the MCA would support rapid intervention without the need to jump through too many hoops if intervention would prove life-saving (Code of Practice, at 3.6). For instance where someone is found in a state of semi-consciousness following a large overdose where life is at stake, the MCA would require that immediate action be taken in the person's best interests. It would not be practical or reasonable to go on an exhaustive fact-finding mission before initiating treatment.

However, beyond the emergency phase, whilst people still lack capacity, the MCA requires a much more concerted assessment of individuals' capacity, the views of their carers or appointed attorneys, formal assessment of their best interests and establishment of any advance decisions. Advance directives are relevant here. In the case of Tracey Wooltorton, the patient used an advance directive to facilitate her suicide bid. Doctors and lawyers deemed her advance directive to be legally binding, and despite suffering from chronic depression secondary to a personality disorder, and despite several accident and emergency visits in the year prior to her suicide, quite shockingly, she was not resuscitated and allowed to die. The principle of self-determination was allowed to run its logical course, but this opened the Pandora's Box for all those who are terminally ill and seeking euthanasia, who are not permitted to kill themselves in law in the UK. The Mental Capacity Act refers to an advance directive specifically as a decision to refuse treatment made in advance and in writing, prepared when the patient had capacity. These features make it legally binding, unless there are legitimate questions as to its validity or applicability. Further guidance is contained in the Code of Practice accompanying the Mental Capacity Act.

The challenge for nursing staff

Nursing staff face a range of challenges in managing this patient group. Not only are they accountable for their actions (or lack of it), they have a responsibility of care as a legal obligation, especially for high-risk out-patients and all in-patients. They are unable to "experiment" with strategies even if non-professional carers can; are bound by confidentiality rules (Tantam and Huband 2009); and are often the victims of serious assaults when trying to prevent acts of self-harm (Sarkar 2010a, b). Whilst there are many documents that provide recommendations on management of self-harm, usually short-term management (NICE 2004, Royal College of Psychiatrists 2004, Kapur 2005, Skegg 2005), they are all "disappointingly inconclusive" (Tantam and Huband 2009). As repetitive self-harm is a behaviour and not an illness, there are no accepted standards for its management. As noted above, NICE guidelines are inadequate, and indeed inappropriate in certain groups and settings. For disengaged and non-compliant personality disordered patients, forensic patients who assault staff, and those in prison and secure institutions, these guidelines leave a lot to be desired. Not surprisingly then, a range of locally developed risk assessment and management strategies are in use (Sarkar 2010a), which are often led by the primary diagnosis of the patient. This may be relatively straightforward with diagnoses such as schizophrenia and affective disorder, but is far more complex in those with personality disorders due to multiple underlying motivational factors (Klonsky 2007). The NICE guidelines themselves highlight this,

> *The evidence base (is) small and tends to recruit fairly specific groups, making generalisations problematic.*

and further

> *people who self-harm are highly heterogeneous, and what works for one sub-group may be useless for another.*
>
> (NICE 2004).

Principles of managing harm to self

It is evident that case law is utterly confusing for busy nurses struggling with suicidal or self-harming patients. Nurses have a clinical duty of care towards their patients. Unless patients are engaging in low-risk self-harming behaviour, i.e. superficial cutting and laceration where risk to life is negligible, and the benefits to them are significant, for instance the capacity to deal, albeit in a maladaptive manner, with intense negative feelings, self-harm is permissible and tolerable. There are many individuals in the community who self-harm, without any intention to end their lives, using this behaviour much like an addiction. Instead of using drugs and alcohol, the "drug" of abuse is self-harm. However when risks to life and limb outweigh any perceived benefits, for instance emotional, psychological or indeed the sanctity of self-determination, and where there is an additional risk of harm to others related to harm to self, staff have a clear duty to intervene.

Three key tasks are necessary in determining whether the self-harm acts are likely to be potentially suicidal. What was the lethality (Skegg 2005) or nature of the injury caused – cutting, stabbing, poisoning or hanging? Second, what was the underlying intention of the self-harmer (Jamieson 1999): to self-harm superficially, seriously or make attempts to kill him or herself? Thirdly, are the prevailing circumstances, or inimicality (Shneidman 1981) within which self-harm occurs, such that it is likely that grave injuries may result and/or detection by others, and thus help, is unlikely to materialise.

Lethality is best understood as the probability that the person's act of self-harm is likely to end in death. It can also be referred to as the "How likely to die?" question (Sarkar 2010c).

Intentionality can be defined as an individual's intensity of desire to die, if the ultimate purpose of a self-harmer is to kill him or herself. It can be also referred to as the "How quickly to death?" question, best inferred objectively from the nature and severity of self-harm (Sarkar 2010c). In that sense it is closely entwined with the lethality of the act. The higher the intentionality, the greater the likely lethality of the act. As patients tend to (a) either not know their level of intention clearly ("Don't know" answers are the commonest responses clinicians get whilst trying to assess reasons for self-harm in the accident and emergency setting); (b) self-harm for inter-personal influence and indeed on occasions emotional blackmail (Klonsky 2007);and/or (c) making seemingly non-lethal attempts despite high intentionality; it is necessary to make the process of determining intentionality as objective as possible. When intentionality is assessed within a set of contextual factors, particularly in relatively controlled in-patient settings, it is possible to determine the real intent as opposed to stated or perceived intent, and to avert serious untoward incidents.

Intentionality is objectively gauged by the nature and severity of injury caused and the following factors help determine it:

- Which site and region of the body is injured?
- What is the type and nature of the tissue damage/injury?
- What is the extent of the injury?

As a general rule, internal tissue damage is more dangerous than external visible damage. Certain body regions are higher risk areas because they contain vital organs, e.g. chest injuries are more dangerous than leg injuries, arterial cuts more dangerous than venous cuts. Finally, the depth and breadth of the injury is often a manifestation of the depth of the intention. The principles of assessing intentionality are summarised in *Table 15.1*.

Table 15.1. Determining intentionality from nature and severity of wound	
Site of injury	*Region of injury*
Internal vs external tissue injury	High-risk body regions: genitals, anal, heart and lung, head, eyes, arterial "spurting"
Depth of injury	*Breadth of injury*
Stabbing vs slicing vs cutting vs "placing" objects in a wound pocket Chemical and fire-burn	Burn: Chemicals, fire, laceration, scratching, mechanical burn

Inimicality refers to those actions of patients that make the prevailing circumstances unfavourable or unduly complicated in order to avoid detection by others, and thus increase the likelihood of serious harm or death. It can also be referred to as the "How to avoid detection?" question, and is best gauged by contextual or environmental factors: where, when, how, who was present, etc. (Sarkar 2010c). This refers to the contextual factors which make it easier for people to successfully kill or cause major injuries to themselves. It is related to:

- Ease of access to implements which can cause significant harm, e.g. sharp implements to cut, slash and stab, ligating material, and chemicals and drugs that can be ingested.
- Access to spaces on ward/off ward with poor visibility e.g. blind spots, lack of cameras or staff constantly covering these areas (e.g. seclusion room) leading to relative lack of observation and risk of engaging in risky behaviour, for in-patients.
- Presence of hanging points within the institution.
- Choice of an isolated spot where the patient is unlikely to be confronted by anyone else. High risk periods are those when staffing levels are low, staff are occupied in handovers or dispensing medications, shifts are staffed with inexperienced staff (time of day/night, day of the week/weekend of incident, etc.).
- Nursing shifts when self-harm is carried out for inter-personal influence (high risk shifts, staff inexperienced, "hated" or "liked" staff). For out-patients, choosing to self-harm in front of other individuals for emotional reasons.

Principles of managing harm to self and others, especially nursing staff

Finally, in this patient group, additional risks may be present, e.g. harm to others including serious assaults and even death, attempts to breach security and abscond, the latter becoming an immediate concern when patients have to be taken to accident and emergency departments in unsecured hospital vans or in ambulances. The dual risks of self-harm in tandem with serious violent assaults on staff are a feature largely of secure institutions, hospitals, detention centres and prisons.

The institution has a duty towards the patient, especially health institutions if the patient is detained for health and safety reasons. Equally the institution has a duty to individual members of staff who provide care and treatment to patients detained for their health and safety and protection of others. The institution and the responsible clinician face the risks of claims of negligence by patients if staff do not intervene for fear of being assaulted or deny access to objects that compromise the patients' basic human rights. They also face legal action by staff for claims of negligence by the hospital authority for not taking adequate care or providing protection to its employees when there is a known risk of serious assault. Chapter 14 of the 1999 Code of Practice states that seclusion "should not be used where there is any risk of suicide or self-harm". However, following successful claims of gross negligence by staff against their employers, case law has now determined that employers have an obligation to consider seriously the use of seclusion to protect staff/others when there is a major risk of serious assault. As a result the new Code of Conduct allows seclusion for self-harmers where there is a risk of serious harm to others. An appropriate balance between ensuring patient safety against staff safety must be struck. The suggested strategies in *Box 15.1* might inform self-harm management policies where dual risks are present (from Sarkar 2010b).

Conclusions

The legal and ethical aspects of management of self-harm are imprecise. This chapter attempts to provide an easy to comprehend and clinically meaningful approach to law and ethics in a most challenging area of nursing skill. The principles enshrined are applicable to work in all nursing settings – from community and outpatient services to in-patient care, to forensic institutional care in secure hospital units and prisons. The Mental Health Act obviously is inapplicable within prisons and as such one would need to rely upon the Mental Capacity Act in that setting.

Box 15.1. Managing dual risks of harm to self and others simultaneously

- Patients must never be secluded simply for managing self-harm
- The nature and degree of risk to others must be documented with evidence listed of injuries caused to others, attempts to manage risk to others using less restrictive means and use of alternatives to seclusion
- Alternatives to seclusion can be
  - o physical restraint by staff although this runs the risk of more frequent staff assaults due to close proximity and ability of patients to spit at, bite and scratch staff
  - o in the most exceptional case there could be the use of mechanical restraint which includes use of restrictive garments, emergency response belts or furniture (specially designed with limb restraints)
- Where head-banging is the major self-harm risk, consideration should be given to the creation of a "padded" seclusion room
- Documentation must be detailed to justify overriding the need to protect staff/others
- The specific risks to self whilst in seclusion (type, severity, probability) should be detailed with reference to past behaviours within or outside seclusion
- Explicit guidance should be available for staff on when to intervene in the event of self-harm when in seclusion
- A second opinion should be sought before engaging in practice that is restrictive as this provides a level of external scrutiny
- Ongoing practice should also be externally reviewed by senior clinicians and national experts who have sufficient experience in the field

References

Appleby L, Shaw J, Kapur NN, et al (2006) *Avoidable Deaths: Five year report of the National Confidential Inquiry into Suicide and Homicide by People with Mental Illness*. Department of Health, London

Glover J (1990) *Causing Death and Saving Lives*. Penguin Books, London

Jamieson KR (1999) *Night falls fast: Understanding suicide*. Knopf Doubleday Publishing Group, Washington DC

Kapur N (2005) Management of self-harm in adults: Which way now? *British Journal of Psychiatry* 187: 497–9

Klonsky ED (2007) The functions of deliberate self-injury: A review of the evidence. *Clinical Psychology Review* 27: 226–39

National Institute of Clinical Excellence (2004) *Self harm: The short-term physical and psychological management and secondary prevention of self-harm in primary and secondary care*. National Clinical Practice Guideline No. 16, National Collaborating

Centre for Mental Health. Royal College of Psychiatrists, British Psychological Association, London

Royal College of Psychiatrists (2004) *Assessment Following Self-harm in Adults*. Council report CR 122. Royal College of Psychiatrists, London

Sarkar J (2010a) From science to services: Developing a neuroscience-based innovative clinical treatment model to manage severe and repetitive self-harm personality. *Mental Health*, in press

Sarkar J (2010b) Short-term management of high-risk repetitive self-harm: Developing a model of risk management Paper under review *Psychiatrist*

Sarkar J (2010c) Management of high-risk repetitive self-harm in secure institutions. Commissioned paper under review in *Psychiatric Treatment*

Shneidman E (1996) *The Suicidal Mind*. New York: Oxford University Press

Skegg K (2005) Self harm. *Lancet* **366:** 1471–83

Tantam D, Huband N (2009) *Understanding Repeated Self-injury: A multidisciplinary approach*. Palgrave-Macmillan, Basingstoke

CHAPTER 16

Ethical aspects of seclusion

Richard Byrt and Satnam Kaur

Love is merely a madness, and, I tell you, deserves as well a dark house and a whip as madmen do.

(Shakespeare: *As You Like It*, Act 3, Scene 2 quoted in Edgar 1970)

Since at least the second century AD (Sees 2009, Yorkston and Haw 2009), individuals with mental health problems have been secluded. Rosamund's comments in *As You Like It* suggest an acceptance of seclusion ("a dark house") as natural, and part of everyday, taken-for-granted reality (Brown 2005). So do Charlotte Bronte's comments in *Jane Eyre* (Bronte 1962, first published in 1847): "Since the medical profession had pronounced her mad, she had, *of course*, been shut up" [present author's emphasis]. Although today, seclusion attracts more controversy, and probably a greater range of opinions regarding its use (Sookoo 2009), research findings and Government inquiries suggest that in some mental health and learning disability services, including those that are secure, seclusion is still sometimes seen as a "taken-for-granted reality" of everyday practice. It is unquestioned, and sometimes ingrained in an organisational culture (Duxbury and Whittington 2005, Meehan et al 2006). However, the literature includes accounts of ways that professionals and managers have sometimes questioned the use of seclusion, and replaced it with alternative interventions (Smith et al 2005, Sullivan et al 2005, Pollard et al 2007, Sees 2009).

Seclusion and the Code of Practice

Each country of the UK has a Code of Practice to guide the implementation of mental health legislation (Office of Public Sector Information 2010). For England, the latest edition of the Code of Practice of the Mental Health Act, 1983 defines seclusion as:

The supervised confinement of a patient in a room, which may be locked. Its sole aim is to contain severely disturbed behaviour which is likely to cause harm to others.

(Department of Health 2008, Section 15.43)

In contrast, in some other countries, the aims of seclusion include treatment and prevention of self-harm (Tardiff and Lion, 2008). The Code of Practice is specific about when seclusion can be used in England, stating that it:

- Is never a therapeutic intervention.
- Must be used only to avoid serious physical harm to others when there is no other way to prevent this – as a "last resort" (Department of Health 2008: 123, Section 15.44).
- Must never be used punitively, or to stigmatise clients.
- Must be a "reasonable, proportionate...response" (Department of Health, 2008: 123, Section 15.44): that is, used only to prevent serious harm to other people in the absence of any other means to do so.

(Department of Health 2008, Section 15.19f)

In England, the use of seclusion should normally be governed by the Code of Practice of the Mental Health Act (Department of Health 2008). This Code, unlike an Act of Parliament, does not have the legal requirement that it should be followed. However, in a court of law, it would usually be expected that the use of seclusion would be in accordance with the Code of Practice (Court of Appeal 2003). The House of Lords (2005) decided that "Ashworth Hospital's seclusion policy [which departed, in some respects, from the Code of Practice] was lawful"; but added: "the Code is guidance to which great weight must be given, and from which hospitals should depart only when they have cogent reasons for so doing" (Department of Health 2007).

Although the Code of Practice clearly specifies good, ethical practice in the use of seclusion, a mismatch has been found between expected and actual practice. The voluntary organisation MIND and the former Mental Health Act Commission (whose functions have now been included in the Care Quality Commission 2010) maintained that "the Code of Practice was being departed from...in a number of hospitals...68% of hospitals surveyed did not have safe seclusion facilities" (Joint Committee on Human Rights 2004). The Mental Health Act Commission (2008: 97f) found that, despite some good practice, a number of patients were secluded in unsafe or insanitary conditions.

It is widely agreed that good practice in the use of seclusion means that, in accordance with the Mental Health Act Code of Practice, a wide range of interventions should be used to prevent and reduce patients' violent behaviours, with seclusion being implemented only when there is no alternative to ensure others' safety (National Institute for Health and Clinical Excellence (NICE) 2005, Muir-Cochrane 2009). Where the latter is the case, nurses and other professionals are faced with a moral dilemma (defined in *Chapter 2*) because research findings suggest that the use of seclusion results in trauma to patients (Abderhalden et al 2006) and some staff (Moran et al 2009). However, trauma can also be a consequence of being assaulted (Needham 2006) or from perpetrating violence (Maden 2007).

A moral dilemma in a high secure hospital

This moral dilemma is highlighted by Chandley and Mason (1995), who consider the nursing care needs of four individuals who were patients in a high secure hospital. These people put others at serious risk because of long-term assaultive behaviours which did not reduce, despite nursing interventions and treatment, and consequently, they were secluded for long periods (Chandley and Mason 1995):

> *By being part of the wider nursing community,* [forensic nurses] *have some of the same basic values. However, in the face of such intense violence, these principles are given a lower priority. The debate in the case of this small group of patients is more profoundly felt, as the need for controlling force is more urgent.*
>
> *In practice terms, the reduction of higher principles to the pragmatics of nursing practice is grounded in reality. This does not mean that those higher values are lost, merely that they are an aspiration, rather than an actuality.*
> (Chandley and Mason 1995: 22)

However, given research findings on the adverse effects of seclusion, and the ethical and legal implications of its use (Abderhalden et al 2006), it can be argued that increases in the use and length of seclusion indicate a problem that needs to be addressed. Consideration needs to be given to the following questions:

- How can seclusion be reduced?
- If patients spend long periods in seclusion, are they in the right service to most effectively meet their needs?

Underpinning ethical principles

Hughes (2009) states that ethical values need to be the basis for considering arguments for and against restraint and seclusion of particular individuals. These involve ethical principles which were considered in *Chapter 2*. They include:

- The duty of care to preserve life, health and safety, and to be beneficent (aiming to achieve positive outcomes) and non-maleficent (avoiding harm to the individual patient and other people).
- Respect for persons (Kant 1969), including valuing and respecting the individual.
- Respect for individuals' autonomy.
- Ensuring justice: the fair treatment of all patients without negatively discriminating on any grounds.
  (Dickenson et al 2000, Beauchamp and Childress 2009, Blochet 2009)

These ethical principles may appear obvious, but Government and other inquiries indicate that they have not always been considered by professionals (Mental Health Act Commission 2008, Sees 2009). There are also ethical concerns related to aspects of the forensic and prison nurse's dual roles of ensuring safety and caring, with various authors arguing that these two components may conflict with, or complement each other (Maeve and Vaughan 2001, Kettles et al 2007, Byrt 2008). A considerable amount of nurses' time may be spent in ensuring physical security in forensic settings (Dale and Gardner 2001, Collins and Davies 2004). In addition, in a study of acute admission mental health wards, "approximately half of all nursing resources [were] expended in managing conflict and deploying containment" (Flood et al 2008: 325). The unethical use of seclusion is indicated in the following account:

Incorrect and unethical use of seclusion: Two student nurses' experiences

Satnam Kaur

During a clinical placement, as a student nurse in an acute admission ward, I became increasingly aware of the use of seclusion being applied to patients who had been identified as liable to display aggression and violence towards other patients and staff. I noticed there also appeared to be a much greater tendency by specific nursing staff to implement seclusion, while this form of coercive intervention was not utilised by other nurses. This disparity took place even when dealing with the same patient displaying exactly the same symptoms. The Mental Health Act Code of Practice states that "seclusion should only be implemented as a last resort when all other reasonable steps have been taken to avoid its use". It also asserts that seclusion cannot be regarded as a form of "treatment", nor should it "be used as a punishment" (Section 15.45).

I felt that there had to be an explanation as to why this inconsistency in the application of seclusion existed. The most obvious conclusion was that the staff who regularly implemented seclusion lacked the necessary skills to build a therapeutic relationship and were incapable of defusing aggressive situations (Kettles et al 2007).

It seemed that perhaps this was too simplistic an analysis and that other factors, such as lack of fully experienced staff (Morrison and Lehane 1995), pressure of work, inadequate counselling facilities, ward environment (Timko and Moos 2004), and not following the trust policy fully (Alty 1997), were all influencing factors. Nevertheless, the onus to avoid implementing seclusion lies with the nursing staff (Alty 1997). The experience of seeing seclusion implemented influenced me to believe that its random application by certain nursing staff was to be condemned, while non-application of seclusion by other nursing staff was to be recommended as the preferred method. Nursing staff who implement patient seclusion as a matter of course should be assisted by the ward management to discuss their reasoning for doing so. They should also be given additional training in alternative interventions, particularly use of de-escalation techniques to reduce patient violence and aggression (Ford et al 2010). However, it is not sufficient merely to educate nurses in seclusion reduction. Everyone involved in mental health nursing needs to be involved in developing the multidisciplinary strategies necessary to achieve successful long-term therapeutic treatment (Curran, 2007).

I had occasion to deal with a patient who was regularly subjected to seclusion when a specific staff member was on duty. The client suffered from severe mental illness caused by alcohol abuse. He often displayed aggressive tendencies, but observation had shown that these were triggered by raised voices directed at him and/or his having to look up to make eye contact with someone. As the staff member who used seclusion most was naturally loudly spoken and taller than the patient, these possible triggers of aggressive behaviour were automatically engaged each time the staff member and the patient encountered each other (Paterson and Leadbetter 1999). Had the staff member simply sat down with the patient and spoken quietly, many of the seclusion periods could have been avoided. It can also be asked why the ward management did not question more closely the reason for the frequent seclusion and implement the necessary corrective action (Mason and Chandley 1999). I have concluded that while, unfortunately, there is a need for seclusion to be applied in specific circumstances, it is all too often misapplied (Alty and Mason, 1994). It is an area worthy of further study to determine whether the concept of seclusion as a coercive intervention of "last resort" ties in with the available research and if not, what causal factors for this failure have been established (Sookoo, 2009).

Another student nurse on her first acute psychiatric ward placement was shocked to witness seclusion, which she described as "barbaric". Blyth (2008) described how a female patient was admitted to the ward for assessment. Because of a shortage of staff, the patient was told that nurses were too busy to talk to her. The patient, who was already in an agitated state, struck the nurse in charge and was immediately restrained and subjected to overnight seclusion. Blyth (2008) felt that seclusion was being used to punish the patient and to compensate for staff shortage. She questioned why no attempt was made to calm the patient as an alternative to seclusion: "After all, de-escalation techniques should be a core skill for mental health nurses working in acute settings" (Blyth 2008: 27).

Blyth (2008) also acknowledged the difficulty in determining whether restraint was an infringement of a patient's rights or a necessary technique to ensure the patient's safety and satisfy the legal obligation on nursing staff to provide a duty of care. The student's quandary was clear when, in her next few paragraphs, she wrote that she believed listening and talking to patients were basic skills which a nurse had to learn and use from day one of training, and a patient's needs had priority over paperwork. The student concluded her article by stating that in her opinion, secluding that specific patient breached ethical and legal guidelines. After reflecting on the matter, she appreciated just how complex an issue managing aggression is, and the diverse factors such as ward environment, staffing and communication which both create and de-escalate violence and aggression (Byrt and Doyle 2007).

In both these examples, the nursing staff did not meet the standards of care required by the Code of Practice of the Mental Health Act, 1983.

Absolutist and utilitarian principles in decisions about seclusion

Decisions about seclusion can be informed by absolutist and utilitarian principles (Adshead 2010), which were considered in *Chapter 2*. A nurse taking an absolutist position might argue that, regardless of the circumstances, "seclusion is always wrong" (or always unnecessary if other interventions are used to prevent violence). Conversely, an absolutist position could be: "seclusion should always be used if there is the slightest chance that a patient could become violent". Some authors have argued that seclusion should rarely or never be used (Alty and Mason 1994). However, research findings have suggested that in some services, seclusion and restraint have been used as a first resort, without the use of therapeutic nurse–patient relationships and communication to prevent or reduce violence (Secker et al 2004, Duxbury and Whittington 2005, Meehan et al 2006).

In reflection on practice (rather than during an emergency), the application of utilitarian principles might help professionals to weigh up arguments for and against the use of seclusion, in relation to decisions likely to result in the greatest good and/or the least harm to the patient and to other patients and staff (Collopy 2006, Adshead 2010). In relation to the Mental Health Act Code of Practice, the decision to seclude or not would be linked to others' rights to be protected from violence; as well as consideration of the effects of seclusion on the assaultive patient, and whether other interventions would be less harmful.

Human rights and the secluded patient's physical health needs

Human rights and other legislation is also crucial in decisions to seclude, and the care of the patient in seclusion. Both the United Nations (2008) Convention on the Rights of Persons with Disabilities, and the Human Rights Act 1998 (HM Government 1998) list various human rights of all individuals. Rights to "liberty", freedom from "exploitation, violence and abuse" and "respect for privacy" relate to the use of seclusion for ethically and clinically correct reasons, in accordance with the Code of Practice of the Mental Health Act, 1983. Article 3: "Freedom from torture, inhumane and degrading treatment and punishment" (HM Government 1998) has implications for ensuring that seclusion is never used as a punishment or to stigmatise the individual (Alty and Mason 1994, Department of Health 2008). (However, regardless of nurses' intentions, patients may perceive seclusion and other measures as punitive: a point made in *Chapter 25*, of this book). Article 3 of the Human Rights Act, 1998 also involves ensuring that nursing and other care is of the highest quality. This includes attempts to assess and meet the individual's safety, physical, psychological, spiritual, cultural, advocacy and other needs; and to enable her/his privacy and dignity (Department of Health 2008). (The difficulties in enabling privacy and dignity for patients in seclusion is considered later in this chapter.)

The Human Rights Act 1998 is also concerned with the "right to life". This is very relevant to secluded patients and their care, as some individuals have become seriously physically ill, and occasionally, died in seclusion (Prins et al 1993). This has implications for the duty of care to ensure physical nursing observations and interventions of a high standard. The duty of care includes awareness that medical emergencies may occur because of heightened physical and psychological arousal (Ford et al 2010); the side effects of antipsychotic medication (e.g. given as rapid tranquillisation); and with some patients, poor physical health (NICE 2005, Tardiff and Lion 2008). *Boxes 16.1* and *16.2* summarise important information related to patients' physical health and the administration of rapid tranquillisation.

The rights of the patient and other people

One problem with applying ethical and rights-based principles is that the rights of the individual who is violent may conflict with those of other patients and staff, particularly their right to be protected from harm. The nurse is faced with responsibilities to ensure the health, safety and well-being of not only the individual who is violent, but also of other patients, and under health and safety legislation, of colleagues and students (Eastman et al 2010). The

Box 16.1. Essential observations, especially if rapid tranquillisation is administered

It is crucial to observe the following, and to provide appropriate nursing care and medical treatment, as needed, to the secluded patient, based on observations and nursing care:

- Airway
- Level of consciousness
- Pulse
- Blood pressure
- Respiratory effort
- Temperature
- Hydration (measure and record fluid intake and output)

(From NICE 2005)

The essential nursing care in medical emergencies includes the following:

- Ensure that oxygen, suction, defibrillation are near at hand if needed
- Contact an emergency ambulance if needed
- Elevate the patient's legs if blood pressure is low
- Cardiopulmonary resuscitation and defibrillation if heart and breathing stop
- Administration of cardiac/respiratory stimulants

(NICE 2005)

Other aspects of nursing care of the individual in seclusion

- Enable the individual to meet hygiene and toilet needs with as much privacy and dignity as possible; and maintain a clean room
- Enable plenty of fluids preferred by the patient
- Provide a nourishing diet
- Ensure plates and cutlery are of safe materials
- Treat any injuries sustained in seclusion

(Dix and Page 2008)

Nursing and Midwifery Council (2008) Code requirement is also relevant: "You must act without delay if you believe that you, a colleague or anyone else may be putting someone at risk". Decisions to seclude are often made in an emergency, with little time for discussion with the assaultive individual or with colleagues. However, in the author's experience, a brief, clear, polite request to patients to stop violent behaviour, with the immediate offer of help, is sometimes effective. For example, when one man was asked to "Please stop what you're doing and tell us what's bothering you", he did so, partly because he was surprised at being asked to do so politely. This individual was able to safely use an opportunity to ventilate his frustration, anger and other feelings verbally, without the use of seclusion or restraint (Ford et al 2010).

Box 16.2. Rapid tranquillisation

Rapid tranquillisation is the use of medication to:

- Calm/lightly sedate the service user
- Reduce the risk to self and/or others
- Achieve an optimum reduction in agitation and aggression

(From NICE 2005)

Adverse effects of rapid tranquillisation:

- Loss of consciousness
- Sedation with loss of alertness
- Loss of airway: unable to breathe
- Cardiovascular and respiratory collapse
- Interaction with medicines already prescribed or illicit drugs taken
- Possible damage to staff–patient relationship

(From NICE 2005)

Some authors consider that seclusion and restraint may be necessary in certain circumstances. Davis (2004) uses his experience as both service user and a mental health nurse to comment on the need for nurses to be self-aware and have positive attitudes and beliefs if seclusion is used. It can be argued that similar attitudes and beliefs should underpin the use of seclusion:

> *There may be times when [seclusion/restraint] is a necessary violent act. A person who knows this, and believes violence to be...wrong, will strive to minimise the violence. A person who thinks restraining [or secluding] a patient is not a violent act, will not. They will also not understand why someone would be upset by being restrained [/secluded], and will not be in a position to deal with that upset in a positive way.*
>
> (Davis 2004, quoted in Leadbetter and Paterson 2009: 116)

However, some critics question the use of seclusion at all (Sookoo 2009). *Table 16.1* indicates how seclusion may be viewed by proponents of sociological conflict and consensus theories.

Holistic care

The next part of this chapter considers ethical issues related to specific aspects of holistic nursing care related to seclusion and its alternatives. Holistic care is concerned with the whole individual and her/his care related to safety (*Box 16.3*), physical, psychological, spiritual, cultural, psychosexual, advocacy

Table 16.1. Consensus via conflict models applied to seclusion	
Consensus model	*Conflict model*
It is possible to combine therapeutic interventions with measures, such as seclusion, to ensure safety	Therapeutic and safety aims conflict – and cannot co-exist
Both therapeutic interventions and seclusion have ultimately beneficial consequences for patients, staff and wider society	"Interventions" are solely to keep individuals under control when they are judged to be "deviant" by people in positions of power; and for the benefit of the latter
The mental health professional has a duty of care to ensure safety of the patient and others. Whilst seclusion is used to protect others, it also prevents the patient from actions which she/he may later regret	Mental health professionals should be concerned only with what the patient perceives to be in her/his interests, not with the safety of others
Not using seclusion may result in considerable harms, not only to others, but also to the patient with violent behaviours	Research shows that seclusion is iatrogenic (Illich 1996), resulting in considerable harm, both short and long-term
	Adapted from Byrt (2008: 102), with kind permission from Quay Books, MA Healthcare, Ltd

and other needs (American Holistic Nurses' Association 2010, Ford et al 2010). In relation to seclusion and its alternatives,

> *...holistic care includes integrating, rather than separating, risk from other aspects of care, and avoiding only concentrating on restrictive methods...without considering the distress of the client.*
>
> (Ford et al, citing Kettles et al 2007: 38)

Secluded patients' psychological needs are considered in *Chapter 17* and their physical health needs on pp 211–213 (*Boxes 16.1 and 16.2*).

The safety of other patients and staff

Unless the safety of the secluded patient and staff entering the seclusion room is ensured, it will be difficult to meet the patient's other needs, or to ensure staff well-being. Research suggests that both seclusion and being a victim of assault have negative consequences for the individual. A high

Box 16.3. Ensuring safety

The following measures may be used to ensure the safety of the secluded patient and other people:

- Three nurses always enter the seclusion room – so that restraint techniques can be used if, sadly, this is the only way to ensure safety, in accordance with local procedure and policy
- A fourth nurse opens the seclusion room door
- Safety is also aided by effective communication with the patient, and attempts to empathise with, and alleviate her/his situation
- An observation panel and CCTV cameras contribute to careful observation/safety

(Dix and Page 2008)

The seclusion room

- All fittings, bedding, washing and toilet facilities must be made of safe, indestructible materials
- Room temperature, ventilation, humidity must be maintained at comfortable levels which are regularly recorded
- A safe inter-communication system enables communication and reduces isolation
- Projection of a clock and television screen onto a wall and music/radio programmes may aid orientation and reduce boredom that may contribute to frustration and aggression

(Curran et al 2005, Dix and Page 2008)

proportion of health professionals, especially nurses, are the recipients of physical or verbal violence (Healthcare Commission 2009), particularly in mental health and learning disability settings (NHS Business Authority Security Management Service 2007). Research findings suggest that both violence to staff and seclusion have generally negative consequences for the individual. Effects of violence on mental health professionals include physical injuries, "anxiety or fear...post-traumatic stress disorder... threats to personal integrity or pride...anger...guilt, self-blame or shame" (Needham 2006: 298f: see *Box 16.4*). These effects are remarkably similar to those experienced by patients who have been secluded (Abderhalden et al 2006) and considered in *Chapter 17*. Such findings can mean that staff are faced with a moral dilemma. Research findings suggest that seclusion could result in harm to the assaultive patient, but equally, harm to others could result from a decision not to seclude if this is the only way to prevent or reduce violence.

Box 16.4. Adverse effects of violence experienced by staff interviewed by Howard and Hegarty (2003)

- *Someone's personally attacked you and it feels really upsetting...*
- *And that's the point where you think, "Oh, I've had enough"*
- *You go over the reasons [for the violence] and nothing seems to work...and that gets me really frustrated*
- *Every time...they can be aggressive and you [think]... "I don't want to be here today"*
- *If they're regularly violent towards you, then it does affect your confidence*

(Staff interviewed by and quoted in Howard and Hegarty 2003: 8f)

Effects of seclusion on staff and other patients

A study by Moran et al (2009) found that secluding patients also had negative consequences for nurses. Those who experienced "enduring suffering" (Morse 1991, cited in Moran et al 2009) became hardened to the use of seclusion, and maintained that it did not bother them. These nurses failed to treat patients as individuals. Moran et al (2009) stated that some nurses "...continuously suppressed their unpleasant emotions" related to the use of seclusion. In addition, Mason (1997) and Curran (2007) reported that nurses sometimes secluded patients because of colleagues' expectations and pressures.

Moran et al (2009) found that other nurses in their study experienced very negative and uncomfortable feelings about secluding patients. These feelings were suppressed in order that nurses could "get by" and manage their work:

> *Sometimes, [nurses] feel they have to be comfortable with [restraint/seclusion] even though they're absolutely quaking with fear.*
>
> *It's against your nursing principles...your caring attitude. You can't help but feel guilty at times. Even though you know you're doing it for...safety.*
>
> (Moran et al 2009, quoting nurses interviewed in their study)

In addition, in the author's experience, patients can experience vicarious traumatisation if one of their peers is secluded. When this occurred in one ward in a secure hospital, a patient who was not secluded experienced flashbacks of times when he had been locked for long periods in a prison cell; and of the ill treatment he had previously received from officers when he was in prison.

Various guidelines, including the Code of Practice of the Mental Health Act, 1983 and the NICE (2005) *Guideline on Violence* emphasise principles to ensure sound ethical and clinical practice in relation to secluded patients. Several authors refer to interventions to prevent, as well as reduce violence and aggression, including the availability of nurses for therapeutic communication and relationships (Ford et al 2010, Richter 2006). This involves a culture in which patients are treated as individuals, with the focus of nursing being on intensive care, as well as observation of patients, instead of preoccupation with paperwork, and only responding reactively to crises, mainly through the use of seclusion and restraint (Duxbury and Whittington 2005, Meehan et al 2006, NICE 2005, Secker et al 2004). It also involves ethical principles related to client autonomy (see *Chapter 2*) and participation, with several authors referring to the importance of involving patients in proactive care plans to prevent and reduce violence; and enabling individuals with capacity to make advanced directives stating their preferred interventions if they are violent in the future (O'Hagan 2004, NICE 2005, Department of Health 2008, Pollard et al 2007).

Privacy and dignity

Another aspect of ethical care relates to ensuring the privacy and dignity of people who are secluded. In the author's experience, the latter can be particularly difficult, especially if the individual, for example, smears faeces round the room, micturates on the floor, or (given the need for intensive observation), masturbates. Smearing faeces may occur, particularly if the individual feels there is no other way of exerting any control over the situation. It may be less likely if she/he is enabled, within safety parameters, to have control in other, less harmful ways (Mason 1996). Part of the Royal College of Nursing (2008) definition of dignity includes the following statement:

> *Dignity is concerned with how people feel, think and behave in relation to the worth or value of themselves or others. To treat someone with dignity is to treat them as being of worth, in a way that is respectful of them as valued individuals.*
>
> (Royal College of Nursing 2008)

One ethical problem with the use of seclusion is the probable clash between the patient's perspective of how she/he is being treated, and the nurse's intent. No matter how hard the nurse tries to treat the secluded patient with dignity and respect, the patient is likely to see seclusion as undignified and possibly, disrespectful. The Code of Practice of the Mental Health Act, 1983 states that seclusion should result in "minimum interference to [patients'] privacy and dignity, consistent with the need to protect the patient and other people"

(Section 15.9). However, the Code of Practice does not entirely indicate how to ensure this. The Royal College of Nursing (2008) states:

> *When dignity is absent, people feel devalued, lacking control and comfort.*

Whilst seclusion may be necessary for others' safety, research findings suggest that it results in loss of "control and comfort" for the secluded individual (Abderhalden et al 2006). However, two of 12 patients in Meehan et al's (2000) study viewed seclusion "as a safe environment in which they could gain control over their actions".

Patients' needs related to quality and diversity

Meeting patients' needs related to equality and diversity is another crucial aspect of ethical practice. The Code of Practice of the Mental Health Act, 1983 stresses the need for staff "to demonstrate and encourage respect for racial and cultural diversity". This needs to be considered in the context of the over-representation of black and minority ethnic individuals secluded in the UK (Sewell 2009) and other countries (Knutzen et al 2007). However, Gudjonnson et al (2004) found that, in one secure hospital, this was not statistically significant when a number of variables was taken into account. These authors concluded that

> *...racial 'stereotyping' was unlikely to have played a major direct role in determining nurses' responses.*
>
> (Gudjonnson et al 2004: 258)

The inquiry into the death of David ("Rocky") Bennett was concerned with the death of a patient in a medium secure unit. This resulted from his restraint in the prone position for about 10 minutes without the maintenance of a clear airway. In addition, the inquiry found that although staff were "kind", they paid insufficient attention to Mr Bennett's spiritual and cultural needs. Shortly before the restraint which led to his death, his complaints about another patient's racist remarks were ignored (Blofeld 2003). Despite "delivering race equality" initiatives since 2005 (Department of Health 2005) and a "single equality scheme" (Department of Health 2010), black and minority ethnic clients have continued to express greater dissatisfaction with mental health services, compared with other clients (Healthcare Commission 2009). This was evidenced from comments of black service users who contributed to the NICE (2005) *Guideline on Violence*. These participants referred to professionals' stereotypical associations of being black with violence. One individual with service user experience said:

> *Most of the time, if you're black, you're going to get bent and twisted up and carried into seclusion.*
>
> (Chandler-Oatts and Nelstrop 2008: 36f, quoted in Ford et al 2010: 118).

Chapter 17 considers patients' experiences of seclusion, and ways to replace its use with alternative interventions.

References

Abderhalden C, Hahn S, Bonner DB, Galeazzi GM (2006) Users' perceptions and views on violence and coercion in mental health. In: Richter D, Whittington R (eds) *Violence in Mental Health Settings. Causes Consequences and Management*. Springer, New York

Adshead G (2010) Principles of ethical reasoning in forensic psychiatry. In: Bartlett A, McGauley G (eds) *Forensic Mental Health. Concepts Systems and Practice*. Oxford University Press, Oxford

Alty A (1997) Nurses learning experience and expressed opinions regarding seclusion practice within one NHS trust. *Journal of Advanced Nursing* 25: 786–93

Alty A, Mason T (1994) *Seclusion. A Break with the Past*. Chapman and Hall, London

American Holistic Nurses Association (2010) Available from: www.ahna.org [Last accessed 16 June 2010]

Beauchamp T, Childress JF (2009) *Principles of Biomedical Ethics*. (6th edn) Oxford University Press, New York

Blochet A (2009) Seclusion in psychiatry: Continuing the debate in order to go beyond the conflicts. (English translation of Abstract) *Schweizer Archiv fur Neurologie Neurochirugie und Psychiatrie* 160(1): 4–11

Blofield J (2003) *Independent Inquiry into the Death of David Bennett. An Independent Inquiry Set Up Under HSG (94) 27*. Department of Health, London

Blyth J (2008) Witnessing 'barbaric' seclusion provided impetus for reflection. *Nursing Standard* 20(35): 27

Bronte J (1962) *Jane Eyre*. Collins London. First published in 1847 by Smith and Elder, London

Brown CG (2005) *Postmodernism for Historians*. Pearson Longman, Harlow

Byrt R (2008) Negative control or life saving? Perspectives on power. In: National Forensic Nurses' Research and Development Group: Kettles AM Woods P, Byrt R (eds) *Forensic Mental Health Nursing: Capabilities Roles Responsibilities*. Quay Books MA Healthcare Ltd., London

Byrt R, Doyle M (2007) Prevention and reduction of violence and aggression. In: National Forensic Nurses' Research and Development Group: Kettles AM, Woods P, Byrt R, Addo M A, Coffey M, Doyle M (eds) *Forensic Mental Health Nursing: Forensic Aspects of Acute Care*. Quay Books MA Healthcare Ltd., London

Care Quality Commission (2010) Available from: www.cqc.org.uk/ [Last accessed 16 June 2010]

Chandler-Oatts J, Nelstrop L (2008) Listening to the voices of African-Caribbean mental health service users to develop guideline recommendations on managing violent behaviour. *Diversity in Health and Social Care* 5: 31–41

Chandley M, Mason T (1995) Nursing chronically dangerous patients. Ethical issues of behaviour management and patient health. *Psychiatric Care* 2(1): 20–3

Collins M, Davies S (2004) The secure needs assessment profile: A multidimensional approach to measuring security needs. *International Journal of Forensic Mental Health* 4(1): 39–52

Collopy BJ (2006) Autonomy in long-term care: Some crucial distinctions. In: Green SA, Bloch S (eds) *An Anthology of Psychiatric Ethics*. Oxford University Press, Oxford

Court of Appeal (2003) *R (on the Application of Colonel Munjaz) v Mersey Care NHS Trust and (i) Secretary of State for Health and (ii) MIND; S v Airedale NHS Trust and (i) Secretary of State for Health and (ii) MIND [2003] EWCA civ 1036*. Cited in: Department of Health (2007) *Mental Health. Briefing on Legal Cases*. Available from: www.webarchive.nationalarchives.gov.uk/+/www.dh.gov.uk/en/Healthcare/Mentalhealth/DH_4077674?PageOperation=email [Last accessed 16 June, 2010]

Curran SS (2007) Staff resistance to restraint reduction. *Journal of Psychosocial Nursing and Mental Health Services* 45(5): 45–50

Curran C, Adnett C, Zigmond T (2005) Seclusion: Factors to consider when designing and using a seclusion suite in a mental health hospital. *Hospital Development* January: 19–26

Dale C, Gardner J (2001) Security in forensic environments: Strategic and operational issues. In: Dale C, Thompson T, Woods P (eds) *Forensic Mental Health: Issues in Practice*. Bailliere Tindall/Royal College of Nursing, Edinburgh

Davis P (2004) Cited in: Leadbetter D, Paterson B (2009) Towards restraint – Free Care. In: Hughes R (ed) *Reducing Restraints in Health and Social Care. Practice and Policy Perspectives*. Quay Books MA Healthcare Ltd., London

Department of Health (2005) *Delivering Race Equality in Mental Health Care: An Action Plan for Reform*. Department of Health, London

Department of Health (2007) *R (on the application of Colonel Munjaz) and the Mersey Care NHS Trust – R v Ashworth Hospital Authority (now Mersey Care National Health Service Trust) (Appellants) ex parte Munjaz*. In: Department of Health. *Mental Health. Briefing on Legal Cases*. Available from:: www.webarchive.nationalarchives.gov.uk/+/www.dh.gov.uk/en/Healthcare/Mentalhealth/DH_4077674?PageOperation=email [Last accessed 16 June, 2010]

Department of Health (2008) *Code of Practice Mental Health Act 1983*. The Stationery Office, London

Department of Health (2010) *Single Equality Scheme 2010 – 2013*. Department of Health, London. Available from: www.dh.gov [Last accessed 4 June 2010]

Dickenson D, Fulford B with Birley JLT (eds) (2000) *In Two Minds: A Casebook of Psychiatric Ethics*. Oxford University Press,Oxford

Dix R, Page MJ (2008) Physical environment. In: Beer MD, Pereira S, Paton C (eds) *Psychiatric Intensive Care* (2nd edn). Greenwich Medical Media, London

Duxbury JA, Whittington R (2005) Causes and management of patient aggression and violence: Staff and patient perspectives. *Journal of Psychiatric and Mental Health Nursing* 50(5): 469–78

Eastman N, Riordan D, Adshead G (2010) Ethical roles, relationships and duties of forensic mental health clinicians. In: Bartlett A , McGauley G (eds) *Forensic Mental Health. Concepts Systems and Practice*. Oxford University Press, Oxford

Edgar IT (1970) *Shakespeare, Medicine and Psychiatry: An Historical Study in Criticism and Interpretation*. Philosphical Library, New York

Flood C, Bowers L, Parkin D (2008) Estimating the costs of conflict and containment on adult inpatient psychiatric wards. *Nursing Economics* 26(5): 325–30

Ford K, Byrt R, Dooher J (2010) *Preventing and Reducing Aggression and Violence in Health and Social Care. A Holistic Approach*. M&K Publishing, Keswick.

Gudjonsson GH, Rabe-Hesketh S, Smukler G (2004) Management of in-patient violence: Patient ethnicity and use of medication, restraint and seclusion. *British Journal of Psychiatry* **184**(93): 258–62

Healthcare Commission (2009) National Survey of NHS Staff 2008. Available from: www.cqc.org.uk/

HM Government (1998) *Human Rights Act 1998*. The Stationery Office, London

House of Lords (2005) Judgments – *Regina v Ashworth Hospital Authority (now Mersey Care National Health Service Trust) (Appellant) ex parte Munjaz (FC) (Respondent)* Available from: www.publications.parliament.uk/pa/d200506/djudgment/jd.051013/ash-1.htm [Last accessed 16 June, 2010]

Howard R, Hegarty JR (2003) Violent incidents and staff stress. *British Journal of Developmental Disabilities* 49(1): 3–21

Hughes R (2009) Putting restraint in context. In: Hughes R (ed) *Reducing Restraints in Health and Social Care. Practice and Policy Perspectives*. Quay Books MA Healthcare Ltd., London

Illich I (1996) *Limits to Medicine: Medical Nemesis: The Expropriation of Health*. Martin Boyars, London

Joint Commission on Human Rights (2004) *Third Report*. Available from: www.publications.parliament.uk/pa/jt200405/jtselect/jtrights/15/1502.htm [Last accessed 16 June, 2010]

Kant I (1969) *The Moral Law: Kant's Groundwork of the Metaphysics of Morals*. Hutchinson London (Translated by Paton HJ; First published 1785.) Cited in: Thompson IE, Melia KM, Boyd KM, Horsburgh D (eds) (2006) *Nursing Ethics*. (5th edn) Churchill Livingstone/Elsevier, Edinburgh

Kettles AM, Byrt R, Woods P (2007) Introduction. In: National Forensic Nurses' Research and Development Group: Kettles AM, Woods P, Byrt R., Addo M A, Coffey M and Doyle M (eds) *Aspects of Forensic Mental Health Nursing in Acute Mental Health Settings*. Quay Books MA Healthcare, London

Knutzen M, Sandvik L, Hauff E, Opjordsmoen S, Friis S (2007) Association between patients' gender, age and immigrant background and use of restraint – a two year retrospective study at a department of emergency psychiatry. *Nordic Journal of Psychiatry* **16**(3): 201–6

Leadbetter D, Paterson B (2009) Towards restraint – Free Care. In: Hughes R (ed) *Reducing Restraints in Health and Social Care. Practice and Policy Perspectives*. Quay Books MA Healthcare Ltd., London

Maden T (2007) *Treating Violence: A Guide to Risk Management in Mental Health*. Oxford University Press, Oxford

Maeve MK, Vaughn MS (2001) Nursing with prisoners: The practice of caring: forensic nursing or penal harm nursing? *Advances in Nursing Science* 24(2): 47–64

Mason T (1996) Scatolia: Psychosis to protest. *Journal of Psychiatric and Mental Health Nursing* 3(5): 303–11

Mason T (1997) An ethnomethodological analysis of the use of seclusion. *Journal of Advanced Nursing* 26: 780–9

Mason T, Chandley M (1999) *Managing Violence and Aggression. A Manual for Nurses and Health Care Workers*. Churchill Livingstone, Edinburgh

Meehan T, McIntosh W, Bergen H (2006) Aggressive behaviour in high-secure settings: The perceptions of patients. *Journal of Psychiatric and Mental Health Nursing* **11**: 172–8

Mental Health Act Commission (2008) *Risk Rights Recovery. The Mental Health Act Commission's 12th Biennial Report*. The Stationery Office, London

Moran A, Cocoman A, Scott PA, Matthews A, Staniuliene V, Valimaki M (2009) Restraint and seclusion: A distressing treatment option? *Journal of Psychiatric and Mental Health Nursing* 16(7): 599–605. Unnumbered version downloaded from Cumulative Index for Nursing and Allied Health Professionals (CINAHL) [Last accessed 15 June 2010]

Morrison P, Lehane M (1995) *Staffing Levels and Seclusion Use*. Journal of Advanced Nursing 22: 1193–202

Morse JM (2001) Negotiating commitment and involvement in the nurse–patient relationship. *Journal of Advanced Nursing* 16: 455–68. Cited in: Moran A, Cocoman A, Scott PA, Matthews A, Staniuliene V, Valimaki M (2009) Restraint and seclusion: a distressing treatment option? *Journal of Psychiatric and Mental Health Nursing* 16(7): 599–605

Muir-Cochrane E (2009) The person who appears aggressive or violent. In: Barker P (ed) *Psychiatric and Mental Health Nursing: The Craft of Caring*. (2nd edn) Arnold, London

National Institute for Health and Clinical Excellence (NICE) (2005) *Violence Guideline*. NICE, London. Available from: www.nice.org.uk

NHS Business Services Authority Security Management Service. (2007) *Violence Against NHS Survey: 2006 Report*. London. Business Services Authority/NHS Security Management Service

Needham I (2006) Psychological responses following exposure to violence. In: Richter D, Whittington R (eds) *Violence in Mental Health Settings. Causes Consequences Management*. Springer, New York

Nursing and Midwifery Council (2008) *The Code: Standards of Conduct Performance and Ethics for Nurses and Midwives*. Nursing and Midwifery Council, London

Office of Public Sector Information (2010) *The UK Statute Law Database*. Available from: www.statutelaw.gov.uk/ [Last accessed 20 August 2010]

O'Hagan M (2004) Force in mental health services: International user and survivor perspectives. *Mental Health Practice* 7(5): 12–17

Paterson B, Leadbetter D (1999) De-escalation in the management of aggression and violence: Towards evidence-based Practice. In: Turnbull J and Paterson B (eds) *Aggression and Violence. Approaches to Effective Management*. Macmillan,

Basingstoke

Pollard R, Yanasak EV, Rogers SA, Tapp A (2007) Organizational and unit factors contributing to reduction in the use of seclusion and restraint procedures on an acute psychiatric inpatient unit. *Psychiatric Quarterly* 78: 73–81

Prins H, et al. (1993) *Report of the Committee of Inquiry into the Death in Broadmoor Hospital of Orville Blackwood and a Review of the Deaths of Two Other Afro – Caribbean Patients: "Big Black and Dangerous?"* Department of Health, London

Richter D (2006) Nonphysical conflict management and de-escalation. In: Richter D, Whittington R (eds) *Violence in Mental Health Settings. Causes Consequences Management*. Springer, New York

Royal College of Nursing (2008) *Dignity. At the Heart of Everything We Do*. Leaflet. Royal College of Nursing, London

Secker J, Benson A, Balfe E, Lipsedge M, Robinson S, Walker J (2004) Understanding the social context of violent and aggressive incidents on an inpatient unit. *Journal of Psychiatric and Mental Health Nursing* 11(2): 172–8

Sees DL (2009) Impact of the health care financing administration regulations on restraint and seclusion usage in the acute psychiatric setting. Archives of Psychiatric Nursing 23(4): 277–82

Sewell H (2009) *Working with Ethnicity Race and Culture in Mental Health. A Handbook for Practitioners*. Jessica Kingsley, London

Smith GM, Davis RH, Bixler EO (2005) Pennsylvania State Hospital system's seclusion and restraint reduction program. *Psychiatric Services* **56**(99): 1115–22

Sookoo S (2009) Therapeutic management of aggression and violence. In: Norman I, Ryrie I (eds) *The Art and Science of Mental Health Nursing*. (2nd edn). McGraw Hill Open University Press, Maidenhead

Sullivan A, Bezmen J, Barron CT, Rivera J, Curley-Casey L, Marino D (2005) Reducing restraints: Alternatives to restraints on an inpatient service – utilising safe and effective methods to evaluate and treat the violent patient. *Psychiatric Quarterly* 76(1): 51–65

Tardiff K, Lion JR (2008) Seclusion and restraint. In: Simon RI, Tardiff K (eds) *Violence Assessment and Management*. American Psychiatric Publishing, Inc, Washington DC

Timko C, Moos RH (2004) Measuring the therapeutic environment. In: Campling P, Davies S, Farquharson G (eds) *From Toxic Institutions to Therapeutic Environments: Residential Settings in Mental Health Services*. Gaskell, London

United Nations (2008) *Convention on the Rights of People with Disability*. Available from: www.un.org/disabilities/convention/conventionfull.shtml [Last accessed 16 June, 2010]

Yorston G, Haw C (2009) Historical perspectives on restraint. In: Hughes R (ed) *Reducing Restraints in Health and Social Care*. Quay Books, MA Healthcare, London

CHAPTER 17

Patients' views of seclusion and the way forward

Richard Byrt

Given research findings that suggest that seclusion has mainly harmful effects (Abderhalden et al 2006), should it ever be used? The minimisation of harmful effects, and avoidance of the wrongful use of seclusion, are required by the Code of Practice of the Mental Health Act, 1983 (Department of Health 2008); the National Institute of Health and Clinical Excellence (NICE) (2005) *Guideline on Violence*; and indirectly, by the Human Rights Act, 1998 (HM Government 1998) and codes of professional conduct (e.g. Nursing and Midwifery Council 2008).

Finke (2001: 186) comments that "the use of seclusion is not evidence-based". In a Cochrane database review, Salias and Fenton (2006) concluded that there is no evidence that seclusion is effective, for example in reducing violent behaviours, and added: "In view of data from non-randomised studies, use should be minimised for ethical reasons". These authors commented: "In the absence of any controlled trials...no recommendations can be made about the...harmful effects of seclusion..." (Sailas and Fenton 2001). However, this conclusion can be questioned, given the large number of (mostly small-scale and often qualitative) studies in which the majority of patients report harmful effects from seclusion. In addition, there are ethical and methodological difficulties in conducting randomised controlled trials in this area; and a possible tendency of Cochrane reviews to see qualitative studies as "lower order" research, regardless of the aims of investigators (Rosen 2009). However, caution is needed in drawing conclusions about patients' experiences of seclusion because many studies involve small samples and are not intended to be generalisable to larger populations (Atkinson 2000).

Patients' report of beneficial and adverse effects

Whilst several adverse effects of seclusion have been described, some patients have reported beneficial effects (Hoekstra et al 2004, Stolker et al 2006, Stowers et al 2002). In Meehan et al's (2004) study 96% of patients reported mainly negative consequences from seclusion, but some identified "potentially positive gains" (Whittington et al 2006: 159, citing Meehan et al 2004). In Kennedy et al's (1994) research 52% of patients said seclusion was "helpful". Veltkamp et al (2008: 209) found that about half the patients in their study preferred seclusion to "forced medication", although it might be argued that neither is an attractive alternative for patients. Two out of 12 patients in Meehan et al's (2000) study viewed seclusion as a "safe environment, in which they could gain control over their actions".

> *I'm glad they put me in seclusion away from everybody else...it made me settle down...there's nothing really good about it, it's just sort of to protect yourself and protect other people in the ward.*
>
> (Meehan et al 2000: 372)

However, overall, in surveys of their views, patients appear to report harmful effects far more frequently than benefits (Abderhalden et al 2006). Adverse effects include the following:

- Fear and anxiety (Hammill et al 1989, Norris and Kennedy 1992, Martinez et al 1999, Meehan et al 2000, Hoekstra et al 2004).
- Isolation (Meehan et al 2000, Holmes et al 2004).
- "Depression" (Hammill et al 1989, Meehan et al 2000).
- Boredom (Meehan et al 2000, Hoekstra et al 2004).
- Humiliation and/or feeling disrespected (Hoekstra et al 2004).
- Loneliness (Hoekstra et al 2004).
- "Lack of privacy" in using toilet and related facilities (Abderhalden et al 2006).
- "Loss of dignity" (Huckshorn 2006: 482).

Anxiety, depression and loneliness

A number of writers of fiction have described the negative effects of seclusion (Ainsworth 2010, Bronte 1962, Graham 1994). In Charlotte Bronte's *Jane Eyre*, first published in 1847, not only is Mrs Rochester, who is said to have a mental illness, incarcerated in an attic, but the 10-year-old Jane is locked in the red room by her wicked Aunt Reed:

> *My courage sank. My...humiliation, self-doubt, forlorn depression, fell damp on the embers of my decaying ire...I was oppressed, suffocated, endurance broke down; I rushed to the door and shook the lock in desperate effort...frantic anguish and wild sobs...my heart again sank; inexpressible sadness weighed it down.*
>
> (Bronte 1962 [Accessed via: www.bibliomania.com])

Anxiety and depression have been described by many patients as consequences of their seclusion (Hammill et al 1989, Norris and Kennedy 1992, Martinez et al 1999, Meehan et al 2000, Hoekstra et al 2004). Holmes et al (2004: 559) refer to "intensification of already existing feelings of exclusion, rejection, abandonment". An individual in a study by Hoekstra et al (2004: 280) described his "terrible feeling of loneliness...I have never experienced such loneliness".

Patient anger

Ironically, given that a commonly stated aim of seclusion is to reduce physical violence, it has been found to increase patient anger. Seclusion may engender a sense of injustice: of being treated badly, with no possibility of doing anything about it. This may:

> *...foster in patients a desire to take revenge and fight back...[This] can engender a grim, vicious circle of coercion and patient aggression, with an increased use of coercive measures.*
>
> (Abderhalden et al 2006: 82, citing Sequeira and Halstead 2002)

This suggests the need for patients in seclusion to have ready access, within safety parameters, to independent advocates. In addition, it can be questioned whether there is a point when seclusion becomes unsafe to others, as well as to the secluded patient. Seclusion may not enable individuals to develop positive coping strategies (Fontaine 2009, Norton and Dolan 1995); and may increase the likelihood that violence continues to be perpetrated (Fontaine 2009). Regardless of nurses' intentions, seclusion may be seen as punitive (see *Chapter 25*). In Meehan et al's (2000: 372) study, "experiences [of force] gave rise to an association between seclusion and punishment". This is reminiscent of Kenneth Graham's (1992) *The Wind in the Willows*, in which Toad is secluded in a bedroom by Badger, Mole and Ratty to prevent behaviours that they infer are both "bad" and "mad". They take it in turns to sit outside his "seclusion room" "for your own good, Toad", but the latter, not surprisingly, sees them as imprisoning him in his own home. Meehan et al (2000) found that seclusion increased feelings of being punished and of powerless and helpless:

> *I couldn't have felt any lower, I thought, until they put me in seclusion, and then I realised you could go lower. But by then, there was nothing I could do about it. They even take away your option to change the circumstances to try to lift your mood.*
>
> (Meehan et al 2000: 373)

"Circumstances" here could include communication and therapeutic activities.

Some authors argue the need to work with, as opposed to against, patients (Rogers and Vidgen 2006: 377 quoted in Byrt 2008: 110; see also Breeze and Repper 1998), thus avoiding the unintended and harmful effects (Illich 1996) of seclusion.

Retraumatisation

Research findings indicate that seclusion can result in retraumatisation: for example, triggering flashbacks of childhood experiences of abuse (Sequeira and Halstead 1997, Frueh et al 2005, Huckshorn 2006, Steinert et al 2007). In addition, seclusion may, itself, result in trauma (Hoekstra et al 2004). In this study, one respondent described how, following seclusion, on his return home, he felt anxious in "enclosed spaces"; and found locking doors in his house and "the sound of keys" stressful. This individual commented of his seclusion: "I'll never forget the sound, the click of this heavy door...It sticks in your mind" (Hoekstra et al 2004: 280).

This has implications, not only for efforts to provide viable alternatives to seclusion, but also for the design of seclusion doors to eliminate unpleasant noises. HM Inspector of Prisons (2009) reports that many prisoners are adversely affected by long periods spent in prison cells, sometimes, because of staff shortages, for as much as 24 hours a day, with limited sensory stimulation or activity, despite research findings that boredom can contribute to violent behaviours (Richter and Whittington 2006, Ford et al 2010). There are mixed findings on whether or not seclusion contributes to hallucinations and sensory deprivation:

> *Kennedy et al (1994)...found no statistically significant differences in the state of hallucination of users, before or during seclusion.*
>
> (Aberderhalden et al 2006: 80)

However, Meehan et al (2000) stated:

> *Respondents recalled a heightened awareness of sounds, difficulty in judging time, dysfunctional thought patterns and fears of losing control... [Noise] seemed to overwhelm a number of participants, and acted as a cue for auditory hallucinations...*
>
> (Meehan et al 2000: 374)

Meehan et al's (2000) findings relate to research that has found that both under-stimulation and over-stimulation (sensory overload) can worsen hallucinations and other symptoms experienced by individuals with schizophrenia (Gamble and Brennan 2006). One of the participants in Meehan et al's (2000) study suggested that "they should have paintings on the walls...anything to keep your mind occupied...I was so bored" (Meehan et al 2000: 374). Seclusion or other causes of sensory deprivation may result in illusions: misinterpretations of external stimuli (Semple and Smyth 2009). For example, when the young Jane Eyre is locked in a dark room, she mistakes a lantern light for an angel:

> *A light gleamed on the wall...but...shaken as my nerves were by agitation, I thought [it] was a herald of some coming vision from another world. My heart beat thick, my head grew hot, a sound filled my ears, which I deemed the rushing of wings...I was...suffocated"*
>
> (Bronte 1962 [Accessed via www.bibliomania.com])

Communication with patients

Adverse effects of seclusion appear to be compounded by lack of staff communication. Several studies have found limited communication between nurses and patients in the following situations:

- Before seclusion needed to be used, with coercive measures as a first resort when de-escalation skills could have been effective (Secker et al 2004, Duxbury and Whittington 2005, Meehan et al 2006).
- During seclusion. "It is not necessarily seclusion per se that impacts on their negative...experience...but the lack of nurse–patient contact" (Holmes et al 2004: 560).
- Following seclusion: to give patients an opportunity to express, and resolve, painful feelings and experiences (Meehan et al 2000, Hoekstra et al 2004).

In Meehan et al's (2000) study, patients said that they needed staff to facilitate discussion and expression of their feelings and experiences after the termination of seclusion. One individual commented:

> *They don't understand the pain I went through in that 12 hours [in seclusion], they've got no idea.*
>
> (Meehan et al 2000: 375)

Horsfall and Cleary (2003: 575) describe the development of a leaflet to explain seclusion to patients: "The provision of...written patient information about seclusion...has the potential to decrease patient anxiety and fear".

These authors argue that giving this information may reduce patients' apprehension.

Alternatives to seclusion: Recommendations

Although Salias and Fenton's (2006) observation on the limitations of research needs to be borne in mind, several studies suggest that seclusion has mainly adverse effects on patients. For this reason, it can be argued that it is essential practice to implement other measures to prevent and reduce physical violence (Ford et al 2010). The following alternatives to seclusion are mentioned in the literature (Donat 2005, Richter and Whittington 2006, Larue et al 2009, Olver et al 2009, Woods and Kettles 2009, Ford et al 2010):

- *Risk assessment* to assess the nature, frequency and consequences of violent and aggressive behaviours; and causative and contributory factors and triggers; and as a basis for ensuring safety, developing preventative measures, and alleviating the individual's distress.
- *Holistic assessment* of the individual's psychological, physical, cultural, spiritual, diversity, psychosexual, social, recreational, legal, advocacy, economic and other needs; as well as her/his strengths and positive attributes and specific problems, all of which may be relevant to interventions that are alternatives to seclusion.
- *Basing nursing and other interventions on risk and other assessments.* Care planning these interventions, with the participation of the patient whenever possible.
- *Establishing, from admission, therapeutic professional–patient relationships* characterised by respect for the individual and her/his unique strengths and needs.
- *Non-verbal and verbal communication skills*, including active listening and attempts to empathise with the client and her/his perspectives.
- *Taking the individual and her/his concerns and complaints seriously*, and responding to them.
- *Preparedness, where possible, to negotiate* and ensure that the individual does not "lose face" (see *Chapter 2*).
- *Providing culturally sensitive and culturally competent care* related to the individual's culture, ethnic group, spirituality, age, gender, (dis) abilities, sexual orientation and gender identity.
- *Valuing patients' perspectives* and enabling their participation and expression of views.
- *Changes in organisational culture/attitudes*: e.g. avoidance of authoritarianism.

- *Providing a safe, therapeutic physical and social environment*, including activities that are meaningful to the client and the reduction of boredom; and space for quiet and exercise.
- *Application of a therapeutic framework* to inform interventions: e.g. cognitive behavioural therapy, therapeutic community principles.
- *Skilful use (or non-use) of antipsychotic and other medication.*

Documentation

In order to ensure that secluded patients' needs are met, it is essential that there is clear recording orally, and in writing, of any physical, psychological, spiritual and other adverse effects experienced by the individual during and after seclusion and/or restraint; and of interventions to alleviate these adverse effects and the outcome (Richter and Whittington 2006). Clear communication helps to ensure that all staff involved in an individual's care are aware of the adverse effects of seclusion and related nursing and multidisciplinary care.

Care plan goals to attempt to reduce the adverse effects of seclusion

The author suggests that the following goals should be included in the care plans of secluded patients, in order to reduce adverse psychological and spiritual effects of seclusion. Aspects of the individual's physical health needs were considered in *Chapter 16*.

- Convey, through non-verbal and verbal communication, concern for, and interest in, patients and their feelings and experiences.
- Give individuals opportunities to safely express their concerns, feelings and experiences, including any adverse effects of the seclusion.
- Convey to patients that their concerns and experiences are taken seriously, with (where possible) appropriate action or an explanation if action cannot be taken (e.g. for safety reasons).
- Explain to them that seclusion is continued only to prevent harm to others; that it will be discontinued when this risk is reduced; and will be regularly reviewed (Department of Health 2008).
- Enable as much choice as is compatible with safety (e.g. food and drink, time for quiet or reflection, under observation).
- Enable patients to have access to activities (such as reading) within safety parameters, and if desired.
- Enable them to receive food and drink, in safe containers, according to their choice and cultural, religious and other dietary requirements.

- Enable patients to have visits or communications from approved visitors, as soon as this is safe.
- Enable them to see, or communicate with, a leader or member of their religion or other important belief system, if they wish this, and as soon as this is assessed to be safe.
- Within safety parameters, enable them to see, or communicate with, a solicitor and/or independent advocate.
- Ensure that care in seclusion protects the patient's dignity as much as possible.

Longer-term interventions after seclusion

- Enable patients to talk further, and express their concerns, feelings and experiences related to seclusion.
- If needed, provide specific interventions to reduce any adverse effects of seclusion.
- Continue to convey to patients that their concerns and experiences are taken seriously, with (where possible) appropriate action or an explanation to the patient if action cannot be taken (e.g. for safety reasons).
- With the patient, plan care interventions to prevent and reduce violence and as alternatives to seclusion.

(Linsley 2006, Richter and Whittington, 2006, Ford et al 2010)

Staff support and reviews of seclusion

Besides reviews with patients, there is a need for staff support after all episodes of violence and aggression (Linsley 2006), especially in view of research findings on the moral dilemmas, and consequent distress encountered by many nurses who use seclusion or other interventions (Marangos-Frost and Wells 2000, Moran et al 2009); and the "hardening" of attitudes that some nurses may develop in order to help them cope with patients who are violent (Moran et al 2009). A distinction needs to be made between staff support and staff reviews concerning whether seclusion could have been avoided, and if so, what alternatives could have been used. Other important areas for review are the length of time an individual has spent in seclusion; and of procedures and policies on this intervention and prevention and reduction of violence and aggression (Larue et al 2009). Clinical audit and research can provide important information on the frequency and length of seclusion episodes, the reasons for its use, and related safety issues. Factors influencing the use of seclusion and its alternatives can be identified, including the number and expertise of staff members and their skill mix; other resources; and relevant cultural and organisational factors (Dale et al 1995, Richter and Whittington 2006). Of crucial importance is the monitoring of the ethnic origin of patients who are secluded, in view of research findings that people who are Black or from minority ethnic groups are more likely to be secluded (Knutzen et al 2007, Sewell 2009, Smith et al 2005). In the author's view, national and international databases and other means are needed to share information on seclusion and its alternatives, including examples of good practice. The latter can be facilitated through consultation with external professionals and organisations for ideas on alternatives/specialist services to replace seclusion and to reduce its adverse effects (Larue et al 2009, Richter and Whittington 2006). Rates of seclusion have sometimes dropped in response to various bodies' mandatory requirements for its reduction (Larue et al 2009, Pollard et al 2007, National Coordinating Center to Reduce and Eliminate the Use of Seclusion and Restraint 2010, Sees 2009).

Other relevant factors in reducing seclusion include clear leadership and commitment (Pollard et al 2007), and ownership of practice development initiatives by all managers, staff, and, where possible, patients, within an organisation, to reduce seclusion (Martin 2009). Enabling opportunities for patients and grassroots staff to share ideas and alternatives to prevent and reduce violence and aggression is important (Bowness et al 2008, Chandler-Oats and Nelstrop 2008). Staff support, clinical supervision, education and training (Kontio et al 2009), and "independent patient advocates" (Kallert 2008) are also said to be crucial.

The extent that seclusion is used may also be related to the availability of a range of services that effectively meet individuals' specific needs and problems (Lester and Glasby 2006). This has implications for the commissioning and funding of appropriate services during a period of economic constraint, such is in existence at the time of writing. It is suggested that, despite the latter, in view of research findings on the serious effects of seclusion (Abderhalden et al 2006), service managers have a duty of care to inform service commissioners, Government departments, inspectorates, advocacy services and other relevant bodies of lengthy episodes of seclusion and any urgent need for alternative services.

However, further research is needed on the most effective interventions and services to replace seclusion and reduce its use. In addition, studies are needed on the extent that patients perceive seclusion as more or less coercive than other interventions such as rapid tranquillisation, control and restraint or intensive nursing care by two or more nurses (Abderhalden et al 2006, DiLustro 2008, Geelan 2008, Whittington et al 2009). Also, is seclusion more or less "effective" than other interventions in preventing and reducing violence and aggression in the short and the long-term (Finke 2001)?

Services that may reduce seclusion include the provision of intensive care areas within secure and other hospitals and in prison healthcare services. Such units would need to be well-staffed, and have sufficient space, including access to a safe garden for fresh air and exercise (Dix and Page 2008). The author suggests that there needs to be a review of the speed with which patients can be transferred, perhaps as "emergencies", between prisons and secure hospitals (see *Chapter 12*); and between hospitals with varying levels of security (Collins and Davies 2005). However, it is not clear that this would necessarily reduce the need for seclusion, at least in the short-term.

In conclusion, the author suggests that if individuals are secluded for lengthy periods during the first few months after admission, this probably indicates that the service cannot safely meet their needs. In view of relevant research findings, reviewed earlier in this chapter, the likely harm to such people should always be considered as a matter of urgency. Non-maleficence is an important ethical principle (Beauchamp and Childress 2009) to guide the work of forensic and prison nurses and their colleagues in other disciplines. To repeat Florence Nightingale's dictum considered in *Chapter 2*:

> *It may seem a strange principle to enunciate as the very first requirement in a hospital that it should do the sick no harm.*
>
> (Nightingale 1992: first published 1859)

Acknowledgement

Thank you to colleagues at Arnold Lodge medium secure unit, Leicester for their many ideas on this topic, to Dr Steve Geelan and Dr Mary DiLustro for thought-provoking examples of patients' experiences of alternatives to seclusion; and to the Abstract Committee for the Custody and Caring Conference, Saskatoon, 2009, for the opportunity to present many of the ideas in *Chapters 16 and 17*. This Conference was hosted by the College of Nursing, University of Saskatchewan and the Regional Psychiatric Centre, Saskatoon.

References

Abderhalden C, Hahn S, Bonner DB, Galeazzi GM (2006) Users' perceptions and views on violence and coercion in mental health. In Richter D, Whittington R (eds) *Violence in Mental Health Settings. Causes Consequences and Management*. Springer, New York

Ainsworth HW (2010) *Jack Sheppard*. Penguin Books Harmondsworth (First published 1839)

Atkinson FI (2000) Survey design and sampling. In Cormack D (ed) *The Research Process in Nursing*. (4th edn) Blackwell Science, Oxford

Beauchamp T, Childress JF (2009) *Principles of Biomedical Ethics* (6th edn) Oxford University Press, New York

Bowness S, "Algy", Byrt R, Ngeh R, Mason L, Wray C (2008) Managing angry creatively:

An overview. In National Forensic Nurses' Research and Development Group: Kettles AM, Woods P, Byrt R (eds) *Forensic Mental Health Nursing: Capabilities Roles Responsibilities*. Quay Books, MA Healthcare Ltd, London

Breeze J, Repper J (1998) Struggling for control: The care experiences of "difficult" patients in mental health services. *Journal of Advanced Nursing* **28**(6): 1301–11

Bronte J (1962) *Jane Eyre*. Collins London. First published in 1847 by Smith and Elder London

Byrt R (2008) Negative control or life saving? Perspectives on power. In National Forensic Nurses' Research and Development Group: Kettles AM, Woods P, Byrt R (eds) *Forensic Mental Health Nursing: Capabilities Roles Responsibilities*. Quay Books, MA Healthcare Ltd., London

Chandler-Oatts J, Nelstrop L (2008) Listening to the voices of African-Caribbean mental health service users to develop guideline recommendations on managing violent behaviour. *Diversity in Health and Social Care* **5**: 31–41

Collins M, Davies S (2005) The secure needs assessment profile: A multidimensional approach to measuring security needs. *International Journal of Forensic Mental Health* **4**(1): 39–52

Dale C, Rae M, Tarbuck P (1995) Changing the nursing culture in a special hospital. *Nursing Times* **91**(30): 33–5

Department of Health. (2008) *Code of Practice Mental Health Act 1983*. The Stationery Office, London

DiLustro M (2007) Personal communication

Dix R, Page MJ (2008) Physical environment. In: Beer MD, Pereira S, Paton C (eds) *Psychiatric Intensive Care* (2nd edn) Cambridge University Press, Cambridge

Donat DC (2005) Encouraging alternatives to seclusion, restraint and reliance on PRN drugs in a public psychiatric hospital. *Psychiatric Services* **56**(99): 1105–8

Duxbury J, Whittington R (2005) Causes and management of patient aggression and violence: Staff and patient perspectives. *Journal of Psychiatric and Mental Health Nursing* **50**(5): 469–78

Finke L (2001) The use of seclusion is not evidence-based practice. *Journal of Child and Adolescent Psychiatric Nursing* **14**(4): 186–90

Fontaine KL (2009) *Mental Health Nursing* (6th edn) Pearson Prentice Hall, Upper Saddle River NJ

Ford K, Byrt R, Dooher J (2010) *Preventing and Reducing Aggression and Violence in Health and Social Care. A Holistic Approach*. M&K Publishing, Keswick

Frueh BC, Knapp RC, Cusack KJ, Grubaugh AL, Sauvageot JA, Cousins VC, Yim E, Robins CS, Mosier J, Hiers TG (2005) Patients' reports of traumatic or harmful experiences within the psychiatric setting. *Psychiatric Services* **56**(9): 1123–33

Gamble C, Brennan G (Eds) (2006) *Working with Serious Mental Illness. A Manual for Clinical Practice*. Elsevier, Edinburgh

Geelan S (2008) Personal communication

Graham K (1994) *The Wind in the Willows*. Penguin Books London (First published 1908)

Hammill K, McEvoy JP, Koval H, Schneider N (1989) Hospitalized schizophrenic patient views about seclusion. *Journal of Clinical Psychiatry* **50**(5): 174–7

HM Government. (1998) Human Rights Act 2008. The Stationery Office, London

HM Inspector of Prisons (2009) *HM Inspector of Prisons for England and Wales Annual Report*. The Stationery Office, London

Hoekstra T, Lendemeijer HHG, Jansen MGM (2004) Seclusion: The inside story. *Journal of Psychiatric and Mental Health Nursing* **11**(3): 276–83

Holmes D, Kennedy SL, Perron A (2004) The mentally ill and social exclusion: A critical examination of seclusion from the patient's perspective. *Issues in Mental Health Nursing* **25**(6): 559–78

Horsfall J, Cleary M (2003) Patients' concerns about seclusion: Developing a leaflet. *Issues in Mental Health Nursing* **24**(5): 575–85

Huckshorn KA (2006) Re-designing state mental health policy to prevent the use of seclusion and restraint. *Administration and Policy in Mental Health and Mental Health Services Research* **33**(4): 482–91

Illich I (1996) *Limits to Medicine: Medical Nemesis: The Expropriation of Health*. Martin Boyars, London

Kallert TW (2008) *Coercion in Mental Health Services*. Conference presentation Royal College of Psychiatrists Faculty of Rehabilitation and Social Psychiatry Annual Residential Conference Prague 13 November 2008. Available from:www.rcpsych.ac.uk/docs/Rehab%20Prague%20coercion%20Kallert.ppt [Last accessed 16 June, 2010]

Kennedy BR, Williams CA, Pesut DJ (1994) Hallucinatory experiences of psychiatric patients in seclusion. *Archives of Psychiatric Nursing* **8**(3): 169–76

Kontio R, Valimaki M, Putkonen H, Cocoman A, Turpeinen S, Kuosmanen L, Joffe G (2009) Nurses' and physicians' educational needs in seclusion and restraint practices. *Perspectives in Psychiatric Care* **45**(3): 198–207

Knutzen M, Sandvik L, Hauff E, Opjordsmoen S, Friis S (2007) Association between patients' gender, age and immigrant background and use of restraint – a two year retrospective study at a department of emergency psychiatry. *Nordic Journal of Psychiatry* **16**(3): 201–6

Larue C, Dumais A, Ahern E, Bernheim E, Mailhot M-P. (2009) Factors influencing decisions on seclusion and restraint. *Journal of Psychiatric and Mental Health Nursing*. **16**: 440–6

Lester H, Glasby J (2006) *Mental Health Policy and Practice*. Palgrave Macmillan, Basingstoke

Linsley P (2006) *Violence and Aggression in the Workplace: A Practical Guide to Risk Management in Mental Health*. Radcliffe, Abingdon.

Marangos-Frost S, Wells D (2000) Psychiatric nurses' thoughts and feelings about restraint use: A decision dilemma. *Journal of Advanced Nursing* **31**(92): 362–9

Martin M-L, Szypula F (2009) *Discovery of a Culture to Support Restraint Reduction*. Presentation Custody and Caring Conference Saskatoon Canada

Martinez RJ, Grimm M, Adamson M (1999) From the other side of the door: Patient views of seclusion. *Journal of Psychosocial Nursing and Mental Health Services* **37**(3): 13–22. Cited in Abderhalden C, Hahn S, Bonner DB, Galeazzi GM (2006)

Meehan T, Bergen H, Fjeldsoe K (2004) Staff and patient perspectives of seclusion: Has anything changed? *Journal of Advanced Nursing* **47**(1): 33–8

Meehan T, McIntosh W, Bergen H (2006) Aggressive behaviour in high-secure settings: The perceptions of patients. *Journal of Psychiatric and Mental Health Nursing* **11**: 172–8

Meehan T, Vermeer C, Windsor C (2000) Patients' perceptions of seclusion: A qualitative investigation. *Journal of Advanced Nursing* **31**(2): 370–7

Moran A, Cocoman A, Scott PA, Matthews A, Staniuliene V, Valimaki M (2009) Restraint and seclusion: A distressing treatment option? *Journal of Psychiatric and Mental Health Nursing* 16(7): 599–605. Unnumbered version downloaded from Cumulative Index for Nursing and Allied Health Professionals (CINAHL) [Last accessed 15 June 2010]

National Coordinating Center to Reduce and Eliminate the Use of Seclusion and Restraint. (2010) In: National Association of State Mental Health Program Directors (NASMHPD) website. Available from: www.nasmhpd.org/NTAC-SRcoord.cfm [Last accessed 16 June, 2010]

National Institute for Health and Clinical Excellence (NICE) (2005) *Violence Guideline*. NICE, London. Available from:www.nice.org.uk

Nightingale F (1992) *Notes on Nursing: What It Is and What It Is Not*. V. Skretkowicz (ed) Scutari Press, London (First published 1859)

Norris MK, Kennedy CW (1992) The view from within: How patients perceive the seclusion process. *Journal of Psychosocial Nursing and Mental Health Services*. Cited in Abderhalden C, Hahn S, Bonner DB, Galeazzi GM (2006) Users' perceptions and views on violence and coercion in mental health. In: Richter D and Whittington R (eds) *Violence in Mental Health Settings. Causes Consequences and Management*. Springer, New York

Norton K, Dolan B (1995) Acting out and the institutional response. *Journal of Forensic Psychiatry* **6**: 317–32

Nursing and Midwifery Council (2008) *The Code: Standards of Conduct, Performance and Ethics for Nurses and Midwives*. Nursing and Midwifery Council ,London

Olver J, Love M, Daniel J, Norman T, Nicholls D (2009) The impact on a changed environment on arousal levels of patients in a secure extended rehabilitation facility. *Australasian Psychiatry: Bulletin of Royal Australian and New Zealand College of Psychiatrists* **17**(3): 207–11

Pollard R, Yanasak EV, Rogers SA, Tapp A (2007) Organizational and unit factors contributing to reduction in the use of seclusion and restraint procedures on an acute psychiatric inpatient unit. *Psychiatric Quarterly* **78**: 73–81

Richter D, Whittington R (eds) (2006) *Violence in Mental Health Settings. Causes, Consequences Management*. Springer, New York

Rogers P, Vidgen A (2006) Working with people with serious mental illness who are angry. In: Gamble C, Brennan G (eds) *Working with Serious Mental Illness, A Manual for Clinical Practice* (2nd edn). Elsevier, Edinburgh

Rosen M (2009) The Aprotinin saga and the risks of conducting meta-analyses on small randomised controlled trials – a critique of a Cochrane Review. *BMC Health Service Research* **9**(34)

Sailas E, Fenton M (2006) *Seclusion and Restraint for People with Serious Mental Illness*. Cochrane Library **1** (CD001163)

Sees DL (2009) Impact of the health care financing administration regulations on restraint and seclusion usage in the acute psychiatric setting. *Archives of Psychiatric Nursing* **23**(4): 277–82

Semple D, Smyth R (2009) *Oxford Handbook of Psychiatry* (2nd edn) Oxford University

Press, Oxford

Sequeira H, Halstead S (1997) Control and restraint in the UK: Service users' perspectives. Cited in Abderhalden Hahn S, Bonner DB, Galeazzi GM (2006) Users' perceptions and views on violence and coercion in mental health. In: Richter D, Whittington R (eds) *Violence in Mental Health Settings. Causes, Consequences and Management.* Springer, New York

Sequeira H, Halstead S (2002) Restraint and seclusion: Service user views. *British Journal of Forensic Practice*.4(1): 9–19. Cited in Abderhalden C, Hahn S, Bonner DB, Galeazzi GM (2006) Users' perceptions and views on violence and coercion in mental health. In: Richter D, Whittington R (eds) (2006) *Violence in Mental Health Settings. Causes, Consequences and Management.* Springer, New York

Sewell H (2009) *Working with Ethnicity Race and Culture in Mental Health. A Handbook for Practitioners.* Jessica Kingsley, London

Shakespeare W (2006) *As You Like It.* J. Dusinberre (ed) Arden Shakespeare Thomson Learning London (First written/produced circa 1600)

Smith GM, Davis RH, Bixler EO (2005) Pennsylvania State Hospital system's seclusion and restraint reduction program. *Psychiatric Services* **56**(99): 1115–22

Steinert T, Bergbauer G, Schmid P, Gebhardt RP, Veltkamp E, Nijman H, Stolker JJ, Frigge K, Dries P, Bowers L (2007) Seclusion and restraint in patients with schizophrenia: Clinical and biographical correlates. *Journal of Nervous and Mental Disease* **195**(6): 402–96

Stolker JJ, Nijman HLI., Zwanikken P-H (2006) Are patients' views on seclusion associated with lack of privacy on the ward? *Archives of Psychiatric Nursing* **20**(6): 282–7

Stowers C et al (2002) How patients and staff view the use of seclusion. *Nursing Times* **98**(42): 38–9

Veltkamp E, Nijman H, Stolker JJ, Frigge K, Dries P, Bowers L (2008) Patients' preferences for seclusion or forced medication in acute psychiatric emergency in The Netherlands. *Psychiatric Services* **59**(2): 209–11

Whittington R, Baskind E, Paterson B (2006) Coercive measures in the management of imminent violence: Restraint, seclusion and enhanced observation. In Richter D, Whittington R (eds) *Violence in Mental Health Settings. Causes, Consequences and Management.* Springer, New York

Whittington R, Bowers L, Nolan P, Simpson A, Neil L (2009) Approval ratings of inpatient coercive interventions in a national sample of mental health service users and staff in England. *Psychiatric Services* **60**(6): 792–8

Woods P, Kettles A (eds) (2009) *Risk Assessment and Risk Management in Mental Health Nursing.* Wiley-Blackwell, Chichester

CHAPTER 18

User-led research project in a medium secure unit

Keith Halsall

User-led research: From start to finish

In 2003 I found myself working at a secure unit in the UK. I was there to pilot a questionnaire that was going to be used by the Healthcare Commission to interview forensic service users. At the same time there was a call for outline proposals from the National Programme for Research and Development in Forensic Mental Health (NPRDFMH), funded by the Department of Health, for (forensic) service users to research their concerns. Having had experience of using forensic services, of mental health journalism, of public speaking and of working with other users, and encouraged by my peers, I put together a proposal with limited help from the research and development manager at the trust.

The call for proposals followed the lead of an NHS research directive in 2000 to have user participation at all stages of research projects in the NHS. This led to my plan being well received. Having access to a secure unit without any formal research credentials, and as an ex-forensic service user, was very unusual. Indeed the fact that this research project was wholly user-led, is something which I have not seen elsewhere. Faulkner and Morris (2003), two service user academics, had written a paper for the NPRDFMH which also provided groundwork for the project.

The fact that the language in the outline research proposal was unlike customary NHS research plans led the director of the unit to state that he could not support the plan – but if it was successful – he would give us the necessary access and support.

Development of the research plan

I re-developed the outline research plan and negotiated with the user forum, the patients group for the unit. This forum is a place where patients and staff discuss policy issues and so on. We were told by a user in this forum that ".. .if there's nowt in it for us – it's not worth doing". After discussion we agreed to pay the participants £5 per unit of participation; we also agreed to pay the sum in cash at the end of each piece of work the participants helped us with. Previous researchers had left the patients waiting for weeks for their rewards, hence this agreement.

One of the stipulations of the NPRDFMH, was that we needed to have an experienced academic supervisor for the qualitative research I proposed to do. To show how inexperienced I was at this stage, I did not understand what qualitative or quantitative research was. However, I began approaching suitable people. Among others that I spoke to, Professor Dawn Freshwater of Bournemouth University inspired me with her belief that a research project needed to be a therapeutic journey for the participants; we were not there to take advantage of them.

I also realised from experiences of being interviewed by mental health professionals that users are frequently "questionnaired out" (i.e. asked to fill in many quality questionnaires) and that the research team needed to tread gently. I felt that there was a need to understand how important respect for one's peers is. This is something that I believe is often missing in mental health circles, not least forensic mental health services. I was also inspired by the Hippocratic Oath's message of "do no harm".

Ethics committee

Quentin Stimpson, a senior lecturer experienced in supervising psychotherapy students studying MAs, accompanied me when I met the ethics committee of the NHS Trust in August of 2004. Having heard horror stories of ethics committees elsewhere in the country "savaging" proposals of researchers, I was relieved to receive what I saw as a fair hearing. The discussion led to three points that needed clarification.

1. There could be no artwork by users because it could identify them. It was understood that to prevent any possible backlash to patients in the unit from staff the users needed to be anonymous. It is also sometimes necessary in forensic services to protect – where possible – newsworthy patients from press intrusion and sensationalism.
2. We needed to make clear to users that while we would interview them in confidence, if they told us they were in danger of harming themselves or others, we would be duty bound to alert the relevant liaison manager.
3. Finally we would only seek consent from the patients if they took an active part in the research, i.e. in one-to-one interviews, group sessions, or in criticism/feedback, but not simply because they were present on the wards or attending the social events we were planning to hold.

One member of the ethics panel suggested that, in paying the participants, we could be accused of "buying" the results we wanted. However, another member of the panel, who worked with service users with learning difficulties elsewhere in the trust, explained that it was customary for users in long-stay hospitals to be rewarded for their efforts. The Department of Work and Pensions also allows in-patient claimants to receive small sums of money as rewards.

It was also standard practice for the Healthcare Commission, when I worked with them, to pay service users for agreeing to be interviewed, and work by Faulkner (2004) laid down guidelines on financial rewards for service users involved in research.

The research team

For the other core service users for the project, I chose people who would enhance the project team. Tina Coldham, a skilled and experienced user worker, gave the women in the women only unit, someone who they might prefer to be interviewed by, rather than a male. Her gender would also help, I assumed, in understanding some of the lived issues that women face in hospital, although she had no experience of secondary mental health services, let alone forensic services.

The other member of the team was a male of African descent and since approximately 70% of the users in the unit were Black or Asian, he was an invaluable member of the team. I am White and both he and I shared the experience of having used forensic services in the past.

Managers protecting and serving patients

We met with managers during 2004 to discuss the project and for them to "keep an eye on us", as one of them put it. Their customary relations with users as patients in the unit meant that they had to learn, as we did, in our new roles. We agreed to begin the project with a pilot on the women's unit. The manager talked of the need to give the female users an equal crack of the whip since, in the past, the women had been left out of activities that the male users had enjoyed.

The two of us were also involved in discussions with a manager from human resources and one of the day managers, to briefly discuss our Criminal Records Bureau (CRB) disclosures. It was necessary that they "check us out" to ensure that no one was at risk. Also all of the core team needed to sign honorary contracts and be covered by the insurance liability certificate of the trust.

Reflective practice and action research

The project then began on the women's unit. This purpose-built unit opened around the year 2000 and holds a total of nine women, when full. It was very clear that we needed to be reflexive (gentle and reflective) in our approach as the women were in a vulnerable state emotionally, in terms of their mental illnesses and with regard to the shame they felt for their particular offending behaviour. My fellow male interviewer turned out to be our key worker, as his charismatic approach and nature was very much appreciated by them. Without him we may not have got the agreement of the five women who participated in the research. He was used as a mentor as well as a carer, relaying the struggles of one of the women to a manager, as was her wish.

At a conference to present case research in medium secure units one of the doctor researchers mentioned the use of charismatic women to interview male users to ensure they gained the necessary sample.

We had planned to interview the women for one hour each, but we soon began to be guided by the women themselves as to how long they felt comfortable to talk to us. One of the participants talked for an hour, another told us all they needed to, in response to our prompting, in 15 minutes. One user declined to be recorded (she was the only one out of the 15 or so male and female interviews we conducted).

The women appeared to be reticence in making themselves available for interview. They felt compelled to agree to be interviewed by mental health professionals (to be good patients) but when we met them they realised we were their peers and that we were not pressurising them.

The social events

As well as paying the participants, we also organised parties on the four clinics (wards) in order to draw clients out and encourage participation. After listening to the women we held the parties on Sundays as the users stated that there was nothing to do at the weekends

We understood the role that food plays in units such as these, providing pleasure in environments which many users experience as lacking meaningful (pleasurable) activities; as they say, the way to a man's heart is through his stomach, and I am sure this also applies to women.

The parties were also a way of celebrating the unusual nature of the project and in showing our appreciation of the users' involvement. This user-led project was, and remains, an unusual departure from the norm in forensic mental health research, and I am grateful for the foresight of the NHS managers. The voices of forensic users are seldom heard, not unlike the experience of women in the past. The freeing of women from restrictive social mores and their emancipation, has echoes of where I believe users of mental health services need to be heading.

The food we provided (by outside caterers) was ethically appropriate and very successful; users "wolfed it down". Some of the Black users had earlier told us about problems with getting the foodstuffs they wanted supplied to the unit when we interviewed them. The four clinics were self-catering.

However, while it was very helpful in getting our messages across, that we valued users' input and respected them, some of the users were, I assumed, uncomfortable to be mixing socially, and ate quickly and disappeared to their rooms. This was not unexpected; people suffering mental ill-health can isolate themselves or may just be more interested in watching the horse-racing on the television (as occurred), or indeed may not like us or trust us.

Four of the men from the three clinics where we worked helped us organise and advertise the social events and we paid them for this help. We also needed their assistance in encouraging users to fill in the questionnaire that was circulated around the male clinics.

Our agenda is your agenda

Our funders' initial calls for users to research their concerns led us to develop three project aims:

1. To research the concerns of forensic service users. This was the primary aim.
2. To research the users' research priorities (as suggested by Faulkner and Morris 2003).
3. To find out what the service users thought of this user-led project.

It was of the utmost importance to us that our agenda was led by the Healthcare Commission as our funding body. As such, at the start of the one-to-one interviews we began by asking, "What I want to know is what matters to you right now?" This meant that we were led by the participants' concerns so that we could not be accused of introducing our own agendas as service users.

Action research: Is this right?

Later, after the one-to-one interviews had been transcribed and analysed by our core team, I worked with the male and female users in several groups to seek clarification and discussion of the themes that had emerged. After this I created the first draft of the report. I then circulated this to about 30 male users, either the entire report (circa 50 pages), a two-page synopsis and/or verbally with groups of users to check we had captured their lived experience. It was unusual for the users to ask to read the full draft, indeed some users could not manage it, although one man was able to speed read the draft and obtained a good grasp of the key themes in minutes. There was approval from the men that the draft was a very accurate description of their lived experience. I gave some of the men a notebook in which they could critically review the draft and add more data, and they did this. This meant that we increased our information base and ensured that the participants did actually review the draft and not just take the money we offered. I produced a separate draft for the women, which was only reviewed by two of them (the other three lost interest). It became clear that the women's experience was different to the men's.

It was important to me to keep participants informed throughout the research process, i.e. by regularly putting up posters on the wards (every three to four months) describing the differing stages of the research. The work at the unit lasted about 18 months, 12 of these were intensive work, with the re-writing of the draft taking additional time. I did not finish the project within the time-frame I had planned, which I discovered was not unusual in research. As the supervisor of the project told me at the start, in his experience, there would be significant obstacles to completing the project.

The questionnaire

The work we had done had given us a rich body of data of what mattered to both the women and the men. It was from the men's report that we created a questionnaire based on the themes that had emerged there. We then asked male users to fill in a questionnaire as to what research they would like to see carried out in the future by other researchers.

Checking frequently (action research) with the participants that their voices were heard accurately was essential. Having only two women at this stage was not a big enough sample to create a questionnaire to ascertain their research priorities.

Project workers' vulnerabilities

As well as treating the participants as gently as I could, I also discovered that I needed to be gentle with myself and the three other team members. It soon became evident that we all had challenging life journeys that I needed to respect and be patient with. My African male co-worker left the project early on and the research supervisor was battling with a large workload, which meant that he was mainly unavailable, which was difficult. However he supplied enough direction initially to keep the project on track, did the necessary analysis of the data and occasionally supervised me carrying out interviews in the unit. Fortunately a friend with academic experience provided the necessary academic support and expertise to help me write the report professionally.

If work is going to continue to develop user-led research I believe it is important that the inherent weaknesses we have are respected and that we receive support both in terms of money and help to enable us to be successful.

Peer-reviewed report

The report was then reviewed by three academics. One thought the report needed to be completely re-written. Another described it as of a very high quality, and the other as of average quality.

More value for money, more voices heard: Thank you NHS

As the project reached the end of its time at the unit, I began to do what I felt was necessary to continue to give value for money for the funding body and the unit and to ensure that the users' voices were heard. I presented the work to the clinic staff, at two of the trust's research and development conferences, and at a trust management meeting. Later I spoke at three other secure units, at the annual research in medium secure settings conference at the Royal College of Psychiatry, at a conference to present the work funded by the NPFRDMH, and at a users' research conference in London.

Without rewarding users for their involvement in the research one user said we would not have had as many participants as we did, while others also thanked us for paying them. We worked with approximately 50 men and women out of the 90 patients (not static) who attended the unit over the year. The respect and social events were much appreciated by the users who reported very positive experiences of the research project.

I also disseminated a hard copy user-friendly synopsis of the project to secure settings nationally, to the users and staff at the clinic, as well as to the ethics committee who had cleared us.

The elephant in the room

In concluding our work, one of the academics who worked on the National Programme (NPRFMH) was perplexed that there was very little reference by us to the interviewees' past offending. We labelled this the elephant in the room. Our agenda was, like the programme, to ascertain the users' concerns. They led us where they wanted, and felt comfortable, to go. Other researchers have concentrated on users' offending behaviour, but that was not our agenda.

The full report is available from: http://www.liv.ac.uk/www/fmhweb/research.htm#cpr

References

Faulkner A (2004) *The ethics of survivor research: Guidelines for the ethical conduct of research carried out by mental health service users and survivors*. Policy Press, Bristol

Faulkner A, Morris B (2003) *User involvement in forensic mental health research and development*. NHS National Programme on Forensic Mental Health Research and Development, Liverpool

CHAPTER 19

On a scale of 1–5 how satisfied are you with the healthcare service you receive?

Paul Godin and Jacqueline Davies

The recent trend towards involving service users in research poses a number of ethical issues, particularly in the area of forensic mental healthcare. There is a propensity for traditional researchers to involve service users in a rather perfunctory, minimal and even tokenistic manner. They might consider asking service users' advice about what questions to include in a questionnaire or interview schedule and might even pay some service users to survey or interview their peers. But, if you were a forensic mental healthcare service user, how would you feel about someone, albeit a fellow service user, shoving a Likert-type scale satisfaction questionnaire through the bars of your cage? What could you convey about your experiences of forensic mental healthcare through the few boxes you ticked? How actively involved or empowered would it make you feel? We contend that such putative user involvement research is morally objectionable as it encourages service users to retain a largely passive, "done to" role. Furthermore, it stands in the way of more genuinely participatory research that can give voice to service users and enable them to bring about change for the better in themselves and the world around them.

Elsewhere, we have given a detailed account of one of the first Department of Health funded research projects to involve forensic mental health service users in the evaluation of their care (Banongo et al 2005). We have also explained how the project adhered to core principles of participatory research and went some way towards facilitating what Habermas (1984) calls "communicative action" (Godin et al 2007). In short, communicative action might be described as free open debate between people concerned to understand and change the world for the better; the basis for deliberative democracy. In this brief account of the project, we reflect on some of the ethical problems and issues that it posed for us as we facilitated it. We hope that our reflections are of use to those who share our values about involving service users in research and aim to advance participatory research in the world of forensic mental healthcare.

As forensic mental healthcare service users are often incarcerated in highly secure environments, they and the people who attempt to undertake research with them inevitably face considerable restraint on what they can do. For this reason, the research project we facilitated recruited forensic mental health service users who were at liberty to come and meet with us at City University to participate in the project.

We were determined that the service users we recruited would be maximally involved in all stages of the research project, from setting the research questions to gathering and analysing data, to disseminating their findings. There was to be no cleavage between the researchers and researched as exists in traditional studies. The service users researched themselves and each other as they gave accounts of their experiences of using forensic mental health services, which they then analysed. As we (academics and service users) talked as a group, sharing our experiences of forensic mental healthcare, we (academics, some with mental health nursing backgrounds) too became subjects within the research.

We, the academics on the project team, attempted to place our expertise at the disposal of the service user researchers to use as they wished in order to evaluate the services they had received. This ideal was never fully realised, not least because it was us who employed the service users rather than the other way around. To obtain funding and ethical approval, the project proposal had to be explained in very open-ended terms, speculating what the service user researchers might wish to do. Fortunately our funders (the National Forensic Mental Health Research and Development Programme) and the ethics committee understood our intention and approved our proposal.

When we began the project, the first task was to recruit service users to it. This posed a number of ethical questions. Were we to be so mindful of their forensic histories that we were to invite psychiatric experts to screen and select a number of "their" patients that they deemed safe and suitable for the project? We thought not and resolved to recruit the service users as other hourly paid researchers. After advertising we interviewed people who contacted us and then sought a reference from somebody that knew the candidate well, usually their key worker. How were we to pay our recruits? Were we to dole out cash to them as a reward each time they came to the group or were we to treat them as proper hourly paid employees of the university receiving a contract of employment and a pay cheque at the end of the month? We went for the second option as we believed that this afforded respect for the service users as employees engaged in a proper job.

As we have explained elsewhere (Banongo et al 2005), recruitment proved difficult as applicants were not readily forthcoming and those that there were proved to be very ambivalent about joining the project. The seven service users that eventually joined came to us largely as a result of encouragement from their key workers. Although we were of course extremely grateful for the efforts of key workers, in one case it appeared that the encouragement was too much. We had contacted, interviewed and accepted one candidate, introduced to us by his key worker. After attending the group a couple of times the service user, an intelligent and thoughtful man, stopped attending. His key worker then phoned us to find out how his client was getting on in the group. On telling the key worker of his client's non-attendance, the key worker expressed disappointment, telling us that he and the consultant psychiatrist had written in the service user's care plan that he should attend the group. We were determined that the group should not be regarded as formal therapy, far less that service users should be compelled to attend. Thus when we next met the service user we explained that although we did not want to lose him we were quite happy for him to discontinue coming to the group if he so wished.

Although we made it clear to the service users that the purpose of the group was to enable them to conduct research rather than for them to receive therapy, there were moments when the service users sought or clearly needed help from us. One of the service users often asked our advice about his health. We listened sympathetically and made suggestions as to from whom he could receive help. Although most meetings were largely convivial, service users often disagreed with each other in group discussion.

At the end of one of the group meetings a service user threatened violence towards another. Fortunately one of the academics managed to mediate between the two to defuse the situation. Just like any research managers, we had a duty of care to the researchers. Perhaps this responsibility is greater when employing people that are users of health services.

Although the project was to be led by the service users, they found it difficult to take the initiative to direct the project. In the early meetings the service users asked us: "What do you want us to do?" We shared our expertise and knowledge of research and explained that we were available to help them undertake any service evaluation research that they wished to do. They then responded by asking us: "So what do you want us to want to do?" Ironically we had to be very directive in getting them to be self-directive.

After a number of meetings the service users set their research questions. The main question they wished to ask was: "Why are services so bad?" With our expertise and knowledge of social science research, we suggested that their question was inappropriately phrased as a leading question. We advised that the normal and recommended style for questions was something more balanced. We suggested they ask what was good and not so good about services. They unanimously agreed that it was quite obvious to all users of forensic mental healthcare that the services they received were inadequate.

In their view, satisfaction questionnaires would only establish what was already known by service users.

Progressively the focus of our weekly meeting shifted from discussion about what research the service users wanted to do and how to do it, towards actually doing the research. In short, the service users converted our meetings into focus groups, which they analysed and recreated in filming. This was complemented by a number of the service users also producing written accounts of their experiences of using services. This material was put together in a glossy report with an accompanying DVD (which can be obtained free of charge on request by e-mail from p.m.godin@city.ac.uk) (Banongo et al 2005). As the service users were actively involved in the research it was only correct that they, along with the academics, claimed authorship of the report. Thus it bears the names, in alphabetical order, of all those involved in its production. The service users also played a very full and active part in disseminating the research in a number of seminar and conference presentations.

Reactions to presentations of the research and the report have particular importance in relation to the ethics of such participatory research in the area of forensic mental healthcare. In one way or another, some people criticised us for ignoring the "elephant in the room". We were told that we were blind to the fact that our service user researchers were "difficult", "manipulative" people with "challenging behaviours", which rendered their voices suspect if not untrustworthy. Furthermore, some critics questioned whether it was right to allow people who had committed serious crimes to have a voice as they had curtailed the freedom of their victims. Lastly, other critics condescendingly suggested that the service users might find the freedom and responsibility of leading the research too much to handle. In essence, all of these criticisms serve to mute or disregard the voice of forensic mental health service users and deny the possibility of open democratic debate with them. In conclusion we suggest that if we (academics and clinicians) really want to involve forensic mental health service users in research then we must be prepared to listen to their voices as they wish to express them, rather than to merely record and add up the ticks they place on satisfaction surveys.

References

Banongo E, Davies J, Godin P, Thompson JB, Lohneis C, Denys C, Floyd M, Fuller S, Heyman B, Reynolds L, Simpson A (2005) *Engaging Service Users in the Evaluation and Development of Forensic Mental Health Care Services*. City University, London

Godin P, Davies J, Heyman B, Reynolds L, Simpson A, Floyd M (2007) Opening communicative space: A Habermasian understanding of a user led participatory research project. *Forensic Psychiatry and Psychology* **18**(4) 452–69

Habermas J (1984) *The Theory of Communicative Action, Volume One: Reason and Rationalization of Society*. Heinemann, London

CHAPTER 20

Moral reasoning: A nurse-led approach in a medium secure unit

David Wilkinson and Sukhbinder Panacer with Stephen Pope, Ryan, Stuart and Pete

Introduction

When faced with moral questions or dilemmas in our daily life, we may not always be aware that the decisions we arrive at are based upon our own view of morality. Sometimes, we appear to act impulsively or even instinctively, based on the situation at hand. Sometimes we may question what we ought to do in these situations without necessarily being aware that we are making a moral judgement. In contrast, Purdy (2002) writes that moral reasoning is essentially responsibly conducted thinking, in which the "reasoner" attempts to reach a well-supported answer to a well-defined question.

In this chapter we discuss how and why two of the authors (David Wilkinson and Suky Panacer) have implemented a nurse-led moral reasoning treatment programme delivered on Cannock and Ridgeway wards, two personality disorder units in Arnold Lodge, a medium secure forensic psychiatric hospital. We also highlight the theoretical approaches that were influential in the development of this programme and discuss how it has been adapted to meet the needs of our focused client group. We also look at the delivery, time constraints and other problems we have encountered through our work and the problems faced regarding a reliable, valid tool for assessment, measurement and evaluation of outcomes.

Why moral reasoning?

Although moral development and moral education are becoming increasingly popular topics in the fields of psychology and education, in our experience they are areas that are covered to a minor extent and appear under-utilised in ward-based treatments in adult forensic psychiatric establishments.

In individuals with personality disorder, the failure to demonstrate the ability for sound moral reasoning may be expressed as rigid, dichotomous thinking (Adshead and McGauley 2010). This is often particularly evident in patients who are newly admitted to the Personality Disorder Units (Cannock and Ridgeway wards) at Arnold Lodge. We observed that this patient group often presents with a host of maladaptive coping strategies, often appearing to derive from difficulties in upbringing during childhood and a lack of social guidance, or from traumatic life experiences coupled with offending lifestyles (Odgers 2009, Adshead and McGauley 2010).

The issue of maladaptive coping strategies and poor social functioning is an area which the therapeutic programme that runs between Cannock and Ridgeway wards attempts to address at the earliest possible opportunity, in terms of introducing the individual to the concept of formalised problem-solving and "Stop and Think" principles (D'Zurilla and Nezu 2006). This exercise appears to have an initial dual function in that it attempts to enable the participant to organise chaotic thoughts, as well as demonstrate to him or her that problems do not necessarily have only one solution (Bowness et al 2008).

Two of the authors, having worked on Cannock ward for some time as staff nurse (David Wilkinson) and clinical team leader (Suky Panacer), felt that the current programme of treatment presented an opportunity for moral reasoning educative work to be conducted with this client group. We therefore began to write and develop a programme of treatment that would complement key skills taught through core programmes and principal theories in problem solving (D'Zurilla and Nezu 2006), social skills (Hargie 2010), anger management (McMurran et al 2001), substance misuse (Corbett et al 1998) and other areas. We assimilated certain core processes from these and other areas into the plan for the new moral reasoning programme; and introduced concepts such as beneficence, non-maleficence, teleology and utilitarianism. (These ethical principles were considered in *Chapter 1*.)

Having submitted the plan to the multidisciplinary team, we were granted a slot in the timetable, and a pilot programme of six two-hour sessions was delivered in the Autumn of 2005 entitled the "Discussion Group". Although the content was well received and positively evaluated by the six chosen participants, the name of the programme was changed to more accurately reflect the content; and the group programme was developed further, to allow for greater scope, into a 15-session programme. This was achieved with the continued agreement and support of the multidisciplinary team. Whilst developing this programme, we drew upon various theories regarding moral reasoning (Grassian 1992, Palmer 2003), offending behaviour (Palmer 2003, Soothill et al 2008) and personality disorder (Howard and Duggan 2010).

Jean Piaget was among the first psychologists whose work has direct relevance to contemporary theories of moral development. This work focused specifically on the moral lives of children (Piaget 1932); and although the client groups at Arnold Lodge are adult, we felt that some of the basic principles could be applied in this instance. Piaget (1932) used a four-stage model of logical reasoning which ranged from birth through to early adolescence. Stage four of this model is particularly concerned with formal operational thinking: the ability to utilise complex, abstract cognitive skills in order to solve problems. This addresses the ability to consider possibilities, rather than actualities, and allows a person to employ consequential thinking skills along with deductive reasoning and logical approaches. Although this stage is primarily linked to adolescence, Piaget noted that not all adults are able to fully utilise these skills (Piaget 1932, cited in Gross 2010). Psychology researchers have found that socialisation in childhood affects individuals' moral development (Ferguson and Cairns 2002, Fung and Smith 2010, Holton 2010: See *Box 20.1*).

Our experiences on Cannock and Ridgeway wards have demonstrated that a large proportion of people diagnosed with a personality disorder have experienced abuse in one form or another. This appears to impact on the individual in terms of developing inappropriate, maladaptive coping strategies and failure to form trusting relationships. It may also be argued that in these cases the individual's capacity to process information may also be underdeveloped to some extent (Aiyegbusi and Clarke-Moore 2009, Adshead and McGauly 2010).

Lawrence Kohlberg (1976) elaborated and expanded greatly upon Piaget's work and laid further groundwork for some of the more current debates on moral reasoning and development. During the initial development of our moral reasoning programme, we were influenced to some extent by Kohlberg's translation of the stages of moral reasoning, outlining basic principal thought processes through the stages of cognitive developmental growth. Kagan (1984: 88) wrote that "...without this fundamental capacity, which 19th Century observers called moral sense, the child could not be socialised". It can be argued that people with personality disorder may, in some instances, lack the moral development that other people begin to acquire at an early age (Adshead and McGauley 2010). For additional discussion on links to culture see *Box 20.1*.

Although during the development of the moral reasoning treatment programme we drew upon some aspects of these theories to offending in individuals with personality disorder, it is important to note that not all who engage in offending behaviour, or who are diagnosed with a personality disorder, will have poor moral reasoning skills; and that poor moral reasoning is by no means a defining factor in offending behaviour (Prins 2010). Our observation suggested that when offending behaviour and personality disorder are common factors, then poor moral reasoning becomes increasingly notable.

Box 20.1. Moral reasoning and the link with culture

Brazier (2003) reported a link between moral development and cultural climate in that moral development might be retarded if young people develop against a backdrop of political conflict. This author cites Ferguson and Cairns' (2002) study, in which samples of young people in Northern Ireland living in conditions of political violence were compared with their peers living in peaceful areas of Scotland and the Republic of Ireland. The researchers accounted for age, gender, urbanisation, education attainment, and religious identification in the Northern Ireland sample. They found that young people living in Northern Ireland in areas of particularly high political violence did show lower levels of moral maturity. They offered explanations for the results of their study by suggesting that there were people who supported the actions of the terrorists and viewed them as heroes; in contrast, other members of the community regarded their actions as unacceptable and completely unjustifiable. Inherent in these areas of high political violence, there were factors such as increased threat, segregation (racial and social), and radical politics. The researchers believed these factors to increase tribal loyalty. It was therefore surmised that young people in these areas tended to support the culture of violence and rely on lower level moral solutions to the issues they faced.

Although Ferguson and Cairns' (2002) study appears to suggest that high political violence produces lower levels of moral maturity, the researchers do not appear to account for the role of socialisation and parental influence. Socialisation, including parental influence, has been shown by numerous studies (e.g. Fung and Smith 2010, Holton 2010), to affect development in many areas of young children's lives. Political bias and racial and religious ideologies tend to be passed from parents to children. Whether this influence extends to adulthood has yet to be fully established.

A further explanation for the low levels of moral maturity found by Ferguson and Cairns is that of the values and truisms hypothesis suggested by Kelman (1974). This hypothesis suggests that values function as truisms and are extensively shared but rarely questioned. By this, the values lack reasonable argument, that is, although relevant issues are debated in a society, the values themselves are extensively shared but rarely questioned. Kelman (1974) argued that individuals adopt values as a means of complying with society's norms or as a means for identifying with important others.

Adapted from Pope (Date unknown)

What is the intent of the moral reasoning group?

The Moral Reasoning Group programme explores and addresses issues relating to a sense of right and wrong and how one arrives at an informed decision, whilst assisting the participant to understand how anger and aggression, verbal confrontation, body language and personal perception may affect situations. This is achieved through various group activities taking the form of debate sessions, discussions, the use of moral dilemma vignettes and to a minor extent, role play. These sessions are conducted within a safe, controlled environment, achieved through maintaining a closed group format and by maintaining the same facilitators throughout the duration of the programme to promote continuity of approach (Freeman et al 2003).

Some of the sessions (where appropriate) run over two consecutive weeks, although the majority of group activities run for a single two-hour session. The programme is divided into a total of 20 sessions; these are conducted in the form of a group therapy programme (one group session per week) with provision made for several extra sessions if required. Unfortunately, the length of the Moral Reasoning programme has been limited to some extent by the timetable of other programmes. Because of the current quantity of therapeutic programmes offered by the personality disorder units at Arnold Lodge, these programmes need to be rotated every few weeks in order for our patients to access the scope of treatment in their two-year stay.

These sessions begin with a collective negotiation of group rules to include maintenance of confidentiality, mutual respect, how participants will conduct themselves if experiencing stress or anger and how support will be provided, etc. This allows the participants a greater ownership and autonomy within the programme. The opening session entitled "Who am I?" is a relatively a simple "ice breaker" session aimed at providing the facilitators with an indication of participants' level of understanding, their core beliefs about themselves, their current environment and their views about their future. The sessions then increase in difficulty and complexity and include moral debate sessions, where set trigger material is provided from a host of topics, including equality, crime and punishment, mental and physical health, self-image, dealing with loss and political issues with one topic being explored each week. Moral dilemma sessions include adaptations of "The Overcrowded Lifeboat" and "A Callous Passerby" exercises (Grassian 1992). For a summary of participant perspectives of attending the group see *Box 20.2*.

Patient participation, understanding and developmental progress are evaluated throughout the course of the programme and at the end. The findings are then presented to the multidisciplinary team. Each session is also evaluated by the participating patients. These evaluations are then utilised to adapt and improve session facilitation and guide ideas for future session content.

Box 20.2. Moral reasoning: Participants' perspectives by Ryan, Stuart and Pete

The following account has been provided by three patients following participation in the Moral Reasoning Programme:

Moral reasoning is to do with thinking outside the box. Most people have what is called black and white thinking styles or another way of putting it is "rigid thinking", which basically means they can put an argument forward and only see one side of it. In this case, the individual is stubborn and their thoughts will not be swayed or turned around by anyone.

Moral reasoning in a treatment group promotes an awareness of moral and social issues by engaging in group discussions and debates. This helps you build on your lateral thinking so it's more appropriate. This helps to gain more of an understanding of what to consider when you are putting moral reasoning into practice and also highlights that there is more than one angle to a discussion; and so to use different approaches to achieve a conclusion that is supported and well defined, without offending other people.

This group helps in enabling individuals to put forward ideas and thoughts that may be controversial and contentious. The group helps to develop skills of assertiveness, as the chances of someone disagreeing with your opinion are high and the need to stay calm and explain your reasoning is crucial in being assertive. The group also challenges your belief system in asking the question, "Why do you hold that belief?" For example, if an elderly person is mugged, it is assumed to be a more heinous offence than that of a young adult male being mugged. This then questions why you hold such beliefs, and where they stem from, in a way that ordinarily you wouldn't consider.

Putting all these together, you get a wider awareness of social and moral issues, which in turn, develops a greater understanding of different beliefs and viewpoints. Moral reasoning also helps to promote confidence and self-esteem when working in group settings and to speak openly in a safe environment. The group will help to show how each member comes across in terms of the language used and the body language displayed when discussing emotional and controversial subjects.

The group is a useful tool in that it connects well with other treatment groups on the Personality Disorder Unit programme, as being able to make decisions that are fair and moral and help in supporting each other in meetings and core treatment groups. It helps to gain an understanding of why others in authority may make the decisions they make, such as to exclude someone who is continually disruptive to a group. It is therefore felt, from a group perspective, that moral reasoning is useful and constructive, encouraging skills that are vital, such as assertiveness, and being able to challenge one's own thinking styles and building skills that are transferable to other groups on the Personality Disorder Unit programme and on release into the community.

For the purpose of running this programme, the guidelines/concepts that we utilised to promote an awareness of basic core principles that govern the concept of moral reasoning, are introduced cautiously into the sessions. As the programme progresses, the participants are expected to appreciate and show a greater awareness for these concepts by demonstration, through discussion and constructive debate, thus showing an increasing capacity to move away from dichotomous thinking and apply lateral cognitive processes to reach a supported answer. The sessions are structured in such a way as to validate the core skills gained from other treatment programmes currently running on Cannock and Ridgeway wards by assimilating these processes.

The key aims of the moral reasoning group programme are to assist the participant to assimilate key skills promoted in the other core groups of the treatment programmes offered on the personality disorder units at Arnold Lodge. Throughout the programme, principles such as utilitarianism, teleology, and deontology are introduced and aspects of beneficence, non-maleficence, autonomy, fairness and honesty are explored to demonstrate how these may impact upon current and past thinking styles. Through key sessions in the moral reasoning programme, a wider awareness of moral and social issues is promoted in the participating patients, in order to facilitate a greater understanding of conflicting beliefs and views. We also encourage the participants to offer considered debate and questioning whilst facilitating a "safe" environment in which these skills may be practised and freedom of speech explored in an appropriate manner, with feedback provided as necessary. This has the added bonus of promoting confidence and self-esteem when interacting in group settings.

With the written permission of the participants, some of the sessions in the programme are video recorded. This material is played back to them in order to develop a greater understanding and awareness of body language when discussing emotional or controversial subject matter.

Among other obstacles encountered during the development and delivery of the programme, a valid, reliable measurement of outcome was found to be problematic. Whilst much of the reporting is down to objective analysis of the participants' development, understanding, and ability to apply theory to practice throughout the course of the programme, we felt the need for a more robust method of assessment, and therefore looked at a number of psychometric tools, many of which were not adaptable to our needs. During our search for a possible measurement tool we came across the Moral Judgement Test (MJT) (Lind 2002); and having contacted Professor Lind personally, we obtained permission to use the test. Results from use of this test have been disappointingly inconclusive as an indicator of change in the moral reasoning ability of our participants; and we continue to search for other alternatives at the time of writing. The use of the MJT has not been ruled out, however; and the inconclusive results to date may be attributed to many different factors. Our development and improvement of the moral reasoning programme is continuous, with later inclusion of more theoretical content to the teaching sessions in order to further validate learning. We look forward to its sustained inclusion in the programme of therapeutic treatment opportunities currently available at Arnold Lodge with a view to expanding the use of this programme throughout the hospital unit.

References

Adshead G, McGauley G (2010) Caring for individuals with personality disorder in secure settings. In Bartlett A, McGauley G (eds) *Forensic Mental Health. Concepts, Systems and Practice*. Oxford University Press, Oxford

Aiyegbusi A and Clark-Moore J (eds) (2009) Therapeutic relationships with offenders. In: *An Introduction to the Psychodynamics of Forensic Mental Health Nursing*. Jessica Kingsley, London

Bowness S, "Algy", Byrt R, Ngeh R, Mason L, Wray C (2008) Managing angry creatively: An overview. In: National Forensic Nurses' Research and Development Group: Kettles AM, Woods P, Byrt R (eds) *Forensic Mental Health Nursing: Capabilities Roles Responsibilities*. Quay Books MA Healthcare Ltd, London

Brazier L (2003) Does conflict affect moral reasoning? *The Psychologist* 16(1): 33

Corbett M, Duggan C, Larkin E (1998) Substance misuse and violence: A comparison of special hospital inpatients diagnosed with either schizophrenia or personality disorder. *Criminal Behaviour and Mental Health* 8: 311–21

D'Zurilla T, Nezu A (2006) *Problem-Solving Therapy: A Positive Approach to Clinical Intervention* (3rd edn). Springer Publishing, New York

Ferguson N, Cairns E (2002) The impact of political conflict on moral maturity: A cross-cultural perspective. *Journal of Adolescence* 25(5): 441–52. Cited in Brazier L (2003) Does conflict affect moral reasoning? *The Psychologist* 16(1): 33

Freeman G, Crawford M, Weaver T, Low J, de Jonge E (2003) *Continuity of Care for People with Severe Mental Illness. A Briefing Paper.* National Institute for Health Research Service and Delivery (NHR SDO): London. Available from: www.sdo.lshtm.ac.uk/continuityofcare.htm

Fung H, Smith B (2010) Learning morality. In: Lancy DF, Bock J, Gaskins S (eds) *The Anthropology of Learning in Childhood*. Alta Mira Press, Walnut Creek CA

Grassian V (1992) *Moral Reasoning. Ethical Theory and Some Contemporary Moral Problems* (2nd edn). Prentice Hall, New Jersey

Gross R (2010) *Psychology. The Science of Mind and Behaviour* (6th edn). Hodder Arnold Hachette UK, London.

Hargie O (2010) *Social Skills in Interpersonal Communication* (5th edn). Routledge Taylor and Francis Group, Hove

Holton RK (2010) Parental cognitive antecedents of child prosocial behaviours. *Dissertation Abstracts International. Section A: Humanities and Social Sciences* 70(7–A): 2749

Howard R, Duggan C (2010) Personality disorders. In: Towl G, Crighton DA (eds) *Forensic Psychology*. Wiley-Blackwell, Chichester

Kagan J (1984) *The Nature of The Child*. (p 88)Basic Books, New York. Available from: http://www.psy.vanderbilt.edu/courses/psy101/notes17.htm

Kelman HC (1974) Further thoughts on the process of compliance, identification, and internalisation. Cited in Maio GR (2002) Values-truth and meaning. *The Psychologist 15*(6): 296–9

Kholberg L (1976) Moral stages and moralisation: The cognitive-developmental approach. In: Lickona T (ed) *Moral Behavior Theory Research and Social Issues*. Holt Reinhart and Wilson, New York. Available from: http://students.usm.maine.edu/bmcpha61/Kholberg_stages_of_morality.htm

Lind G (2002) Moral Judgement Test (MJT) Available from: http://www.uni-konstanz.de/ag-moral/

McMurran M, Fyffe S, McCarthy L, Duggan C, Latham A (2001) Stop and Think! Social problem-solving therapy with personality disordered offenders. *Criminal Behaviour and Mental Health* 11(4): 273–85

Odgers CL (2009) The life–course persistent pathway of antisocial behaviour: Risks for violence and poor physical health. In: Hodgins S, Viding E, Plodowski A (eds) *The Neurological Basis of Violence: Science and Rehabilitation*. Oxford University Press, Oxford

Palmer E (2003) *Offending Behaviour. Moral Reasoning, Criminal Conduct and the Rehabilitation of Offenders*. Willan Publishing Uffculme, Cullompton

Piaget J (1932) *The Moral Judgment of the Child*. Routledge and Kegan Paul London. Cited in Gross R (2010) *Psychology. The Science of Mind and Behaviour* (6th edn). Hodder Arnold Hachette, UK

Pope S (Date unknown) BSc psychology dissertation. Full details unavailable at the time of going to press

Prins H (2010) *Offenders Deviants or Patients?* (4th edn) Routledge Francis and Taylor Group, London.

Purdy L (2002) Moral Reasoning in a Nutshell. Wells College, Wells. Available from: aurora.wells.edu/~lpurdy/moral.htm [Last accessed 27 May, 2010]

Soothill K, Rogers P, Dolan M (eds) (2008) *Handbook of Forensic Mental Health*. Willam Publishing, Uffculme, Collumpton

CHAPTER 21

Mind, brain and forensic psychiatry

Tim Hardie

Introduction

There is a presumption in the law, in psychiatry, and particularly in forensic psychiatry, that human beings can make "true choices", influence their behaviour by mental processes, and be held responsible for their own actions. Most offences require a guilty mind or *mens rea* which, if not proven, means the offence was not committed for the purposes of the law: but what does this actually mean? If a person commits an offence as a result of the direct influence of delusions, hallucinations or other symptoms of mental illness, the law allows that they are not guilty or have a case for saying that they were not fully responsible. Psychiatrists are often asked to "assist" the courts in deciding how much of a true choice was made by the defendant when he or she broke the law. There are other areas where this true choice problem arises for mental health professionals, and it is not uncommon for those involved to disagree, feel a sense of confusion, or resort to professional guidelines, Acts of Parliament or simply pragmatism to resolve the matter.

What, therefore, is a "true choice"? This can be defined as a choice that has been freely made, and not influenced by factors that could reduce this freedom. Influences that might reduce the true ability to make a free choice include brain problems, such as dementia or a learning disability, and major mental illness. Other influences might include the effect of childhood experiences. It is not uncommon to recognise that patients have apparently learned behaviour or attitudes from experiences in early life and to conclude that this is clouding their judgement in some way. Another important influence might be other people. For example, a vulnerable in-patient who is being bullied and gives his possessions to another, may be viewed as vulnerable and not necessarily able to make a true choice. It might also be argued that the effect of outside influences is mitigated by such things as strength of character or a religious conviction.

When thinking about choice in this way there is a sense that there is something separate from the brain that can decide what it actually wants and that certain influences can get in the way of this. However, given the many possible influences, a choice that is made completely free of outside influences must be a rare thing indeed.

The use of language plays a part in confusing things more. One meaning of the word "mind" is to describe that which is separate from the brain but which can be affected by brain abnormalities. On the other hand, legal frameworks sometimes refer only to disorders of the mind, clearly including brain disease. There are many other words that are used in this context, such as consciousness, spirit, and soul. Although they are sometimes referring to the same thing, these words also have the potential for different meanings, increasing the risk of confusion or misunderstanding when they are used. Although different words for "mind" are used below, the intention is to refer to that part of mental experience that involves self-awareness, thought and emotions.

If a patient on a ward assaults a nurse, the reaction of the victim and his or her colleagues can be complicated. In the mix of factors that will determine the reaction there will to be something about whether or not the patient was in his or her right mind. A patient who has a clearly identifiable clinical problem, that is perceived as contributing directly to the assault, will be viewed differently from one for whom this is not the case. A patient who has no history of violence, and attacks another in the context of post-ictal confusion, is likely to engender a different reaction from the patient who hits in the same way but out of racist motives. The latter is more likely to be seen as blameworthy, responsible and accountable for the behaviour. In the clinical context, there is more to this than the ascertainment of criminal behaviour. The perceived motivation will inevitably, and should, affect the response of staff. Although rarely expressed explicitly, some concepts or assumptions are being made about the ability of the person to make true choices, and it may be useful to examine some of these underlying assumptions more carefully.

It feels impossible to disentangle the clinical problems from three old philosophical questions. Firstly, whether or not mind and brain are the same thing, or two (or even more) things; secondly, whether true choice can exist versus the view that all "choices" are completely determined (i.e. made inevitable) by what has happened before; and, thirdly, how this should be related to a person's responsibility for his or her own actions. Over the last few decades the discipline of "consciousness studies" has emerged, some of which has experimental work which is relevant to this; neuroscience is increasingly showing the workings of the brain; and genetics is finding relationships between certain genes and behaviour (e.g. Mayfield et al 2008).

Despite the enormous growth of science in the area, there is still a real question as to whether or not neuroscience can ever really unpick how mind relates to brain. Revonsuo (2001) believes that this is theoretically possible but not with current techniques. He draws a distinction between "images of mind", which are produced by modern neuroimaging techniques such as positron emission tomography (PET) and functional magnetic resonance imaging (fMRI), and actually "seeing the mind". He asserts that it is possible to "see" the mind directly, but that current imaging techniques do not do this, they only reveal what he calls "neural correlates of consciousness". Barba (2001), in the same edition of the *Journal of Consciousness Studies*, argues that neuroscientific advances can only ever find something that is equivalent to an objective experience of consciousness, not the actual subjective experience of feelings and emotions. The reason for this is that "consciousness in its entirety defines itself precisely as what is not object". Science, from his perspective, can therefore only ever discover a kind of "degraded" version of true consciousness.

The philosophical and scientific work that addresses the mind–brain problem is attempting to answer these very real issues but has not resolved them. The question remains as to whether knowledge of this work can assist nurses when they are assessing their patients' ability to make a true choice. At first glance, it feels as if it should, because mental health professionals often make assessments of a patient's ability to make choices, and so it should be directly relevant. Although it needs to be recognised that these questions have yet to be resolved by philosophy or science, there are legal, professional, religious, moral and social frameworks that exist for addressing these issues. Whether or not these are explicitly recognised, they are what tend to be used in everyday situations.

Legal, medical, political and social factors in true choice

Mental capacity

Day-to-day decisions on psychiatric wards demand that nurses, and other mental health professionals, make decisions about whether or not they should act against patients' expressed wishes or without directly seeking their agreement. Frequently this is done on the basis of common sense. For example, it is not necessary to seek express consent every time medication is dispensed. Psychiatry, and particularly forensic psychiatry, comes up against this even more than general medicine because patients are often detained, and it is necessary to take more account of security or risk management. From a medical point of view, there is a consensus that people have a right to self-determination unless they are incapable of making decisions for themselves, and when patients are incapable of making decisions then it is appropriate to act in their best interests.

It is easy to assume that this means mental health professionals, who are often nursing staff, are basing their decisions on a "true" assessment of how much patients are able to think for themselves. In an ideal world, it might be said, this is exactly what should be being done, and if it is, then the issue of whether or not true choice is actually possible is of paramount importance. However, mental capacity to consent to or decline medical intervention is legally defined, and in this sense does nothing to address the ultimate issue.

When the Mental Capacity Act 2005 directly addresses the issue of true choice, it does so by reference to mind and brain, giving an impression that it is examining the ultimate issue:

> *For the purposes of this Act, a person lacks capacity in relation to a matter if at the material time he is unable to make a decision himself in relation to the matter because of an impairment of, or a disturbance in the functioning of, the mind or brain.*
>
> Mental Capacity Act 2005: s2(1)

The Mental Capacity Act was a long time in the making and was preceded by considerable common law, a number of consultation documents produced by the Law Commission, and political debate. The aims of the original consultation, leading to the Act had nothing to do with resolving the essential problem of the truth of true choice. The consultation was intended to address potential conflicts within the law as it stood at that time (Law Commission 1991: 6–8).

Nonetheless, in the first Law Commission report (1991: 103), consistent with the current medical consensus, there was a presumption that people could make choices for themselves, giving them a right to determine their own affairs if capable. It should be noted though that even this principle was not always held in such regard. Eugenics is the science of racial improvement and, following the activities of the Nazis in the Second World War, is now a virtually obsolete science. In the first decades of the 20th century, however, it was an important factor in determining public policy, even in the UK. The Mental Deficiency Act 1913 allowed for the segregation of "mental defectives" in colonies with the clear aim of preventing them from breeding and thus avoiding "national degeneration" (Fennell 1996). Following this, there was a vigorous debate (supported by some doctors) about whether these people should be legally sterilised for eugenic purposes. It is an odd paradox that Nazi atrocities, by effectively discrediting eugenics, might have given support to the principle of self-determination.

Although the self-determination is usually stated as being a "right" for those who are able to make valid choices, the principle is not as fixed as it might appear. Even now there are circumstances that mental health professionals frequently see, where the ability of people to make decisions about themselves is not what determines whether patients can be treated against their wishes. The amended Mental Health Act 1983 allows for detention and forcible treatment of people with a mental disorder, for three months, without reference to their capacity to make decisions for themselves; and after three months of detention, even if they have capacity, if it is "appropriate" to do so (Amended Mental Health Act 1983: s58(3b)).

Another example occurred in the late 1990s, when, amid increasing political concern about dangerous people with personality disorder, there was a move by the Government of the day to detain these people on the grounds of risk alone, again without reference to capacity to agree or even benefit from treatment, under mental health legislation (Department of Health and Home Office 1999). This was followed (as with the eugenics proposals described above) by vigorous debate, and although the majority of doctors were against the proposals, a significant number supported them (Haddock et al 2001). This ultimately led to the new wording of the criteria for detention in the amended Mental Health Act, removing the necessity for "treatability" for people with personality disorder, and increasing the emphasis on risk management.

Personality disorders also raise issues directly in relation to mental capacity. It can be very unclear as to whether or not personality disorder can influence capacity to make true choice, and if it can, then under what circumstances. The case of Ian Brady (Dyer 2000) at Ashworth Hospital makes it clear that the law does accept that this is potentially possible, as the law sanctioned the forcible saving of his life when he was protesting on hunger strike about his circumstances. This of course does not mean that personality disordered patients always lack legal capacity in all circumstances, and there is a legal process for clarifying the interpretation of the law in individual cases.

Mental capacity for medical treatment is therefore a legal concept, based on legal precedent and now an Act of Parliament. Further, the principles underlying this legal concept have been hugely influenced by social and political pressures.

Does this mean that nurses, when deciding whether to act against a patient's wishes, should be engaging in a purely legal exercise to ensure that they are acting within the law? This is after all what the courts will do if presented with such a problem. Naturally, mental health professionals should act within the law, but it is also necessary to act within professional codes and the constraints of personal conscience. This requires more than an interpretation of the legality of a situation, particularly if the law appears to force the individual into doing something to a patient that the individual does not believe to be right.

Criminal responsibility

It sounds straightforward to say that mental illness or brain damage can mitigate criminal responsibility. How can you be held liable if your mind or brain is not working properly? Legal insanity allows that a "defect of reason from disease of the mind" can reduce criminal liability, and murder can be reduced to manslaughter by an "abnormality of mind" under the Homicide Act 1957. This seems only fair.

Legal problems arise, though, when individual cases raise the issue of degree of abnormality and how much this affects decision making ability. New law is still being made on the question of intoxication with drugs or alcohol, which the courts seem reluctant to allow as mitigation even though most people would agree that brain function is clearly impaired by intoxication. Even more strikingly, imaging studies have allowed visualisation of how the brains of those with psychopathic disorder tend to differ from those without. In one sense this might be seen as evidence that psychopathic disorder is a true "disease", because physical "pathology" has been found. On this basis, psychopaths could be construed as being unable to help themselves, which might allow for legal mitigation. This is the basis of what has been described as "neurolaw" (Tallis 2007). The problem, then, is where this will end. It seems likely that all patterns of thinking and behaviour have biological correlates which will one day be identified by increasingly sophisticated techniques. In the case of criminal patterns of behaviour, this raises the possibility that much, if not all, of criminal behaviour will one day have identified physical correlates that might be labelled as pathological and therefore potentially mitigating.

In relation to criminal responsibility the legal system must be making a number of assumptions about the relationship of some potentially free-thinking mind and influences on this, firstly, that true free choice decisions are possible; secondly, that other factors such biology, abnormal psychology, or influences from outside the person's body can reduce this freedom; and, thirdly, that this reduction is quantifiable. Although there is no scientific evidence to support these assumptions, without them, criminal law as we know it would fail.

What is not known

It is not known if the mind and the brain are distinct from each other. In other words, it is not known if there is a mind substance of some sort that is different from the physical brain substance. Without a distinct mind substance the possibility of life after death as an individual is excluded, as is the possibility of experiences such as true spirit possession or genuine out-of-body movement. Religious belief often accepts the validity of these things and whilst there is no proof in the scientific sense, there is also no disproof. Nonetheless, from a clinical perspective, religious matters often have great significance for patients and require recognition, understanding and respect from healthcare professionals. Apart from this observation, religious approaches to the mind–brain problem are not discussed further below.

If there are two substances, it is not known how they would interact. There is a possibility that such interaction might breach the physical law of conservation of energy, and a possibility that quantum mechanics might allow this not to be so. It is also not known how, if there is only one substance, it is possible to have an experience of consciousness that feels separate or at least different from the body.

For the purposes of true choice issues, it is not known if true choice is possible at all. If there is only one substance, the physical stuff of the body, then the principles of physics, chemistry and biology may completely determine what happens. If this is the case, then all decisions, thoughts and feelings might be as inevitable as hydrogen being produced when magnesium is placed in a sulphuric acid solution, and choice is an illusion.

One substance or two?

Two substances

The idea that there are two substances is called dualism. Dualism usually implies that the mind or consciousness is comprised of something that is not the same as the physical substances that make up the body. This other substance is just as real as physical substance, but has different properties. If this is the case, then it is clear that the physical substance must relate in some way to the mind substance.

Descartes (1596–1650) is famous for believing in dualism and his ideas have been hugely influential. He started off with a principle of doubting everything: using the logic that if somehow a demon was able to mislead him about things he thought he knew, then these things must be cast in doubt (Russell 1984). It was out of this that he concluded that the only thing of which he could be certain, and of which he could not be deceived, was that he was thinking: hence, "I think, therefore I am." He therefore started from the position that there was a mind substance or soul which is easier to know than the body. He speculated that the mind substance could influence the body through interaction at the pineal gland. This kind of theory is called interactionist dualism because the mind and the body are believed to interact with one another, each being able to affect the actions of the other.

Another version of interactionist dualism comes from Eccles (1990) who believed that mind matter is comprised of mind units that he called psychons. He believed that these could interact with each other directly but were also uniquely associated with individual dendrons in the brain. Hence, there are approximately 40 million dendrons and 40 million psychons. He believed that these psychons could cause changes in the neurons that were so small that they were within the limits of quantum uncertainty. He believed this was enough to alter the likelihood of a nerve cell discharging and therefore cause physical brain events.

Another version of dualism, known as epiphenomenalism theorises that physical matter is the primary substance and that mental substance exists only as a by-product or side effect of what happens physically. According to this, mental events do not alter brain events and the impression that we have true choice, or in fact any form of mental freedom, is an illusion. Parallelism is the view that mental events and physical events run completely separately from each other and do not interact directly at all.

Problems with dualism

Eccles' theory illustrates one of the primary problems and potential solutions with interactionist dualism. The first law of thermodynamics states that energy (i.e. energy or matter) cannot be created or destroyed. Dualism proposes that there is something else other than physical matter, and, in interactionist dualism, that this other substance can make changes to physical matter. The problem is that energy is required to make something happen in the brain because it is a physical system. The energy is needed to do something chemically or physically to make nerve cells function or at least trigger a response. If mind substance is indeed different from physical substance, it cannot do this without creating energy. In other words, the first law of thermodynamics is violated. This has caused some people to argue that interactionist dualism is impossible.

Eccles' response to this comes from the finding in quantum theory that the position or momentum of the smallest particles, such as electrons, can be indicated by a probability. The argument goes that it is not necessary to use energy to change something in the physical world, only influence probability, which then might influence the position or momentum of a quantum size of particle. There is, however, some evidence against this. Wilson (1999) has calculated the energy required to make the smallest possible changes in neurons, such the opening of a sodium channel for long enough for a single atom of sodium to pass through. Sodium channels are proteins in cell membranes that mediate the passage of sodium ions across those membranes. The passage of sodium ions is necessary for many cell functions including the electrical functioning of neurons in the brain. He found that the minimum energy required to do this is many millions of times greater than could be explained by quantum variation. Another solution deriving from quantum mechanics comes from Stapp (1999), who used the notion that in quantum mechanics an observer seems to be essential to make measurements. He noted that when these measurements are made, they can only be resolved mathematically by introducing probabilities rather than absolute measurements. He draws a parallel between this and what appears to be a similar problem in looking at mind and brain at the same time, and suggests that this could be used as a means of explaining interactionism.

There are other problems with dualism. It is well known that brain damage can affect consciousness. Although this does not make dualism impossible, it does imply that the brain is required for consciousness, which is not implicit in interactionist dualism or parallelism. There is also the observation that at some point in animal evolution consciousness must have appeared. If mind substance is different from physical substance, where did it come from, when in evolution, and why? A similar argument has been put forward in relation to the development of consciousness in each developing human being, from sperm and egg to conscious being. Although raising difficult problems does not amount to disproof of dualism, it does appear to increase the likelihood that science that attempts to look at these problems will eventually find a genuine disproof.

One substance

The idea that there is only one substance is called monism, and there are number of versions of this. If the one substance is physical then the form of monism is called physicalism and if the one substance is mental then it is called idealism. If both mind and brain are constituted of the same substance it is called neutral monism.

The psychological discipline of behaviourism illustrates a physicalist approach. It is based on the belief that only behaviour, not thoughts or emotions, are relevant to the understanding of psychology. This view is now rare in British psychiatry and psychology, and it is much more common for thoughts and feelings to be part of a behavioural approach. The term "cognitive behaviour therapy" reflects this view.

Anomalous monism, an approach put forward by Donald Davidson, uses a linguistic approach to address how mental and physical events are related whilst maintaining the view that everything is physical (Yalowitz 2008). Although strict "laws" govern how physical events are related to each other, this does not apply to connections between mental and physical events. The term "supervenience" is used to describe how mental events relate to physical events by being "properties" of some sort.

Table 21.1. Use of terms in relation to free will and determinism		
	Free will	*No free will*
Determinism	Compatibilism	Hard determinism
Indeterminism	Libertarianism	

Is true choice possible?

If everything is determined by physical processes and the mind cannot intervene to change this, then (in theory at least) everything is inevitable. It also raises the uncomfortable possibility that when we think we are making choices the outcome of each decision is inevitable because it is determined by the outcome of the physical processes in the brain. The view that everything is determined in this way is called determinism.

Determinism, surprisingly, does not necessarily exclude the possibility that choices are made, even if the outcome of those choices is inevitable. Free will can be defined not by the possibility of more than one outcome but by the feeling that the choice exists and, from the individual's point of view, that choices are made. This means that it is possible to argue that free will exists even if determinism is true: freedom being defined as the "absence of restraint" on choices (Gomes 2007). This approach is called compatibilism. A criticism of compatibilism would be to say that it is semantics to call this free will if in fact there were no real possibility of different choices being made. Use of terms in relation to free will and determinism are shown in *Table 21.1*.

This appears to be relevant to the issue of whether or not individuals should be held responsible for their actions. It might be argued that if everything is determined, and all behaviour is an inevitable result of the physical processes that precede it, then people should not be held responsible for their actions. Put this way, it is not only those with an abnormal brain or a mental illness who cannot be held responsible, but everybody.

There are a number of responses to this, which allow not only a determinist approach, but also an argument for retaining the idea of criminal responsibility. Morse (2007) argues that although there is a genuine debate to be had about whether free will truly exists this is not relevant to the law because the various definitions of legal responsibility do not involve a consideration of free will. He writes that legal responsibility is, for example, about "capacity for rationality" which he says is defined by "moral, political, and, ultimately, legal judgement": i.e. it is not about a consideration of true free will. It can also be argued that people being held legally responsible and therefore subject to sanctions is part of the chain of determinist causes that leads to the desired outcome in criminal cases. In this sense it is vital to accept that criminal responsibility exists even if determinism is true, in order to allow society to function.

Science and true choice

Despite the unresolved issues around whether or not mind and brain are the same or different, and whether or not true free will exists, it is possible to find genuine science that takes understanding of these matters beyond theoretical debate.

Free will can be an illusion

Wegner and Wheatley (1999) performed an experiment which showed just this. The set up involved an experimenter, a subject and a computer screen with a number of objects showing on the screen. Both the subject and the experimenter had control of a mouse which allowed them to move a single cursor to select objects on the screen. At the same time the names of the objects were spoken into a set of headphones. Subjects were allowed to select whatever object they chose, irrespective of what was said into the headphones. They showed that merely hearing the name of an object did not cause the subjects to choose that object. However, if the name of the object was spoken at about the same time as the experimenter selected the object, an illusion was created in the subjects that they, not the experimenter, had made the selection.

They concluded that free will is an illusion which is set up when an apparent action is linked to an outcome by timing, the compatibility of the action with the outcome, and a reduction in the apparent available possibilities (which they called "exclusivity of thought"). This conclusion is an argument for determinism, but the fact that we can be mistaken about what is real should come as no surprise to psychiatric nurses who work daily with patients who have delusions and hallucinations. It will be equally apparent that the fact that we can be mistaken about reality does not necessarily mean that we are always so mistaken. That we can be fooled into thinking we have made a free choice does not necessarily mean that free choice does not exist.

Neuroscience, consciousness studies and choice

Benjamin Libet (1916–2007) was an important contributor to this area and his work has been replicated by others. He undertook numerous electrophysiological experiments from the 1950s onwards, involving brain or nerve stimulation and the recording and relating of these to subjective experience (Libet 2004).

In his earlier work he investigated the workings of the sensory pathway from the brain, which includes the sensory cortex, the thalamus, the medial lemniscus (midbrain), spinal cord and receptors in the skin. Using direct stimulation of the brain on conscious subjects during brain operations he was able to show that by stimulating the brain an experience of touch could be produced. He also showed that this stimulus had to be about half a second long or it would not result in a skin sensation.

This work was followed by further experiments that led to the remarkable conclusion that the brain detects skin stimuli about half a second after they happen, and that the brain then retimes the experience to the precise time of the skin stimulus. In other words consciousness is actually experiencing events that happened about half a second in the past, which is a remarkably long time. The evidence for this was as follows:

- Brain stimulation up to about half a second after a skin sensation can make that skin sensation appear stronger than if brain stimulation is not applied.
- If two skin stimuli are applied within half a second of each other, the second one can mask the first, giving the impression that it was not given at all.

If we are experiencing things in "real time" these first two observations should be impossible: it would mean the future "re-writing" the past.

- Minimum reaction times to any stimulus are about one-fifth of a second. This applies, for example, to applying the brakes in a car to avoid an accident. In an experimental setup, if subjects are asked to lengthen their reaction time just a little (for example by one-tenth of a second) they are unable to consciously do this. It appears that the minimum length of time that reactions can be consciously extended is about half a second.
- Skin sensations produce electrical activity in the brain. It is only if this electrical activity lasts for at least half a second that the skin sensation becomes conscious.

It is understandable that there is a delay between sensations and those sensations being brought to consciousness, because it must take time for the brain to process the data. What is remarkable is the length of the processing time and that from a subjective point of view we are living in "real time". In other words that brain is able to retime or "antedate" the experience by half a second for the purposes of conscious awareness.

In his really groundbreaking experiment Libet (1983) showed that there is unconscious brain activity up to about 350ms before a conscious choice is made. This seems to suggest that conscious choice is initiated by a brain rather than a mind event, because electrical activity precedes any awareness of the choice being made. The experiment was designed around a choice made by an experimental subject to move his wrist at any time he wanted. The timing of the first moment that the subject became aware of any intention to move his wrist, was a crucial part of the experiment. This was made by the subject noting the position of a dot on an oscilloscope, which took about 2.5 seconds to move in a circle. Muscle movement was timed with electromyography (EMG), and an electroencephalograph (EEG) timed brain activity. He found that the EEG activity preceded the first awareness of a choice being made by about 350ms. In other words there was about one-third of a second of unconscious brain activity before any conscious awareness of a decision to move.

This experiment, and others like it, have been used to justify determinism on the basis that the electrical activity preceding the decision is unconscious and therefore presumably arises from the chemistry of the brain as opposed to being initiated by a purely mental activity. Surprising, though, Libet was not a determinist, and he was very careful to avoid making statements which could not be supported by evidence. He took the view, quoting Karl Popper, that only hypotheses which could be potentially refuted had any scientific value (Libet 2001). He proposed a hypothesis that neural activity produced a "unified field" which was consciousness and would be equivalent to "mind". This field he described as an "emergent" phenomenon of brain activity. He was very clear that this was not a physical field like a magnetic or electrical field, and that thoughts could move through this field without using connections within the brain. He was then able to devise an experiment which could potentially refute the hypothesis, thus meeting requirements of Popper's good scientific method. This experiment involved isolating a slice of brain, such as sensory cortex, from its neural connections whilst maintaining its blood supply to keep it alive. If external stimulation of this cortex failed to produce a conscious sensation the hypothesis would be refuted.

The theory sounds like epiphenomenalism, but in his case he also speculated that this emergent phenomenon of a unified field was not just a passive by-product of the brain and could itself affect the physical brain. This ability would be strictly limited to vetoing action only on brain activity. His evidence for this came from the observation that his subjects could be aware of a choice to move their wrist in the above experiment, and time this as above with associated EEG activity: but they could also consciously stop themselves from actually moving so no EMG activity was recorded.

Conclusions

Nurses often make assessments of a patient's motivation, level of responsibility and the ability to take valid decisions for themselves. It is important to appreciate the context of these assessments and make them using the appropriate knowledge framework. A knowledge of mental capacity legislation can help inform decisions where this is relevant and a knowledge of the law can help understand the limits of criminal responsibility. A knowledge of the biological and psychodynamic basis of behaviour can help nurses understand a patient's behaviour in this sense, and formulate appropriate care plans or treatments. Finally, professional guidelines indicate the current consensus about best practice, and all of this is coloured by moral or religious beliefs.

The mind–brain problem is therefore relevant to forensic psychiatry because there is a risk that those making decisions about patients might oversimplify issues relating to choice by making assumptions about how mind and brain work without an understanding of what is not known. An understanding of the possibilities and limitations of current knowledge is important to nurses and other clinicians simply because it should cause us to reflect on the actual basis on which we are assessing our patients. When serious clinical decisions are being made, it is particularly important to be clear about how much we are applying legal, moral, religious or professional frameworks; and how much (or how little) is truly based on scientific evidence. This will help avoid pointless and circular arguments when clinical teams discuss the problems, and ensure that we are treating our patients fairly, and in the best possible way.

References

Barba GD (2001) Beyond the memory trace paradox and the fallacy of the Homunculus: A hypothesis concerning the relationship between memory, consciousness and temporality. *Journal of Consciousness Studies* **8**(3): 51–78

Department of Health and Home Office (1999) *Managing Dangerous People with Severe Personality Disorder: Proposals for policy development*. Department of Health and Home Office, London

Dyer C (2000) Force feeding of Ian Brady declared lawful. *British Medical Journal* **320**(7237): 731

Eccles J (1990) A unitary hypothesis of mind–brain interaction in the cerebral cortex. *Proceedings of the Royal Society of London B* **240**: 433–51

Fennell P (1996) *Treatment Without Consent. Law, psychiatry and the treatment of mentally disordered people since 1845*. Routledge, London

Gomes G (2007) Free will, the self, and the brain. *Behavioural Sciences and the Law* **25**: 221–34

Haddock A, Snowden P, Dolan M, Parker J, Rees H (2001) Managing dangerous people with severe personality disorder: A survey of forensic psychiatrists' opinions. *Psychiatric Bulletin* **25**: 293–6

Honderich T (1982) The argument for anomalous monism. *Analysis* **2**(2): 59–64

Law Commission (1991) Consultation paper no 119. *Mentally Incapacitated Adults and Decision Making: An overview.* HMSO, London

Libet B (1983) Time of conscious intention to act in relation to the onset of cerebral activity (readiness potential). *Brain* **106**: 623–42

Libet B (2001) Consciousness, free activity and the brain: Commentary. *Journal of Consciousness Studies* **8**(8): 59–65

Libet B (2004) *Mind Time*. Harvard University Press, Cambridge MA

Mayfield RD, Harris RA, Schuckit MA (2008) Genetic factors influencing alcohol dependence. *British Journal of Pharmacology* **154**(2): 275–87

Morse S (2007) The non-problem of free will in forensic psychiatry and psychology. *Behavioural Sciences and the Law* **25**: 203–20

Revonsuo A (2001) Can functional brain imaging discover consciousness in the brain? *Journal of Consciousness Studies* **8**(3): 3–23

Russell B (1984) *A History of Western Philosophy* (first published 1946) George Allen and Unwin (Publishers), Boston MA

Stapp H (1999) Attention, intention and will in quantum physics. *Journal of Consciousness Studies* **6**(8–9): 143–64

Tallis R (2007) Why blame me? It was all my brain's fault. *The Sunday Times* 24 October. Available from: www.timesonline.co.uk/tol/comment/columnists/guest_contributors/article2766643.ece

Wegner DM, Wheatley T (1999) Apparent mental causation: Sources of the experience of will. *American Psychologist* **54**(7): 480-92

Wilson DL (1999) Mind–brain interaction and violation of physical laws. *Journal of Consciousness Studies* **6**(8–9): 185–200

Yalowitz S (2008) "Anomalous Monism. In Edward N. Zalta (ed) *The Stanford Encyclopedia of Philosophy* (Fall 2008 Edition) Available from: http://plato.stanford.edu/archives/fall2008/entries/anomalous-monism/>.

CHAPTER 22

Dementia and offending behaviour

Chris Knifton

Introduction

Dementia is a condition that is gathering increasing concern in today's society. As many as 700 000 people are estimated to be diagnosed with this condition, increasing by the year 2021 to 940 110 (Knapp et al 2007). However its relevance to forensic mental health nursing and the associated implications in meeting challenges within care of the elderly and dementia care in general has been largely neglected. Developments in this area however are beginning to emerge, with an increasing interest towards the older offender (Fazel 2008). Although projections suggest that the elderly in England and Wales account for less than 1% of all criminal convictions (Hindley and Gordon 2000), there remains uncertainty regarding the true extent of crime committed by this group (Nnatu et al 2005). In addition, it has been suggested that nearly half of all older persons charged with a crime suffer from a mental illness (Yorston 1999, Taylor and Parrot 1988) and the total number of all elderly mentally disordered offenders will increase (Curtice et al 2003, Coid et al 2002). Indeed when compared to the projected rise in cases of dementia, and findings that the most common psychiatric diagnosis within this group includes psychosis, personality disorder and dementia (Heinik et al 1994), the possible relationship may be of increasing significance for forensic mental health settings. The purpose of this chapter is to suggest some key points to aid our understanding of this area, and propose a need for increasing service recognition.

Understanding dementia

The use of the word dementia is in fact as an umbrella term that includes a wide range of causes. It is typically viewed as a

> *...global cognitive impairment, which represents a decline from previous level of functioning, and is associated with impairment in functional abilities and, in many cases, behavioural and psychiatric disturbances.*
> (NICE/Social Care Institute for Excellence 2006: 67)

Box 22.1. Some forms of dementia

- Alzheimer's disease
- Vascular dementias
- Dementia with Lewy bodies
- Frontotemporal lobe dementia
- Korsakoff psychosis

Box 22.2. Common symptoms

- Memory and cognition problems
- Disorientation to time, place, and/or person
- Communication difficulties
- Inability to maintain usual levels of activities of daily living
- Behavioural and psychological symptoms of dementia may also in some cases (but not all) include: Aggression, delusions, depression, hallucinations, mental ill-health, personality changes, psychosis, sexual disinhibition, shouting/excessive vocalisation, and what may appear as inappropriate walking/restlessness ("wandering")

Box 22.3. Policy documents and guidance papers

- Department of Health (2001) *National Service Framework for Older People*. The Stationery Office, London
- NICE/Social Care Institute for Excellence (2006) *Dementia: Supporting people with dementia and their carers in health and social care*. The Stationery Office, London
- Knapp et al (2007) *Dementia UK: The full report*. Alzheimer's Society, London
- National Audit Office (2007) *Improving Services and Support for People With Dementia*. The Stationery Office, London
- Department of Health (2009) *Living Well With Dementia: A national dementia strategy*. Department of Health, London

Some of the common causes of dementia (but not all) are shown in *Box 22.1*. Although it is usually associated with older age, young onset dementia (where it develops before the age of 65) can also occur.

Some of the more common symptoms usually associated with most forms/types of dementia are shown in *Box 22.2*, although symptoms will still vary according to the person, the form of dementia, and stage of disease progression.

Given the projected increase in people with dementia over the next decade, it is perhaps all the more important that all services, including forensic services, take time to reflect if they are able to meet the challenges that this may represent. A range of policy documents and guidance papers has been written on supporting people with dementia and their carers. Some of these are shown in *Box 22.3*. A common theme is the recognition for greater awareness and training about dementia for all staff working with older people, for co-ordinated health and social care and for improving the quality of services.

How far, if at all, is this of any relevance to forensic services? Our starting point perhaps is to consider if there is any clear association between crime or offending behaviour and dementia, and thus the potential likelihood of involvement from forensic mental health services.

Crime and dementia

Reports of people with dementia engaging in offending behaviour are rarely documented. Jacoby (1997: 749) cites the work of Dankwarth and Püschel (1991) who note the case of a 90-year-old man suffering from dementia following a stroke who strangled his 79-year-old wife and then committed suicide. More recently, in 2008, a range of national newspapers reported the case of a 74-year-old man with dementia being found guilty of culpable homicide after strangling his wife when she refused to give him money to go out drinking (*Times Online* 2008, *The Independent* 2008). Whilst a range of reasons may be offered for why offences such as these are committed, the potential impact of any mental disorder, including dementia, must also be considered a key factor. Understanding, therefore, any potential relationship between crime and dementia warrants further attention.

Initial epidemiological evidence however has suggested no clear statistical association between dementia and crime (Jacoby 1990), although organic brain disease has in the past been linked to antisocial or criminal acts (Hindley and Gordon 2000). However it is acknowledged that for some minor offences, people may not be charged and instead directed into the medical/health service, for example, in the case of shoplifting (Jacoby 1997). In addition, there may be a clear reluctance to report people to the police who appear to be unwell or frail (O'Sullivan and Chesterman 2007). The true picture therefore will no doubt continue to remain unclear.

A recent study however suggests a possible relationship. O'Sullivan and Chesterman (2007) identified 282 patients aged 60 years or older subject to restriction orders in England and Wales. Taking a patient sample of 37 who committed offences when aged 60 or over, the authors found them significantly more likely to be diagnosed with a delusional disorder, depression or dementia. Such findings are similar to Coid et al's (2002) that found depression, delusional disorder and dementia as the most prevalent diagnoses of elderly patient admissions to a secure forensic psychiatric service over 7 years. The authors found that for elderly patients, often their first appearance in court coincided, and led to, their first psychiatric hospital admission. In connection with dementia, Fazel et al (2001) carried out a study of 203 male prisoners in England and Wales aged over 60, and identified two cases of dementia, and later, Fazel and Grann (2002) found 19 (0.3%) people referred for forensic psychiatric assessment in Sweden had a diagnosis of dementia. Additionally, Murray (2004) cites the work of Fazel and Jacoby (2002), who looked at a number of studies where dementia was viewed as a catalyst to criminal behaviours. These numbers, although appearing relatively small, still have notable implications for service provision. Although the connection between dementia and crime may however appear at best anecdotal, these studies do reflect that people with dementia may still engage in offending behaviour and thus are at risk of becoming part of the criminal justice system and/or the forensic mental health services.

Examples of offending behaviour carried out by people with dementia, and reported to the authorities have included sexual offences, violence, and arson (Curtice et al 2003), shoplifting (Edwards-Lee et al 1997), and homicide (Dankwarth and Püshchel 1991).

Sexual offences

The Sexual Offences Act 2003 lists a range of differing sexual offences, which include both non-contact offences (such as voyeurism) as well as contact offences (such as forms of rape). Curtice et al (2003) found evidence of dementia in six (19%) cases of patients admitted to a regional medium secure unit. Notably, the highest offences by this group of patients included three sexual offences (rape of a minor, unlawful sexual intercourse, and inappropriate sexual behaviour), two offences against the person (grievous bodily harm and attempted wounding) and arson.

This relationship between dementia and sexual offences is often considered strong (Heinik et al 1994), although Jacoby (1997) argues there remain insufficient data from published studies on any association, a view also supported by Dinniss (1999). Indeed, Fazel et al (2002) suggests that sex offending in the elderly on the whole is more likely to be associated with personality rather than organic brain disease. However, an association between dementia and personality change as a cardinal feature might itself then warrant consideration, particularly where personality changes involve disinhibition, aggression or other seemingly negative characteristics. Oppenheimer (2008) reviewed a number of published studies in considering evidence for findings of personality change in dementia. Her conclusions argue for the existence of a pattern of personality changes in some people with dementia to support the idea that this may be an essential feature of the disease itself. In people, however, with frontotemporal dementia, evidence for personality change, she argues, is much stronger. Although no direct association is made between criminal behaviour and a personality change in dementia, the need for future study may warrant further investigation. Neary (2005) notes, for example, that for a small percentage of people with frontotemporal dementia, there may be a preoccupation with sex, an increase in sexual demands on partners or an interest in mild sexual perversions. Higgins et al (2004: 1331) cite the work of Kuhn et al (1998) who suggest that hypersexuality or inappropriate sexual expression may be a rare but disturbing behaviour in some individuals. Despite this, however, as noted by Warner (2005), criminal proceedings regarding inappropriate sexual activity among people with dementia do remain rare. However, 16% of sexual offences in Curtice et al's (2003) study were from patients with a diagnosis of dementia; a similar prevalence of 14% was noted in another study of 43 elderly sex offenders by Hucker (1984), cited by Curtice et al (2003). Reasons for any possible connection between sexual offences and dementia may in part be due to disinhibition, which Jacoby (1990) has suggested may result in sexually inappropriate behaviour. However, Warner (2005) discusses a number of studies that suggest low rates of sexual disinhibition among people with dementia ranging from 3% (Devanand et al 1992) to 7% (Burns et al 1990).

Violence

Practitioners working with people with dementia in healthcare settings may encounter individuals who exhibit complex or challenging behaviour, including aggression and potential violence. Usually in dementia, the underlying cause is often attributable to communication difficulties and/or the environment. The consequences of violence or aggression should not be underestimated for either party. Aside from any physical health consequences, the effects on emotional well-being should also be considered. Victims may include practitioners, informal carers, or fellow patients and are likely to experience a range of emotions and differing reactions. For the person with dementia, the risk of social exclusion, labelling and stereotyping are likely.

Dinniss (1999) suggests, however, that dementia itself is rarely associated with violent crime, and that violence may rather be due to other conditions, such as depression or paranoia. Depressive symptoms are however also common in dementia (Shanmugham and Alexopoulous 2005), with the true relationship between dementia and depression argued as complex (Eastley and Wilcock 2005). There is a suggested mean comorbidity of 20% (Ballard et al 1996, cited by Eastley and Wilcock 2005: 39). Depression and paranoia then are also features that may make up the behavioural and psychological symptoms of some people's dementia, and thus need to be carefully considered.

Hindley and Gordon (2000) cite the work of Petrie et al who reported that in a geriatric unit in the United States, patients with a diagnosis of dementia committed more unarmed acts of violence than other patients. Indeed, Jacoby (1997) notes that although serious violence is rare in people with dementia, it does occasionally occur.

Minor offences

Other examples of criminal activity or offending behaviour associated with dementia have included shoplifting (Edwards-Lee et al 1997) and possibly nuisance offences, noted in *Box 22.4*. It is not surprising that offences such as nuisance and anti-social behaviour may occur as a result of poor cognition, faltering memory or disorders of perception (including delusional beliefs about neighbours), perhaps made all the more likely if the person is living alone. Such behaviours however are often effectively managed through community psychiatric and social services, and rarely if at all directly involve the criminal or forensic services.

Relationship between forms of dementia and offending behaviour

As noted at the beginning of this chapter, dementia is an umbrella term that includes a range of differing types or forms of conditions. Whether or not offending behaviour in dementia is attributable to specific forms may be an important concern. See *Box 22.5* for the forms of dementia that have been associated with criminal activity. In a recent study, Curtice et al (2003) collected data from a 30-bedded regional medium secure unit. The most common diagnosis was that of dementia in six (19%) cases, with the average age of this group being 73.5 years. The types of dementia included Alzheimer's disease, vascular dementia, Huntington's chorea, two accounts of early/pre-senile dementia, and one described merely as moderate/severe dementia. Although a small sample, it does suggest that no one particular form was particularly associated with offending behaviour. However, Miller et al (1997) argue that

Box 22.4. Nuisance and anti-social behaviour offences that may be associated with dementia

- Noise
- Fumes and smells such as smoke, burning rubbish
- Failure to clear litter/refuse
- Dogs left uncontrolled
- Damage caused by domestic animals
- Harassment/intimidating behaviour, including paranoia/delusions about neighbours

criminal behaviour is more common in patients with frontotemporal dementia than in those with Alzheimer's disease. These findings are similar to that of Strip (1995) as cited by Brower and Price (2001) who found higher rates of antisocial behaviour, that included stealing, physical assault and sexually offensive behaviour, in patients with frontotemporal dementia. In addition, Edwards-Lee et al (1997) describe examples of "obsessive visual attention" in frontotemporal dementia leading to shoplifting in six cases, arguing that this may reflect a visual preoccupation with small objects in this condition. They discuss the example of a man who became "obsessed with coins" who went out every day, intentionally passing phone booths, cash registers, busy city streets and restaurant tables, all places where he might find and pocket coins. This behaviour was associated with efforts to steal pens, wallets and tips from restaurant tables (1997: 1038). This perhaps suggests consideration of a relationship between offending behaviour and disinhibition, especially as disinhibition may be recognised as a cardinal symptom in frontotemporal dementia. Jacoby (1990) further has suggested that disinhibition may be a factor in sexually inappropriate behaviour. Finally, Brower and Price (2001) argue that clinically significant frontal lobe dysfunction is associated with aggressive dyscontrol. However, the authors found that no study showed that disorders of pre-frontal cortex would predict violent crime.

It is of interest to note that despite the association between criminal activity and substance misuse, including alcohol consumption, there remains at present little empirical data on the association between criminal activity and dementia associated with alcohol dependence/excessive consumption. Atkinson (1997: 661) suggests that research demonstrates alcohol dependence in the elderly may remain a public health problem of moderate proportion in some societies. Indeed, despite the relative increase in dementia associated with alcohol dependence (Bowden and Ritter 2005), including Wernicke-Korsakoff syndrome, this as of yet does not appear to be associated with criminal activity. Reasons for this lack of association may be related to problems with obtaining a clear diagnosis, or a greater propensity for family and caregivers to under-report. Such difficulties may indeed suggest that alcohol misuse as a precursor for dementia, and any consequent associated criminal conduct, may indeed remain hidden from clinical and legal scrutiny.

Box 22.5. Forms of dementia associated with criminal activity

Greatest association

- Frontotemporal lobe dementias

Lesser association

- Alzheimer's disease
- Huntington's chorea
- Vascular dementia

In addition, there appear to be no published data of dementia with Lewy bodies and offences (including anti-social behaviour), despite the fact that this form of dementia includes visual hallucinations and fluctuating cognitive disturbances.

Discussion

Although there is no direct correlation between having a diagnosis of dementia and then engaging in offending behaviour, there is some limited evidence that shows why criminal behaviour may nonetheless occur in some rare instances. The purpose of this chapter was to bring to the attention this relatively neglected and under-researched area of the connection between forensic and dementia care. Small however as it may be, this concern will continue to remain of importance for the range of staff working with people with a diagnosis of dementia who have engaged in offending behaviour and those who find themselves caring for them in forensic or other mental health services.

Nurses are expected to engage with an ever diverse client group (Nursing and Midwifery Council 2008). Can, however, the absence of a comprehensive detailed discussion on the forensic aspects of dementia care be ethically and legally justified? Does it imply that the needs of people with dementia who may commit criminal offences are not worth discussion, debate or research? Indeed as the number of elderly mentally disordered offenders steadily increases, forensic mental health nursing may have to accept an emerging and growing responsibility for the needs of this relatively small, but important, client group.

There remains a greater propensity for practitioners, family and caregivers, and the public in general, to under-report offending behaviour carried out by vulnerable adults, including people with dementia. As such, any consequent associated criminal conduct by people with dementia may indeed remain hidden from clinical and legal scrutiny with only isolated or extreme cases, as shown, coming to the attention of the forensic services. There remains a need to fully understand the diversity involved in dementia care, including the provision of appropriate care management in the most suitable setting. To ignore or to fail to recognise that people with dementia may, in extreme circumstances, also engage in offending behaviour cannot be ethically justified. As we end this chapter, we perhaps return to our starting place – a growing recognition of this area of practice; the next step will be to scrutinise service provision and care management across health and social care, forensic mental health services, and the criminal justice system and the ability of these services to adequately support and respect the needs, rights, equality and diversity of people with dementia who have engaged in offending behaviour.

Further reading

NICE/Social Care Institute for Excellence (2006) Dementia. Supporting People With Dementia and Their Carer's in Health and Social Care. The Stationery Office, London

Department of Health (2009) Living Well with Dementia: A national dementia strategy. Department of Health, London

References

Atkinson RA (1997) Alcohol and drug abuse in the elderly. In Jacoby R, Oppenheimer C (eds) *Psychiatry in the Elderly* (pp. 661–87). Oxford University Press, Oxford

Ballard CG, Bannister C, Oyebode F (1996) Depression in dementia sufferers. *International Journal of Geriatric Psychiatry* **11**: 507–15

Bowden SC, Ritter AJ (2005) Alcohol-related dementia and the clinical spectrum of Wernicke-Korsakoff syndrome. In Burns A, O'Brien J, and Ames D (eds) *Dementia* (3rd edn) Hodder Arnold, London

Brower MC, Price BH (2001) Neuropsychiatry of frontal lobe dysfunction in violent and criminal behaviour: A critical review. *Journal of Neurology, Neurosurgery and Psychiatry* **71**: 720-6

Burns A, Jacoby R, Levy R (1990) Psychiatric phenomena in Alzheimer's disease. IV: disorders of behaviour. *British Journal of Psychiatry* **157**: 86–94

Coid J, Fazel S, Kahtan N (2002) Elderly patients admitted to secure forensic psychiatric services. *Journal of Forensic Psychiatry* **13**(2): 416–27

Curtice M, Parker J, Wismayer FS, Tomison A (2003) The elderly offender: An 11-year survey of referrals to a regional forensic psychiatric service. *Journal of Forensic Psychiatry and Psychology* **14**(2): 253–65

Dankwarth G, Püschel K (1991) Straftaten gegen das Leben – alte Menschrn als Opfer und Täter. Zeitschrift für Gerontologie **24**, 266–270.

Department of Health (2001) *National Service Framework for Older People*. Stationery Office, London

Department of Health (2009) *Living Well With Dementia: A national dementia strategy*. Department of Health, London

Devanand DP, Brockington CD, Moody BJ et al (1992) Behavioural syndromes in Alzheimer's disease. *International Psychogeriatrics* **4**(suppl.2): 161–84

Dinniss S (1999) Violent crime in an elderly demented patient. *International Journal of Geriatric Psychiatry* **14**: 889–91

Eastley R, Wilcock GK (2005) Assessment of dementia. In Burns A, O'Brien J, Ames D (eds) *Dementia*. (3rd edn). Hodder Arnold Publishers, London

Edwards-Lee T, Miller BL, Benson DF, Cummings JL, Russell GL, Bonne K, Mena I (1997) The temporal variant of frontotemporal dementia. *Brain* **120**: 1027–40

Fazel S (2008) Psychiatric aspects of crime and the elderly. Cited in Jacoby R, Oppenheimer C, Dening T, Thomas A (eds) *Oxford Textbook of Old Age Psychiatry*. Oxford University Press, Oxford

Fazel S, Grann M (2002) Older criminals: A descriptive study of psychiatrically examined offenders in Sweden. *International Journal of Geriatric Psychiatry* **17**: .907–13

Fazel S, Hope T, O'Donnell I, Jacoby R (2001) Hidden psychiatric morbidity in elderly prisoners. *British Journal of Psychiatry* **1769**: 535–9

Fazel S, Hope T, O'Donnell I, Jacoby R (2002) Psychiatric, demographic, and personality characteristics of elderly sex offenders. *Psychological Medicine* **32**: 219–26

Fazel S, Jacoby R (2002) Psychiatric aspects of crime and the elderly. In Jacoby R, Oppenheimer C (eds) *Psychiatry in the Elderly*. (3rd edn). Oxford: Oxford University Press

Heinik J, Kimhi R, Hes JP. (1994) Dementia and crime: A forensic psychiatric unit study in Israel. *International Journal of Geriatric Psychiatry* **9**: 491–4

Higgins A, Barker P, Begley CM (2004) Hypersexuality and dementia: Dealing with inappropriate sexual expression. *British Journal of Nursing* **13**(22): 1330-4

Hindley N, Gordon H (2000) The elderly, dementia, aggression and risk assessment. *International Journal of Geriatric Psychiatry* **15**: 254–9

Hucker SJ (1984) Psychiatric aspects of crime in old age. In Newman ES, Newman DJ, Gewirtz ML, et al (eds) *Elderly Criminals*. Cambridge: Oelgeschlager (cited by Curtice et al (2003) *op cit*)

Jacoby R (1990) Senile dementia and crime. Cited in Bluglass R, Bowden P (eds) *Principles and Practice of Forensic Psychiatry*. Churchill Livingstone, London

Jacoby R (1997) Psychiatric aspects of crime and the elderly. In Jacoby R, Oppenheimer C, (eds) *Psychiatry in the Elderly* 2nd edn). Oxford University Press, Oxford

Knapp M, Prince M, Albanese E, Banerjee S, Dhanasiri S, Fernandez JL, Ferri C, McCrone P, Snell T, Stewart R (2007) *Dementia UK: The full report*. Alzheimer's Society, London

Kuhn DR, Greiner D, Arseneau LA (1998) Addressing hypersexuality in Alzheimer's disease. *Journal of Gerentological Nursing* **24**(4): 44–50

Miller BL, Darby A, Benson DF, Cummings JL, Miller MH (1997) Aggressive, socially disruptive and antisocial behaviour associated with front-temporal dementia. *British Journal of Psychiatry* **170**: 150-5

Murray A (2004) Prisoners who develop dementia: What we need to know. *Journal of Dementia Care* **Jan/Feb**: 29–33

National Audit Office (NAO) (2007) *Improving services and support for people with dementia*. The Stationery Office, London

National Institute for Clinical Excellence and Social Care Institute for Excellence (NICE/SCIE) (2006) *Dementia. Supporting people with dementia and their carer's in health and social care*. The Stationery Office, London

Neary D (2005) Frontotemporal dementia. In Burns A, O'Brien J, Ames D (eds) *Dementia*. (3rd edn). Hodder Arnold Publishers, London

Nnatu IO, Mahomed F, Shah A (2005) Is there a need for elderly forensic psychiatric services? *Medicine Science and the Law* **45**: 154–60

Nursing and Midwifery Council (2008) *The Code: Standards of Conduct Performance and Ethics for Nurses and Midwives*. NMC, London

Oppenheimer C (2008) Personality in later life: Personality disorder and the effects of illness on personality. In Jacoby R, Oppenheimer C, Dening T, Thomas A (eds) *Oxford Textbook of Old Age Psychiatry* (pp. 605–16). Oxford University Press, Oxford

O'Sulivan PCJ, Chesterman LP (2007) Older adult patients subject to restriction orders in England and Wales: A cross-sectional survey. *Journal of Forensic Psychiatry and Psychology* **18**(2): 204–20

Shanmugham B, Alexopoulos G (2005) Depression with cognitive impairment. In Burns A, O'Brien J, Ames D (eds) *Dementia*. (3rd edn, pp.731–7). Hodder Arnold, London

Strip E (1995) Compulsive disorder and acquired antisocial behaviour in frontal lobe dementia. *Journal of Neuropsychiatry Clinical Neuroscience* **7**: 116

Taylor PJ, Parrot JM (1988) Elderly offenders: A study of age related factors among custodially remanded prisoners. *British Journal of Psychiatry* **151**: 340-6

Times Online (2008) Judge bans Edward Flaherty, who killed his wife, from going to pub, by Charlene Sweeney. August 4. Available from:www.timesonline.co.uk/tol/news/uk/crime/article4459498 [last accessed 6 January 2009]

The Independent (2008) Pensioner who strangled wife is sentenced to one-year ban, by Ian Johnson. 5 August. Available from: www.independent.co.uk/news/uk/crime/pensioner-who-strangled-wife-is-sentenced-to-one-year-ban-Crime,UK [last accessed 16 January 2009]

Warner J (2005) Sexuality and dementia. Cited in Burns A, O'Brien J, Ames D (eds) (2005) *Dementia*. Hodder Arnold, London

Yorston G (1999) Aged and dangerousness. *British Journal of Psychiatry* **175**: 193–5

CHAPTER 23

The care programme approach and recovery

Tony Earp and Richard Byrt

This chapter considers ethical and other aspects of the care programme approach (CPA) and recovery principles.

> *Yesterday's "scandals" of the institution have already been replaced by today's scandals of the community.*
>
> (Rose 1986: 206, quoted in Crichton and Sheppard 1996: 65)

CPA and other community care "reforms", such as community treatment orders and related central Government legislation and policy, appear to have been initiated partly because of media and political pressures related to scandals and moral panics, rather than in response to service users' perceived needs (Lester and Glasby 2006). Concerns for public, and sometimes client, safety appear to have been the main policy drivers (Fawcett and Karban 2005, Lester and Glasby 2006). CPA was introduced in England and Wales in 1991 after Ben Silcock, a young man with a diagnosis of schizophrenia, was seriously attacked by a lion after getting into its cage at London Zoo (Fawcett and Karban 2005, Jones 1993).

According to Thornicroft and Szmukler (2001), quoting and citing Department of Health (1999b) CPA has involved:

> - *Systematic arrangements for assessing the health and social needs of people accepted by the specialist psychiatric services.*
> - *The formulation of a care plan which addresses these needs.*
> - *The appointment of a keyworker to keep in close touch with the [client] and monitor care.*
> - *Regular review, and if need be, changes to the care plan. Multi-agency and interagency working is stressed. Care plans should be agreed with users and their carers, as far as possible.*
>
> Thornicroft and Szmukler (2001: 557)

CPA also aimed to "minimise the risk that [clients] lose contact with services" (Department of Health 1990).

Subsequent reviews of the CPA saw the introduction of care co-ordinators, "the integration of the CPA and case management"; and a shift from CPA being used solely in the community to "residential settings, including prisons" (Department of Health 1999a, and page 4). In March 2008, a further review of CPA introduced a "set of values and principles" intended to underpin its implementation, and assist in the introduction of the recovery approach (Department of Health 2008, and page 2).

The above is only a thumbnail sketch of some aspects of CPA. There is also a wide range of standards and principles to be considered, which include the integration of risk assessment into CPA, and consideration of carers' needs. However, in this chapter, the focus is on the values and principles of recovery and social inclusion and related ethical and other concerns.

The term recovery appears to have many meanings in the literature. A distinction has been made between "clinical recovery" as a "cure" for illness (Whitehill 2009) or a reduction of its signs and symptoms (Davidson et al 2006); and recovery, which, amongst other things, involves "the restoration, rebuilding, reclaiming or taking control of one's life" (National Institute for Mental Health in England 2005, quoted in Watkins 2007: 3).

Recovery approaches, in this sense, argue for a move away from seeing individuals only as "mental health clients", and from only concentrating on the reduction of signs and symptoms, problems and "deficits", to a recognition that people who have used mental health services have other more crucial roles and identities, as well as aspirations and goals, talents, abilities and positive attributes (Tew 2005, Watkins 2007, Slade 2009).

> *Recovery involves the development of new meaning and purpose in one's life as one grows beyond the catastrophic effects of mental illness.*
>
> (Anthony 1993, quoted in Perkins and Repper 2009: 86)

The term recovery, in this sense, refers to "the ability to live well in the presence or absence of one's illness (or whatever people choose to name their experience)" (Mental Health Commission New Zealand 2001: 1).

The application of recovery principles by professionals means that service users are seen as having much to offer other people and society from their unique experiences. In addition, they are perceived as individuals with a range of physical, psychological, spiritual, cultural, psychosexual, economic and other needs and aspirations; rather than as someone whose only identity is that of "patient" or "client". Professionals' recognition of a wide variety of needs related to recovery lends itself to multi-disciplinary and inter-agency team working (Davidson et al 2006). Recovery also includes the recognition that individuals with service user experience have rights to social inclusion, with an absence of negative discrimination and access to the same life opportunities as other people. Above all, recovery principles are about valuing, validating and affirming the individual and her/his experiences and perspectives (Watkins 2007, Helm 2009, Perkins and Repper 2009, Whitehill 2009), similar, in some respects, to the application of the ethical concept "respect for persons" (Kant 1969), considered in *Chapter 2*.

There are difficulties in implementing recovery principles in secure hospitals and for clients of forensic community mental health services. Firstly, recovery appears to receive limited consideration in the forensic mental health and forensic nursing literature; and at first sight, there appears to be little research in this area. This means that there is an apparent lack of a theoretical or evidence base, or published examples to inform the implementation of recovery principles in secure hospitals or forensic community services. However, to many people who have been clients of mental health services (Helm 2009, Whitehill 2009), the values on which recovery is based (Fulford 2004) may be of more salience than "evidence". Davidson et al (2006) argue, in relation to recovery principles in general:

> *In [one] respect, it makes no sense to ask whether recovery or recovery-oriented care is "evidence based". There is ample evidence, documented extensively over 30 years, that people can and do learn how to live with and recover from serious mental illness...The question about evidence-based practices, is which interventions, provided by whom, are most effective at promoting which of...various forms of recovery under what circumstances?*
>
> (Davidson et al 2006: 643)

However, Davidson et al (2006: 643) report that, in the USA, the President's New Freedom Commission on Mental Health (2002) proposed that recovery be the principal goal "of all mental health services (with the exception of forensic services...the primary aim of which may be containment or community safety)". Arguably, the political and other requirements for safety may conflict with recovery principles. Mezey and Eastman (2009: 503) outline the difficulty of increasing the social inclusion of forensic patients, given Government requirements for "public protection within an increasingly risk-averse society", in which individuals with both mental health problems and histories of offending are widely stigmatised (Bartlett 2004). Patients' social exclusion may be compounded by the social isolation of secure hospitals and prison healthcare services, especially if there are few links with local communities and patients are admitted long distances from their partners, families and neighbourhoods (Harner 2004, Lester and Glasby 2006, Byrt et al 2008).

In the authors' experience, the often pressing concerns related to assessing, preventing and reducing risk to others can also affect the implementation of recovery principles in secure hospitals. This is partly because nurses and other professionals may perceive the duty of care to ensure safety to outweigh the ethical imperative to enable patient autonomy (Adshead 2010). (Duty of care and autonomy were considered in *Chapter 2*.) If patients are subject to restrictions with which they disagree, this conflicts with recovery principles of individuals achieving their goals and aspirations (Watkins 2007), at least in the short-term. In addition, in some settings, so much of nurses' energy and time may be devoted to reducing risk, that there can appear to be little opportunity to consider recovery principles, including assessing and meeting individuals' needs related to spirituality, culture and aspects of diversity. And yet, risk may be increased if there is neglect of these areas, and a failure to provide holistic care (Byrt 2008). Aiyegbusi (2009) questions the extent that recovery principles can be applied in secure settings, when many patients are there for long periods of time, but concludes:

> *It could be argued that the principles of recovery are applicable to this population because recovery is defined as an internal process involving a personal and hopeful journey that the patient makes at their own pace, towards reclaiming a meaningful life from the despair of mental ill health...However, the mental health practitioner can, by their behaviour, either assist or obstruct the patient in their recovery.*
>
> (Aiyegbusi 2009: 27)

Some therapies used in secure hospitals and prisons incorporate values and principles that may contribute to patients' recovery. Examples include psychosocial interventions for individuals with mental illness, dialectical behaviour therapy and therapeutic community principles, all of which may enable healing from trauma, an emphasis on the individual's strengths, and validation of her/his experiences (Jeffcote and Watson 2004, Aiyegbusi and Clarke-Moore 2009, Bartlett and McGauley 2010).

Recovery is not only a positive, hopeful approach for people who use services, but provides managers and professionals with alternatives to traditional psychiatry. In recovery approaches, service users are enabled to find their own solutions to problems (Allott 2005). There is, however, much debate about what the term recovery means, particularly in relation to the delivery of services and the development of policy (Davidson et al 2006). In terms of healthcare delivery in the United Kingdom, the concept of recovery has been said to have different meanings:

- A spontaneous and natural process.

- A response to effective treatments.
- A way of growing, despite disability.

(Repper and Perkins 2003)

The National Service Framework for Mental Health referred to recovery with reference to the effects of mental ill health on individuals' "social, emotional and physical well-being" (Department of Health 1999b: 14). This document stated:

> *Health and social services should promote mental health for all, working with individuals and communities combating discrimination against individuals and groups with mental health problems, and promote their social inclusion.*
>
> (Department of Health 1999b, Standard One: 14)

Documents that followed underpinned this thinking. The NHS plan identified the resources that would be required for changes to enable social inclusion to occur (Department of Health 2002). The *Ten Essential Capabilities: A Framework for the Whole Mental Health Workforce* (Sainsbury Centre for Mental Health 2004) highlighted the importance of skills that assist the implementation of a recovery approach to care and how it is essential that it is embedded into practice. The Chief Nursing Officer's review of mental health nursing stated clearly how this could be achieved (Department of Health 2006a), but without specific reference to forensic or prison nursing. *Our Health, Our Care, Our Say* (Department of Health 2006b) considered preventative approaches to care, and supported recovery approaches through multi-agency working across health and social care services. This thinking was supported by Darzi (2007), who referred to multi-agency working and personalised care. The New Horizons policy initiative (HM Government 2009, 2010), which has replaced the National Service Framework for Mental Health (Department of Health 1999b, 2004), emphasises "public health and well-being", social inclusion and recovery. These policy documents adopt a public health approach, and stress the relevance of mental health to many areas of life, including economics, employment, education and accommodation; and conclude that mental health is "everybody's responsibility". Shifts in thinking towards recovery and public health perspectives have required an examination of current working.

However, in spite of this positive drive to change the face of the delivery of mental healthcare, there are concerns. These go back to definitions of recovery and what it means. Some professionals state that it implies cure rather than the promotion of the optimum functioning of the service user and the opportunities that this might afford (Davidson et al 2006). It is a paradox that some clients have expressed fears that services would be provided only if they were committed to notions of recovery (Frak 2005). This raises the issue of how the concepts of recovery are understood and actioned in service provision.

The way ahead

When discussing the concept of recovery, it is essential to understand that we are referring to an approach to, rather than a model of, care (Perkins and Repper 2009). Appreciating this enables the application of recovery approaches to models of care that meet the needs of service users, as well as the goals of mental health services (Mental Health Commission New Zealand 2001). Nevertheless, some contemporary models of care and treatment may enable recovery to be understood more effectively (Allott 2005). To expand on this, there needs to be an understanding of what need is, and the application of current frameworks that try to explain the origins of mental ill-health. Service users' needs can be considered in relation to the elimination of factors causing social disablement or discrimination; or considered more narrowly, and only in relation to professionals' perspectives concerning services, treatment, care and risk reduction (Davidson et al 2006, Perkins and Repper 2009).

Ryan and Morgan (2004a: 157) describe the importance of the service user in the "strengths approach" to care planning, in which care is based on the service user's needs and wants, which, in turn, would be linked directly to the care plan. This sounds simple enough, but raises the whole issue of engagement of not only the service user, but also the service provider. Morgan and Ryan (2004) go on to discuss the importance of engagement and assessment through a psychosocial interventions approach. The process of engagement needs to be responsive to the needs of service users and carers. This means that it is not just a process that we go through but is an activity that has value and meaning. The role of the service provider is initially to foster a therapeutic environment and relationship, where hope for the service user can be expressed (Campbell 2001). Many service users present themselves for care in a distressed state, often with an absence of hope. In times such as this, it is the responsibility of the service to keep hope alive for the service user when she/he is in crisis (Morgan and Ryan 2004).

Repper and Perkins (2003) explain the importance of following a "strengths approach" to assessment, as opposed to a symptoms approach. To follow a symptoms approach implies that the service user is unable to function until symptoms have subsided. This is essentially incorrect, as some service users may be able to function in the presence of symptoms (Davidson et al 2006). One of the purposes of care planning is "translating identified needs and wants" of the service user "into real actions" (Ryan and Morgan 2004b:175, citing Morgan and Akbar-Khan 2000). This requires the service to work with service users when setting goals based on their needs and wants. Care panning can have a number of functions, including:

- A method of trying to achieve a goal.
- A safety-net for when the service user is in crisis (crisis management plan).
- Checking where the service user is on her/his journey.

(Ryan and Morgan 2004b)

In care planning, goals can be broken down into small steps (Repper and Perkins 2003). If a service user wants to live in the community, there may be a number of steps that have to take place, such as arranging housing, looking at benefits, managing risks and taking medication. This can be a focus for conflict between professionals and the service user, as it may not be what she/he wants, but may be required by the service. This can result in the service user's understandable disengagement (Ryan and Morgan 2004b). Service users who enter care against their wishes, including forensic patients, may find themselves experiencing this level of disempowerment, as conditions with which they disagree may be put in place as part of their discharge pathway (Gamble et al 2009).

For the service user who is using inpatient services, the goal of discharge symbolises something more than just leaving hospital, but that of reclaiming her/his sense of belonging in the community (Repper and Perkins 2003). Stickley (2005) outlined the benefits of social inclusion for service users. Not only does it enable individuals to lead fulfilling lives and make a valuable contribution to society, but also it challenges some of the constructs that lead to stigma. Traditional service provision tends to be focused on the maintenance of the person's identity as a service user. This has led to the development of drop-in centres and day hospitals which, although having a possible role in service provision, can also be seen as reinforcing the sick role (Brooker and Repper 1998). These authors, in referring to Maslow's (1970) hierarchy of needs, point out that although some needs may be met in traditional settings, more creative methods should be undertaken to promote social inclusion and tackle stigma.

This raises the issue of equality and diversity and reinforces that people need to be treated with respect. For the service, this means that the professional needs to work with the service user when identifying what is available. This can provide empowerment, as service users may be able to make choices with regard to what they want and what they do not want to do (Perkins and Repper 2009, Slade 2009, Watkins 2007). An example of this is the service user who has experienced a number of hospital admissions with a diagnosis of schizophrenia. After a period of assessment, he identified that he wanted a job, friends and a home of his own. Initially and with assistance, he found a job, and started to make friends whilst still in hospital. However when he found a place of his own, he became withdrawn and both his social life and his work life began to suffer. After discussion with his worker, he identified that his main goals were work and social life. As a consequence he moved into supported living and his functioning improved (Brooker and Repper 1998).

What this demonstrates, is that, with good engagement and involvement, the service user was able to achieve his goals with some adjustments to the plan. Care planning requires both services users and the service being able to negotiate the objectives and stages of the plan (Ryan and Morgan 2004b, citing Kisthardt 1992).

Example of the application of recovery principles

Bob (a pseudonym) is a 42-year-old independent man and father. He is creative and describes himself as having an interest in nature. Bob was an adopted child who found out at an early age that his adoptive parents were not his own. His formative years were spent in and out of care.

Bob has had a number of negative experiences in his life which have led to offending behaviour, ranging from theft and substance misuse to violence, which led to custodial care. Bob eventually found himself in receipt of mental health services, following a diagnosis of schizophrenia. His last offence resulted in his admission to a secure hospital under Part 3 of the Mental Health Act 1983.

Whilst in hospital, discussions with his key worker revealed that he did not feel that he required a recovery programme. However, in spite of this, he did agree to carry on discussion with his key worker regarding his needs and aspirations. The discussions revealed the following:

- His life on the ward is mundane.
- He enjoys walking dogs and caring for animals.
- He describes himself as being strong-willed, broadminded and having common sense. This, he feels, people see as a strength.
- Things that he feels people do not like are that he can, at times, be callous and not willing to change his point of view.
- With regard to his mental health, he is of the opinion that medication does not help him. He does not know how he copes, but he feels he does. When discussing his diagnosis, he does not feel he has mental health problems.

Bob's future plans are to get married and have kids, to have a house and seek employment.

The plan

In the past, Bob has proved that although his life was chaotic, he has been able to self-care. In terms of vulnerability factors, Bob has a history of substance misuse and a diagnosis of mental illness. Clinically, it appears that he is doing well and is currently engaged in using escorted leave to go and work for a charitable animal welfare organisation.

Interestingly enough, although Bob does not agree that he has mental health problems, he has made attempts at completing an advance statement (Mandelstam 2009). In this, he highlights what would be the early warning signs of his becoming unwell, and has suggested what people should do. This is of some use when looking at providing opportunities for support on discharge.

A care plan for Bob would include the aim of moving to a council house or other accommodation with a garden. This would involve specifying what Bob "is aiming to achieve towards long-term goals" (Ryan and Morgan 2004b: 183). The latter could include Bob's application for accommodation; identifying what benefits and community support are available; and attending housing interviews. The care plan would also identify the roles of Bob and specific members, and deadline dates to achieve specific goals.

This is only an example of what could be done, and is a very broad care plan. Further detail would be needed when considering various components, such as risk assessment and crisis management plans (Department of Health 2007, 2008). What this plan does demonstrate, is that the focus is on Bob's aspirations. The challenge for the service is to operationalise the aspirations with Bob. There may still be areas for conflict: for example, regarding the need to stay on a medication regime. Earlier, this was raised as a potential barrier but is also something that can be negotiated (Healy 2010), since, in his advance statement, Bob did acknowledge the place for medication. It is important for the success of care planning that the service user is involved in goal setting. This has the potential to encourage ownership of the plan (Moore-Kirkland 1981). In terms of the CPA process, Bob will need to be introduced in advance to the persons who will be working with him once in the community. This would initially be raised in the reviews of his care plan. Clinical teams must not treat this process as a bureaucratic exercise, but rather as an opportunity to check where they are in the process of Bob's reintegration into the community (Ryan and Morgan 2004b).

Bearing in mind Bob's past life experiences, stigma is something that may always be in evidence (Morris 2006). However, this should not prevent Bob from attempting to realise his aspirations. The discharge process into the community is fraught with risk. However, the clinical team, in partnership with Bob, will need to take therapeutic risks. This is emphasised by Davidson et al (2006), who point out that some professionals see risk as a factor that inhibits the application of recovery principles. In relation to Bob, there is a number of risks that need to be addressed. These include the risk of absconding, and the risk of not being able to find someone who is prepared to allow Bob to engage in dog-walking and other animal care activities. The latter could be perceived by Bob as failure. The worker would have to prepare Bob for the various responses to his wish. With regard to absconding, this would have to be managed carefully by the clinical team. The team would have to undertake a risk assessment which would need to examine the history of prior absconding and the relationship that Bob has with the team (Department of Health 2007). Because of the circumstances surrounding Bob's admission, the Ministry of Justice would need to be involved and a plan of how the trips would be managed would have to be presented to them. One of the principles of positive risk taking is to examine the risk and look at how an activity can take place. Repper and Perkins (2003) explain that there comes a time when practitioners need to recognise the service user's skills and abilities; and that at times, risks need to be taken. In this case, the trip would have to be escorted; however, over a period of time, as the relationship improves and trust is developed, the role of the escort would diminish.

Conclusion

The journey for recovery can only be touched on in this chapter. The real question for the authors is how do we apply such principles in a secure setting? Mezey and Eastman (2009) discuss the difficulty that clinical teams and services users from secure settings are likely to experience when trying to engage in the social inclusion agenda. They highlight the issue of lack of choice and social stigma that may be experienced by the service user. Some of these barriers will come from historical and out-dated views of mental illness (Repper and Perkins 2003). Other barriers can come from clinical teams who are unwilling to take on patients who are ready for discharge from a forensic service because of concerns regarding perceived lack of compliance. This can occur even though the clinical team responsible for the patient concludes, based on risk assessment, that she/he is ready for discharge from the forensic service (Adshead and Sarkar 2005). This raises ethical issues related to ensuring justice to individuals and their right to be cared for within the minimum amount of security and restrictions commensurate with their assessed level of risk (Lester and Glasby 2006).

Health services tend to be underpinned by the ethical principle of beneficence: engaging in a process that is providing benefit for others. The duty of care is extended to a number of stakeholders: the service user, the carer, the survivors/victims of the patient's offence, and other members of the public, as well as professionals (Nursing and Midwifery Council 2008). If clinical teams, which include nurses, subscribe to the principles of beneficence, we have to think about how we can implement the values and principles of recovery and social inclusion within forensic and prison health services, whilst being true to our own professional values and beliefs (Aiyegbusi 2009). When individuals' liberty is taken away, there is the danger that they will lose hope as well. During the time that people are patients in secure hospitals and prison health services, service providers have the responsibility to provide opportunities for recovery from admission. This includes enabling each individual's fulfilment and empowerment, as much as is possible within a secure environment. This, in turn, can keep hope alive for the service user.

Acknowledgement

Thanks to Dr Michael Coffey for drawing Slade (2009) to our attention, and for copies of his review of this text.

References

Adshead G (2010) Ethical issues in secure care. In: Bartlett A, McGauley G (eds) *Forensic Mental Health. Concepts Systems and Practice*. Oxford University Press, Oxford

Adshead G, Sarkar SP (2005) Justice and welfare: Two ethical paradigms in forensic psychiatry. *Australian and New Zealand Journal of Psychiatry* 39: 1011–17

Aiyegbusi A (2009) The nurse–patient relationship with offenders: Containing the unthinkable to promote recovery. I: Aiyegbusi A, Clarke-Moore J (eds) *Therapeutic Relationships with Offenders. An Introduction to the Psychodynamics of Forensic Mental Health Nursing*. Jessica Kingsley, London

Aiyegbusi A, Clarke-Moore J (eds) (2009) *Therapeutic Relationships with Offenders. An Introduction to the Psychodynamics of Forensic Mental Health Nursing*. Jessica Kingsley, London

Allott P (2005) Recovery from "mental illness": One vision, many views. *A Life in the Day* 9(4): 4–8

Anthony WA (1993) Recovery from mental illness: The guiding vision of the mental health system in the 1990s. *Innovations and Research* 2(3): 17–24. Cited in: Norman I, Ryrie I (eds) *The Art and Science of Mental Health Nursing. A Textbook of Principles and Practice*. McGraw Hill Open University Press, Maidenhead

Bartlett A (2004) Fashions in psychiatric care: Implications for sense of self. In: Crisp AH, (ed) *Every Family in the Land: Understanding Prejudice and Discrimination Against People with Mental Illness*. Royal Society of Medicine Press, London

Bartlett A, McGauley G (2010) Introduction to the psychotherapies for mentally disordered offenders. In Bartlett A, McGauley G (eds) *Forensic Mental Health. Concepts Systems and Practice*. Oxford University Press, Oxford

Brooker C, Repper J (1998) *Serious Mental Health Problems in the Community. Policy, practice and research*. Bailliere Tindall, London

Byrt R (2008) Negative control or life saving? Perspectives on power. In: National Forensic Nurses' Research and Development Group: Kettles AM, Woods P, Byrt R (eds) *Forensic Mental Health Nursing: Capabilities Roles Responsibilities*. Quay Books MA Healthcare Ltd, London

Byrt R, Hart L, James-Sow L (2008) Patient empowerment and participation: Barriers and the way forward. In: National Forensic Nurses' Research and Development Group: Kettles AM, Woods P, Byrt R (eds) *Forensic Mental Health Nursing: Capabilities Roles Responsibilities*. Quay Books MA Healthcare Ltd, London

Campbell P (2001) The role of users of psychiatric services in service development – influence not power. *Psychiatric Bulletin* 25, 87–8. Cited in Repper J, Perkins R (2003) *Social Inclusion and Recovery*. Bailliere Tindall, Edinburgh

Crichton J, Sheppard D (1996) Psychiatric inquiries: Learning the lessons. In: Peay J (ed) *Inquiries After Homicide*. Duckworth, London

Darzi A (2007) *Our NHS, Our Future. NHS Next Stage Review. Interim Report*. Department of Health, London

Davidson L, O'Connell M, Tondora J, Styron T, Kangas K (2006) The top ten concerns encountered in mental health system transformation. *Psychiatric Services* 57(5): 640–5

Department of Health (1990) Guidance on the Care Programme Approach. HC (90) 23. Department of Health London.

Department of. Health (1999a) *Effective Care Coordination*. Department of Health, London

Department of Health (1999b) The *National Service Framework for Mental Health*. Department of Health, London

Department of Health (2002*) The NHS Plan***.** Department of Health, London

Department of Health (2004) *The National Service Framework for Mental Health. Five Years On*. Department of Health London

Department of Health (2006a) *Our Health Our Care Our Say*. Department of Health, London

Department of Health (2006b) *From Values to Action: The Chief Nursing Officer review of mental health nursing*. Department of Health, London

Department of Health (2007) *Best Practice in Managing Risk*. Department of Health, London

Department of Health (2008) *Refocusing the Care Programme Approach. Policy and Positive Practice Guidance*. Department of Health, London

Fawcett B, Karban K (2005) *Contemporary Mental Health: Theory Policy and Practice*.

Routledge Taylor and Francis Group, London

Frak D (2005) *Recovery Learning*. Rethink, London

Fulford KWM (2004) Facts/values: Ten principles of values-based medicine. In: Radden J (ed) *The Philosophy of Psychiatry: A Companion*. Oxford University Press, Oxford

Gamble C, Ryrie N, Curthoys J (2009) Psychosocial interventions. In: Norman I, Ryrie I (eds) *The Art and Science of Mental Health Nursing. A Textbook of Principles and Practice*. McGraw Hill Open University Press, Maidenhead

Harner HM (2004) Relationships between incarcerated women. Moving beyond stereotypes. *Journal of Psychosocial Nursing and Mental Health Services* 42(1): 38–46

Healy D (2010) *Psychiatric Drugs Explained* (5th edn). Elsevier Churchill Livingstone Edinburgh

Helm A (2009) Recovery and reclamation: A pilgrimage in understanding who and what we are. In: Barker P (ed) *Psychiatric and Mental Health Nursing: The Craft of Caring*. Arnold, London

HM Government (2009) *New Horizons: A Shared Vision for Mental Health*. Department of Health, London

HM Government. (2010) *New Horizons. Confident Communities Brighter Futures*. Department of Health, London

Jeffcote N, Watson T (eds) (2004) *Working Therapeutically with Women in Secure Settings*. Jessica Kingsley, London

Jones K (1993) *Asylums and After: A Revised History of the Mental Health Services: From the Early Eighteenth Century to the Nineteen Nineties*. The Athlone Press, London

Kant I (1969) *The Moral Law: Kant's Groundwork of the Metaphysics of Morals*. Hutchinson, London (Translated by Paton HJ; First published 1785) Cited in: Thompson IE, Melia KM, Boyd KM, Horsburgh D (eds) (2006) *Nursing Ethics* (5th edn). Churchill Livingstone/Elsevier, Edinburgh

Kisthardt WE (1992) The strengths model of case management: The principles and functions of a helping partnership with persons with persistent mental illness. In: Saleeby D (ed) *A Strengths Perspective for Social Work Practice*. Longman, New York. Cited in: Ryan P, Morgan S (2004) Care planning and care coordination. In: Ryan P, Morgan S (eds) *Assertive Outreach*. Churchill Livingstone, Edinburgh

Lester H, Glasby J (2006) *Mental Health Policy and Practice*. Palgrave Macmillan, Basingstoke

Mandelstam M (2009) *Safeguarding Vulnerable Adults and the Law*. Jessica Kingsley Publishers London

Maslow A (1970) *Motivation and Personality* (2nd edn). Harper and Row, New York. Cited in Brooker C, Repper J (1998) *Serious Mental Health Problems in the Community. Policy, practice and research*. Bailliere Tindall, London

Mental Health Commission New Zealand (2001) *Recovery Competencies for New Zealand Mental Health Worker*. Mental Health Commission New Zealand, Wellington

Mezey G, Eastman N (2009) Choice and social inclusion in forensic psychiatry: Acknowledging mixed messages and double think. *Journal of Forensic Psychiatry and Psychology* 20(4): 503–7

Moore-Kirkland J (1981) Mobilising motivation: From theory to practice. In: Maluccio A (ed) *Promoting Competence in Clients*. New York Free Press, New York. Cited in: Ryan P, Morgan S (2004) Care planning and care coordination. In: Ryan P, Morgan S (eds) *Assertive Outreach*. Churchill Livingstone, Edinburgh

Morgan S, Akbar-Khan S (2000) Individual care planning in the UK. In: Bassett T (ed) *Looking to the Future: Key Issues for Contemporary Mental Health Services*. Pavilion/Mental Health Foundation, Brighton. Cited in: Ryan P, Morgan S (2004) Care planning and care coordination. In: Ryan P, Morgan S (eds) *Assertive Outreach*. Churchill Livingstone, Edinburgh.

Morgan S, Ryan P (2004) Using psychosocial interventions with the service user. In: Ryan P, Morgan S (eds) *Assertive Outreach*. Churchill Livingstone, Edinburgh.

Morris G (2006) *Mental Health Issues and the Media: An Introduction for Mental Health Professionals*. Routledge Taylor and Francis Group, London

National Institute for Mental Health in England (2005) NIMHE Guiding Statement on Recovery. London. Department of Health. Cited in: Watkins P (2007) *Recovery. A Guide for Mental Health Practitioners*. Churchill Livingstone, Edinburgh

Nursing and Midwifery Council (2008) *The Code: Standards of Conduct Performance and Ethics for Nurses and Midwives*. Nursing and Midwifery Council, London

Perkins R, Repper J (2009) Recovery and social inclusion. In: Norman I, Ryrie I (eds) *The Art and Science of Mental Health Nursing. A Textbook of Principles and Practice* (2nd edn). McGraw Hill Open University Press, Maidenhead

President's New Freedom Commission on Mental Health (2002) *Final Report to the President*. Cited in: Davidson L, O'Connell M, Tondora J, Styron T, Kangas K (2006) The top ten concerns encountered in mental health system transformation. *Psychiatric Services* 57(5): 640–5

Repper J, Perkins R (2003) *Social Inclusion and Recovery*. Bailliere Tindall, Edinburgh

Rose N (1986) Law, rights and psychiatry. In: Miller P, Rose N (eds) *The Power of Psychiatry*. Polity Press, Cambridge, in association with Basil Blackwell, Oxford. Cited in: Crichton J, Sheppard D (1996) Psychiatric Inquiries: Learning the Lessons. In: Peay J (ed) *Inquiries After Homicide*. Duckworth, London

Ryan P, Morgan S (2004a) Strengths assessment. In: Ryan P, Morgan S (eds) *Assertive Outreach*. Churchill Livingstone, Edinburgh

Ryan P, Morgan S (2004b) Care planning and care coordination. In: Ryan P, Morgan S (eds) *Assertive Outreach*. Churchill Livingstone, Edinburgh.

Sainsbury Centre for Mental Health (2004) *The Ten Essential Shared Capabilities: A framework for the whole of the mental health workforce*. NIMHE and Sainsbury Centre for Mental Health, London

Slade M (2009) *Personal Recovery and Mental Illness: A Guide for Mental Health Professionals*. Cambridge University Press, Cambridge

Stickley T (2005) Developing a social inclusion strategy for people with ongoing mental health problems. *Mental Health Practice* 8(6): 12–15

Tew J (ed) (2005) *Social Perspectives in Mental Health: Developing Social Models to Understand and Work with Mental Distress*. Jessica Kingsley, London

Thornicroft G, Szmukler G (eds) (2001) *Textbook of Community Psychiatry*. Oxford University Press, Oxford

Watkins P (2007) *Recovery. A Guide for Mental Health Practitioners*. Churchill Livingstone, Edinburgh

Whitehill I (2009) Recovery: A personal perspective. In: Barker P (ed) *Psychiatric and Mental Health Nursing: The Craft of Caring*. Arnold, London

CHAPTER 24:

"Boots and saddles" My experience as a special hospital patient

"Billy B"

"Boots and saddles" called the nurse, and we knew it was time for us to exercise in the airing court. This is an account of my experience, from the early 1980s, as a former patient in three maximum security hospitals and related ethical and legal issues. Maximum security hospitals used to be called special hospitals, and this term will be used in this chapter.

In the olden days in special hospitals, physical control was ethically wrong, but it worked. Staff ran a tight ship. There was the threat of physical violence: some patients witnessed it; others were subjected to it. However, most people never or rarely saw the violence, although they knew it happened. It was never on public display. During my time in three special hospitals, the existence of a specific ward was a deterrent and staff were quick to send people there. Physical intervention replaced talking therapies up to a point.

Rule by fear

You can get used to being a patient in a special hospital. In the mid-1990s, I lived in a 22-bedded dormitory with no privacy and no comforts. But patients and staff became conditioned into accepting it. The ethics were like a public school: you didn't cause them hassle, and they didn't cause you hassle. In my first special hospital in the 1980s, staff were of the old school, and you got punished if you did anything wrong. I used to refer to it as a "psychiatric borstal". There was a work ethic: keeping the place clean through polishing the floor, and a rule by fear: there was a threat of something happening if you didn't behave. Staff wore white coats and there was a distance between staff and patients. But this wasn't 100%. Surprisingly, charge nurses had a more mature outlook. They would sit and watch telly and read the papers with patients, but the nursing assistants were more heavy-handed; they did the kickings, literally. The scariest moment I recall was when someone went off, and the nursing assistants dragged him into a room. You could hear what was going on. It was very scary. The man was crying for his mother. They were beating him up. I used to talk to a patient who had suffered this treatment, who said that a staff member had said, "We all get frayed tempers occasionally."

In my first special hospital, you were told to call staff "Sir" or "Mister". In this hospital, there were no women staff on male wards until the 1990s, compared with another special hospital where this had been the case since the 1960s. In my first special hospital in the 1980s, there were no legal people at all. The aim was mostly to police the hospital, to make sure everything was intact. There was no therapeutic work. Prayers were compulsory; you had to do that.

One thing I remember about my first special hospital is floor scrubbing duties. We all knelt in the corridor with buckets and scrubbers. On one occasion, I looked up and saw this row of patients scrubbing, to-ing and fro-ing in unison, with a nursing assistant going up and down to ensure we were doing it. It was to keep the patient in a vulnerable position, to make it easier to give them a kicking. I used to hear staff saying, in relation to patients' offences: "Don't sit near him, he'll set fire"; "he'll stab you". The nursing assistants were egged on in this way by the trained staff, who realised that nursing assistants were just doing the job for the money.

Running a tight ship

My first special hospital was run according to the ethics of the 1950s and 1960s. Someone once told me that a lot of nurses were from a military background. They were not all bad: they ran a tight ship. What got people discharged was fear. It would be reported: "He conforms to everything" or "No management problem". This was not surprising because of patients' fear. So fear does work up to a point, even if it's unethical. The staff could claim they got results. People suppressed their symptoms because of their fear. If you got into that, you'd accept that was the norm: the cold painted corridors, no carpets, "Yes, Sir, no, Sir". Everyone was conditioned. For staff, that was how things were, and the patients accepted it. Twenty-five patients were showered at a time. In one special hospital, "boots and saddles" referred to getting ready for the courtyard. The nurses who'd been in the armed forces had a policing role which patients accepted, but they'd look after you: feed and water you; make sure the wards were heated at the right temperature. Even though you were banged up, it was compassionate because of an institutional feeling that they were looking after you.

There was a school element to the special hospitals. When I smell food, even here in the medium secure unit where I'm now a patient, I'm reminded of the institutional times of meals: at eight, midday and five, always fish on Fridays. There are lots of similarities between boarding school and high security hospitals, although a public school doesn't need a wall round it. Another similarity to school was education and learning. Education gives people in institutions an opportunity physically and mentally to stretch themselves, and this never stops.

In my first special hospital, patients were not allowed to have emotions: they were a punishable offence. This hospital ran such a tight ship, they only needed a small intensive care ward. The security was amazingly high. You were strip searched every day, and searched every time you went anywhere. The security fed into the idea, "You must watch him." I heard a nurse say to a student nurse: "You can't trust a mental patient. You never know what they're going to do." But you can't trust everybody.

"Can I have a kicking for Christmas?"

A kicking was the best thing, because you were elevated if you said nothing: then your quality of life improved. You were paid for your silence. There was a gang culture, where you knew the kicking existed. If you kept it under wraps, you had your reward: you were moved to a better ward. The patients kept quiet, because they didn't want to suffer the same fate: to be kicked to death. And staff, as well, could be complicit with each other. It's amazing how you can accept things that are unethical, and see them as normal behaviour. You accept that the people who are lower down the hierarchical system will get a slap; you accept that the staff will make the decisions about your care.

I've sometimes wondered if staff behaved as they did, kicking patients, because they deserved it because of their crimes. It's similar with nursing notes. Two things seem to have changed. The brutalisation of some patients became less when female staff started working on male wards. The other factor is that more people were watching, and there was nowhere to take people for a kicking. Also, there are now more legal people: different bodies like the Mental Health Act Commission (now part of the Care Quality Commission 2010), and visiting advocacy groups, so the opportunity for unethical behaviour has been reduced. In addition, there may be better ethical nursing practice. And there's less nepotism with things being kept in the family. At one time many nurses were related to other staff in the hospital, there was a "You don't grass on Uncle Joe", sort of attitude.

"Can I have a kicking for Christmas?" a patient once said in jest. This was almost an acceptance: a reminder of how both patients accepted the kicking, and staff were prepared to give it. However, I never received a kicking.

Therapy didn't exist in the 1980s. Medication and group work existed, as did the "electric breakfast" (electroconvulsive therapy or ECT). Another special hospital, to which I was transferred, was very liberal. But in all three special hospitals, there was bad treatment: what you're dealing with is a policing ethic. The staff were conditioned from day one: "You don't tell them this"; "You lock that...because these are nasty buggers". It suppresses a natural relationship. You're friendless, because they can't tell you where they've been on holiday.

A relaxed and laid back approach

In my second special hospital, there was a massive wall. There was exterior security, but internally, it was not as secure as my first special hospital. The time I was there, they didn't do a "pat down search" in visits or at other times, so alcohol was brought into the hospital. A patient offered me a pina colada. He saw my disbelief. That's how lax it was in the mid-1980s. Patients could keep alcohol as there were no room searches. People demonstrated symptoms of mental illness, but there was a relaxed and laid back approach. It was a holiday camp. We strolled off to the canteen; the staff consulted you about the television and videos; staff wore civilian clothing; patients called staff by their first name and vice versa. There were en-suite baths and showers in patients' rooms. There was a trading ethic, to a greater extent than in my first special hospital, and some patients would sell anything in their room.

In a therapeutic community in one special hospital, the patients saw themselves as an elite. They wore gold chains, flashy clothes, and never spoke to other patients. There was a hierarchical system, as there was in other wards. Some patients held sway, and others were picked on. In all the wards I've been on, except in my first special hospital, the hierarchical structure was based on patients' strength of personality, not money. Generally, people with personality disorders were top of the tree. They could shout the loudest, and sought out the movers and shakers amongst those staff who mirrored their behaviour. These patients made the staff drinks, got them to allow particular television programmes and various favours.

There have been times when I've had to work out how to keep fit physically. They openly discouraged it in one special hospital. There was no gym, and exercise had to be done secretly. You had to work in bricklaying or gardening in order to get exercise. Staff said, "We can't have patients physically or mentally fitter than us."

Comfort in institutions

I wonder if institutions can sometimes become comforting, reassuring. Even if you got a kicking, you knew you could always have a Christmas, with gifts, and not be lonely. You had a shop in the hospital, no bills to pay, you knew you were fed: a true nanny state. Each staff member was in the same comfort zone: perks and fiddles, a secure job in a recession. The culture of institutionalisation permeates both patients and staff to some extent, which is why staff work in the same institution for 40-odd years. Institutionalisation is insidious, and affects both patients and staff to the same level. The "us and them" culture is not necessarily a bad thing. It means both parties can co-exist. Maybe staff don't always remind themselves of people's crimes. Through social interaction, they do not see someone as a patient; they see him/her as just a person. I've experienced it where staff, in relation to their security role, say to patients, "Nothing personal"; and patients say, "Yes, my offence has nothing to do with staff. It's in the past."

In one special hospital, we smuggled in food and had feasts at night, just like in a boarding school. The staff turned a blind eye. When they "patted us down", they ignored cakes and biscuits. Being human, they wanted an easy life too. They didn't rock your boat if you didn't rock theirs. Once when a meal was being served on a ward, I requested chicken. There was one portion of chicken left, but I was told there wasn't any. I realised it was for the staff, so I chose the other option. You knew what "There's no chicken" meant.

People once said: "How can you get used to the bars?" But the bars on the windows don't represent punishment or authority; they're only bars. I didn't see them as a suppressive instrument. Because, over time, I got used to them. But I've thought: yes, I can see how they work to suppress people. I used to count the layers of paint on bars that were chipped away and repainted. But they were not a threat to my freedom. Doctors and tribunals were a greater threat. However, I saw special hospitals as places of comfort, familiarity and structure. Although I thought it was ridiculous having meals at eight, midday and five, there was a comfort element to this.

I do wonder if institutionalisation encouraged the creation of this sort of comfort, so that the mind would be less ravaged and would fit into it. If you remove the stresses, it becomes home, somewhere you want to be. People from outside, visitors, seem shocked at the vile kinds of crime that patients have committed, and ask, "Why doesn't he/she commit the same crime inside?", "Why don't the patients throw the snooker balls?", etc. But they don't because of the structure and what becomes a holding environment (Aiyegbusi and Clarke-Moore 2009) where pressures don't exist.

One private medium secure unit has a very low fence, no cameras and a very relaxed attitude to security. They've created a "gilded cage" environment, where no-one wants to leave. Patients and staff eat together, and there are amazing choices. People I've known stay there 10 years. If an institution has a swimming pool and a golf course, patients are there for a long time. But if there's nothing, no facilities, patients are generally there a short time. People refuse to go from this "gilded cage" medium secure unit to hostels because their lives in the latter are not as good. If you give people everything they would like: enough money, a good quality of life, tuck in bed at night, who would want to leave? It's like in the armed forces' song "Kiss Me Good Night, Sergeant Major" (Pelosi and Noel 1939), which took the mickey out of the Army. One patient used to sing the following song at one high security hospital. It went:

Red brick asylums are the best.
Doo dah, doo dah.
Red brick asylums are the best.
Oh the doo dah day.

Scrubs the floors all night,
And scrubs the floor all day.
Red brick asylums are the best.
Oh the doo dah day.

(Anon, undated. The Editors acknowledge the unknown author of this song)

The water's evaporated off the soap

The above song is an example of conditioning to being in a special hospital: a way of coping. You wouldn't sing it when cleaning the corridors. But it was subversive, it got you through the game. I was a bit subversive. I didn't agree with polishing the floor. I was once asked to clean the dormitory loo, but all I did was stand and look at my watch, and I came out and looked busy when I had done nothing. Eventually, the nurse sussed it out.

He said "Did you clean that toilet? Why is that soap dry?"

"The water's evaporated off the soap," I replied.

But saying all this, I had lots of happy times, even in my first special hospital, despite the swearing and the mental cruelty. Although this was psychological abuse, I got the impression that some nurses were testing us to see how we would respond. Some staff were abusive. But the main thing was to have a happy family. If you were seen as non-aggressive and toed the line, if you weren't anti-system and, generally speaking, not a threat to the general public, you could be in a group of patients who'd direct and act in a play. This was a pretty major therapeutic thing: a comfortable sociableness. I never went into tribunals in a strong way because of the positive aspects of the hospital: the drama group, education. These were good things.

I think patients come to an acceptance of the institution's rules. Once it becomes a norm, it's not a problem. It reduces patients' identification of the lack of freedom because it's replaced by other things. They give you a world, with opportunity for relationships, work, socialising, a relative type of home life, but have separated you from the outside world. However, you were never lonely ever, and you developed your routines and rules, just like people in a street. I'd be surprised to see how many people would leg it if the walls came down because they'd be running from a comfort zone. The ones who did escape were all tall, wiry people, with athletic build, like long-distance runners. And all, without exception, were anti-institution, which urged them not to be there. They didn't buy into the comfort zone, and had a burning hatred of what was around them.

One man who escaped from a special hospital had certain political and anti-institutional beliefs. The institution couldn't get through to him, and staff protected themselves from him. This patient exerted power and control; he came up with all sorts of reasons for resisting staff. He made himself politically unpopular: his threat to the institution was political. A former manager of the hospital made links with other agencies to help him get what he wanted. Such patients, who are immune to the institution, are very rare. For most of us, the comfort zone erodes our independence, with the provision of things which some patients have never had as children. However, certain individuals don't want to admit their dependence on comforts, and make complaints as a sort of smoke screen.

Social environments and their demise

In the main, most patients are affected by comfort aspects of the institution. When one special hospital stopped its social programme (discos and recreation) there was the loss of the comfort zone and it became more prison-like. When the pre-discharge ward closed, this removed the gentlemen's club and the status patients had, and dismantled our reason for being there. We no longer wanted to stay.

In one special hospital, many patients were transferred to other organisations such as medium secure units. Special hospitals can appear to be awful institutions. However, a lot of people didn't really want to leave, but it was organised for them to do so. Social environments were dismantled because many patients left, including, in two hospitals, all the women. In addition, security increased, and it was more difficult to provide some facilities when there were fewer patients. Field, sports and gym facilities were reduced.

The hospital's patients with personality disorder or psychopathy helped create a social environment. Each ward for these people had a patient on a committee who promoted this. These wards were more relaxed, but the staff tightened up on wards for patients with a mental illness. On a ward I was on, we all followed the rules to get more comfort items. Important rules were adhered to because no-one wanted to rock the boat. But you sailed on an even keel. Staff knew minor rules were broken, but turned a blind eye. And you had events on the ward passed by senior staff. Visitors came to events during Christmas, Easter and over the summer, and there were relatives' parties. We saw ourselves as a bit above the other patients. There was always something to live for. Of course you said, "I don't want to be here", but in reality, you had reasons to stay. Patients would organise social events, raise money for a good Christmas with food, goodies, etc. As Chair of an organising committee, the staff gave me an allowance for this.

Patients' use of power

Although there were power struggles with staff, with shouting at times, if you could convince them they were right, doors would open. This was the patients' use of power. Staff would sometimes turn a blind eye to what patients did. For example, if I wanted one particular nurse to make a phone call for me (e.g. about whether a patient on another ward was going to a social event), he would do this instantly if I gave him a can of coke. Whereas usually, staff took their time, frustratingly saying, "Wait a minute". But the coke meant that this particular nurse made a phone call instantly: it was value for money. I had some power there: I wanted a phone call made, he wanted a coke. To me, it was highly efficient; it worked. There's a "blind eye" thing, "I'll do this if you give me that". The staff think, "You don't rock our boat, we'll think about not rocking yours."

In one special hospital, there was brutality at one end of the scale on some wards, and at the other extreme, a gentlemen's club. There were only two staff to 100 patients. You chose the good or the bad route. Patients called the refractory block the "punishment block". You were admitted to a really bad ward, and worked your way up; and then you went to the general population of the hospital. But at the other extreme, you could have parole from eight in the morning to eight at night, and the gentlemen's club. In learning disability services, "high grades" and "low grades" were treated differently. It was a world of extremes, but this is no longer the case.

Peter Taylor, who became Chair of the Matthew Trust (Matthew Trust 2010, Thompson 1972), advised that when you go outside the hospital, only tell the people who need to know about the past because of stigmatisation. He also said whatever you do in the special hospital, such as hobbies, continue with them outside because then you've got some sort of connection, an anchor, something to do outside.

Charge nurses could control power in relation to patients. One patient said, "People only get beaten up if they deserve it." But that form of power abuse is kept low profile. Even so, I can't believe that managers in charge of these abusers didn't know. If abuse becomes too obvious, staff jobs are on the line.

Lawyers' involvement in secure hospitals

Nurses and lawyers are bound by different ethics: nurses by professional and work ethics; lawyers by legal ethics, like knights in shining armour. Patients are bound by institutional ethics. When I was first in a special hospital, we accepted bad behaviour from staff, as staff did from us, and then, later, lawyers came along and questioned it. Staff saw lawyers as an enemy: someone to check them out.

Legal and ethical aspects are interwoven. In my experience, the legal people see it as their ethical right to involve themselves with the welfare of patients in secure hospitals; but morally, the nurses who work there see it as unnecessary to what they're doing. Lawyers' involvement can be seen as a thorn in the side of the therapy. Mental health professionals and legal professionals have different motives. It's almost like political correctness. Maybe sometimes a patient can be distracted and torn between the therapy and legal issues. A solicitor might say, "We can get you discharged", and you can get wrapped up in that, and believe that this is in your best interests. Solicitors want to get people out because they think the mental health staff are *not* doing their job. Whereas mental health professionals want to get people out because they *are* doing their job. Solicitors and mental health professionals are not necessarily singing from the same hymn sheet. They use different language.

I enjoy seeing lawyers hammer doctors at tribunals. I think the patient sees it as a battle: the legal white knight rescuing the patient from the bad hospital. Solicitors sometimes see nurses as gaolers. Patients get used to the keys, but the legal people see them as oppressive. I've come from the days when tribunals were not automatic. But with the 1983 Mental Health Act, they were. Lawyers didn't have a say, didn't exist when I was admitted to high secure hospitals in the early 1980s.

Us and them

There was an "us and them" thing in the special hospitals. Nurses created this by means of security, anonymity and limiting information that patients needed. "Us and them" was inevitable. It existed, not as an authoritarian approach, but was probably necessary because of the environment. It created an ethical gulf between patients and staff: more of a prison-style milieu. There were therapies, but in my early days in special hospitals, the nurses did not pursue therapeutic interventions. But there was token economy and privileges. It was mainly about good behaviour, which meant you could progress from a 22-bedded dormitory to a single room. Once you were in a single room, there was pressure to maintain good behaviour, to not break rules; and a risk of becoming an informant to staff.

The institution, rather than the patients, creates an "us and them" environment. But how far does the institution itself, or staff, managers and the training provided contribute to this? From a patient's point of view, "us and them" is indicated partly by rules and regulations and partly by over-policing.

I firmly believe staff create a climate of 'us and them', mainly because staff read patients' notes and because of their attitudes. Patients are stigmatised and traumatised by staff. The opportunity to stigmatise people is there. OK, they're trained to shut out stigmatising thoughts, but they're only human. And the emphasis on secrecy is negative: "You must not give information about your private life because patients will misuse it." I can understand the reasons, but the outcome is that it develops an "us and them" situation and "personality disorder" and "mental illness" labels. And staff are influenced by how they've been brought up and, for example, by films like *Psycho, Marnie, Vertigo,* and *One Flew Over the Cuckoo's Nest* (Byrt with Dooher 2006, Wedding and Boyd 1999).

In addition, patients may self-stigmatise; they may feel unworthy, or labelled "bad" or "ill", and this creates a barrier. From a patient point of view, it's how the "us and them" can show itself through antagonism. In the past, "us and them" was created through staff beating patients up; and from staff uniforms of white coats and black ties. And also, from what staff said, "Don't sit next to him, he'll set fire to you", or if there was a patient who was on the news. "There he is, you sat next to him." Barriers between patients and staff were created by making us clean and polish as part of a Victorian ethic. With that ethic came brutality because of dehumanisation. When a group of people are polishing the corridor, and staff are walking up and down, it's bound to create more remoteness. "Us and them" showed itself in brutality, dehumanisation, a morbid sense of humour and putdowns. But patients and staff grew to accept the culture. Patients could get good reports and the culture of remoteness gave few opportunities to do things wrong.

I've experienced being lined up naked with other patients to go to our rooms at night. Our mouths, hands and feet were checked, then we'd enter our rooms and have our pyjamas thrown after us. There was no "Good night" from staff; we would step into our rooms in silence. The nurses slammed the door shut, a bolt was thrown and the spy hole opened. At Christmas time, they would say, "Merry f***ing Christmas", and walk away.

However, a lot of staff wanted to make Christmases good. My experience is that the vast majority of staff were quite good, and a small percentage were very bad. When I was first in a special hospital, some staff found it easier to be nasty, but the majority would bring professional and family values into their work.

Patient and staff power

There were varying amounts of power amongst patients in the special hospitals. For example, in a learning disability service, the term "low grade" indicated no power and those designated "high grade" had the most power. In another special hospital, "psychopaths" were seen as having more freedom and responsibilities, and individuals with "mental illness" as having less freedom. In a ward for people with personality disorders, there were patients who ruled by personality. Other patients ruled by physique and physical presence.

Staff always had complete power, and protected their interests. You wouldn't mess staff about. In certain circumstances, you'd curry favour with staff: you wouldn't go out of your way to upset them. With some staff in the past, there was the power of the boot: "Black pills or Dr Martin." I prefer the power of the boot to the power of the pen because the latter has longer-lasting effects, and there's nothing personal about the power of the boot.

How power is wielded and displayed depends on personality. In addition, patients are at the lowest end of the power system because we vary in personality factors which influence how much power we have. In one special hospital ward, there were breaches of security, but these were allowed to happen because the power balance between staff and patients was changed slightly. There was less power for staff, and a bit more for patients. In a therapeutic community, there was a relaxation of rules to enable trust, so this resulted in a shift in power. However, some patients saw it as a reason to escalate their own power needs, and staff were eventually "used" by patients. It was seen by some people as going too far. The old adage, "The lunatics have taken over the asylum" can apply. Whereas, if power structures are fairly rigid, and everyone knows where they stand, it keeps everyone in line. When charge nurses had more power, things were done far quicker.

What I don't understand is how, in one special hospital where patients were allowed a large amount of freedom, the power was abused. But in another special hospital, the gentlemen's club flourished under the same amount of power. Eventually, this hospital had an independent living unit which was freer than some low secure units, but there was no abuse of power.

Informants

Is it ethically right to use informants? Where there are locks and bars and physical security, there are inevitably going to be patients who are recruited to act as informers, which means that a small group of patients have power over larger groups of their peers. The use of informants is inevitable. Is it appropriate for patients to be informants to staff in return for favours? It may help staff to have a wider view, but is it ethical? A nurse once said, "We don't call them informants, but helpers."

There are many reasons why patients decide to become informants. One patient's religious conviction drove him to report things because he saw it as the righteous point of view. Other patients had malicious intent: knowingly going out of their way to make mayhem for people. On the mental illness side, patients acted as informants as a manifestation of symptoms of their illness. Other people informed for reasons of personal gain, or to play one person off against another. Then there's the professional informant: the person who knows how to do it. He/she gains information by befriending people, which may be encouraged by staff. This was the main system of information gathering when I was a patient. Some patients are encouraged to report on their peers: "It's good for all of us to share information." Here, informing is seen as therapeutic. An example is Chamberlin's (1988) report that residents in a therapeutic community in which she was involved were encouraged to "rat" on each other. Some patients inform on others because of a mixture of some or all of the above reasons.

In therapeutic communities, does acting as an informant stem from patients' interpretation of how they see their role? How ethical is this? From my experience, the more severe and secure the environment, the less need there is for informants. I found that in my first special hospital, staff had control over things, a constant presence. Using fear kept patients in check, so staff could report that there was "no management problem". Fear was ethically wrong, but kept people in special hospitals for a shorter time, and there was less use of informants.

Everywhere where there is intensive care, there is a danger of malpractice. Staff may be required (e.g. because of an institutional culture and colleagues' expectations) to be heavy-handed, with the risk of straying beyond acceptable limits. Volatile patients may meet hard resistance, hard restraints. There may appear to be a need for meaty, muscular, no-nonsense, heavy-handed staff, but authoritarian attitudes and communication result in patients being seen only as a challenge (Morrison 1992, Ford et al 2010).

In my first special hospital, fear won in terms of results. Fear was so strong in those days, that there was a very small intensive care ward. The other wards were intimidating. This was unethical, but gave results. Where there was a freer, less authoritarian environment, you had more informants who were used more often. It was risk management by stealth because of the high degree of using informants. Is this ethical, and is the information gained accurate? There were situations where informants eavesdropped on patient exchanges.

If a hospital is very secure, you don't need information via informants. If it is less secure, you get more information by finding various ways of gaining it. If there is physical security, why would a patient want to give information to people locking him/her up?

If we look at secure services today, where we try to be as ethical as possible, informants are used more. Staff maintain an authoritative, powerful position. A number of questions need to be asked: Are informants used and abused? Do they feel they're being used to operate the system? Is there a weakness in nursing staff's need to use informants? I'm referring mainly to maximum secure hospitals (formerly special hospitals), but what I'm writing applies to all forensic services.

Power and staff records

Nursing evaluations can become a potential abuse of power. One thing that has changed is that brutality has been replaced by the pen. Instead of a kicking, you get a bad report in your record. It's gone from a physical to an intellectual approach. "He came to me today, and told me to f***-off, then saw the error of his ways." In the old days, a patient would have got kicked. I'd prefer a slap to having stuff reported. A nurse in one special hospital said: "If we lose the argument, there's always the notes.".You can see the venom in the wording. How do you police the nursing notes? If the nurses are in a bad mood, they're going to write in the notes.

Staff can exert power over patients through their records about them. It is crucial that nurses have the ability to be aware of the power they have; the capacity to use that power wisely; and to recognise and reflect on their possible abuses of power (Nursing and Midwifery Council 2002, 2008).

Nursing staff operate psychological games by getting people to change. We're told, "You must learn by this," but I've never known a nurse thank me if the errors of their ways are pointed out by advocacy. They see it as effrontery, they don't accept it. They wonder why patients are complaining. It's okay for nurses to challenge patients' behaviour, but not vice versa.

Some staff feel that everything that patients say or do must be recorded. They may feel they must take their training literally, and see psychopathy in every word and action. It would be nice for nurses to know that we're intelligent too. They may feel we don't get it, but we do.

Staff testing patients

I'd like to know if there's a proper name for "testing". It's rare to come across a member of staff who says, "Yes, we mess about occasionally to see if patients can cope" or "We test if patients are in touch with emotions to see if groups work." But staff would shoot themselves in the foot if they admitted this because people would be on the watch for such testing.

There's always been this thing of staff testing patients. Some staff used to test patients by frustrating them, by not responding to their requests, unlike the nurse (previously described) who, if you gave him a coke, would do what you wanted immediately.

There is a range of psychological evaluations (tests) which staff are good at; and some that they are clearly not good at. Usually, these tests are designed to stretch patients in particular directions. There are certain ways that staff have of saying "No", e.g. some nurses will delay something to see how patients will respond. They may delay putting a key in a lock. Staff might say a letter has not arrived when it's in front of them.

I can't prove it, but is it ethical for staff to use their personality as a form of testing of patients? Does it tell staff anything? And does it actually work? But what better way of seeing how a patient would react than by testing him/her by pushing a few buttons. However, nurses' views may vary on whether or not testing patients is ethical.

Staff testing patients out can be viewed within the regime of power and control, the nature of which may encourage the consideration of various options, as with the police, in order to get results. But is it ethically right, for purposes of risk evaluation, to get better results by testing patients? This is something student nurses could be asked to consider.

References

Aiyegbusi A, Clarke-Moore J (eds) (2009) *Therapeutic Relationships with Offenders. An Introduction to the Psychodynamics of Forensic Mental Health Nursing*. Jessica Kingsley, London

Byrt R with Dooher J (2006) The social consequences of a personality disorder diagnosis. In: National Forensic Nurses' Research and Development Group: Woods P, Kettles AM, Byrt R, Addo M, Aiyegbusi A, Coffey M, Collins M, Doyle M, Garman G, Watson C (eds) *Forensic Mental Health Nursing: Interventions with People with 'Personality Disorder'*. Quay Books MA Healthcare Ltd, London

Care Quality Commission (2010) Available from: www.cqc.org.uk [Last accessed 16 May 2010]

Chamberlin J (1988) *On Our Own. Patient Controlled Alternatives in the Mental Health System*. MIND Publications, London

Ford K, Byrt R, Dooher J (2010) *Preventing and Reducing Aggression and Violence in Health and Social Care: A Holistic Approach*. MK Publishing, Keswick

Matthew Trust (2010) Available from: www.matthewtrust.org/index.htm [Last accessed 16 May 2010]

Morrison EF (1992) A coercive interactional style as an antecedent to aggression in psychiatric patients. *Research in Nursing and Health* **15**: 421–31

Nursing and Midwifery Council (2002) *Client-Practitioner Relationships and the Prevention of Abuse*. Nursing and Midwifery Council, London.

Nursing and Midwifery Council (2008) *The Code: Standards of Conduct Performance and*

Ethics for Nurses and Midwives. Nursing and Midwifery Council, London

Pelosi A, Noel A (1939) *Kiss Me Goodnight Sergeant Major*. Song. Available from: www.Answers.com [Last accessed 20 May 2010]

Thompson P (1972) *Bound for Broadmoor.* Hodder and Stoughton, London

Wedding D, Boyd MA (1999) *Movies and Mental Illness. Using Films to Understand Psychopathology.* McGraw-Hill, Boston

CHAPTER 25

How to prevent abuse in secure hospitals

Richard Byrt and "Billy B"

How can the abusive practices, described by "Billy B" in the last chapter, be prevented? This chapter considers this question, and some of the ethical implications of Billy B's narrative. There are many explanations for the perpetration of abuse in high security hospitals and other institutions, as reported by Billy B and other authors. This will be considered in relation to ideas concerning power, discourse, institutional cultures and conformity. The chapter concludes with a consideration of ways that abusive practice can be prevented, with reference to the management of change.

Abuse related to power

Onyskiw (2005) refers to lack of agreement concerning definitions of abuse. One definition is:

> *A violation of an individual's human and civil rights by any other person or persons.*
>
> (Department of Health 2010a: 14)

The Nursing and Midwifery Council (2002) included the comment:

> *Abuse within the practitioner–client relationship is the result of the misuse of power or a betrayal of trust, respect or intimacy between the practitioner and client, which the practitioner should know would cause physical or emotional harm to the client.*
>
> (Nursing and Midwifery Council 2002: 5)

Parts of Billy B's account are concerned with power, its uses and abuses. He comments: "It is crucial that nurses have the ability to be aware of the power they have; the capacity to use that power wisely; and to recognise and reflect on their possible abuses of power." Billy emphasises that, in the special (high secure) hospitals where he was a patient, the distribution of some aspects of power was mixed. On some wards, "staff had almost total power; with a rule by fear". On others, patients had greater power, for example, to organise social events and to get away with minor rule-breaking.

Byrt (2008a, b) considers aspects of power in forensic nursing. In Billy B's chapter, "power" refers particularly to "the ability to make other people do what you want them to do" (Masterton and Maslin-Prothero 1999: 212). "Having status or social position" and "having the means to influence others economically, politically and ideologically" (Byrt 2008a: 78, citing Westwood 2002), as aspects of power, are also indicated in Billy's narrative.

Important aspects of nurse–patient relationships involve establishment of trust (Kirby and Cross 2002) and awareness of power imbalances (Barker and Stevenson 2000, Byrt 2008b, Nursing and Midwifery Council 2002, 2009). The Nursing and Midwifery Council (2002) includes the statement:

> *...Registered Nurses...should be aware of the potential imbalance of power in this [professional] relationship...This is generated by the client's need for care, assistance, guidance and support...*
>
> (Nursing and Midwifery Council 2002: 4)

Sadly, some aspects of "Billy B's" account reflect other narratives by service users about the misuse and unnecessary and sometimes appalling impositions of power by some staff in high secure hospitals in the past (Thompson 1972, Laing with McQuarrie 1989, George 1998, Anonymous 2000, Parry-Crook 2000). This was also highlighted in two central Government inquiries into special hospitals (Department of Health and Social Security 1980, Department of Health 1992a, b). However, Harry (1999) writes positively about his experiences, as a patient, of improvements in a high secure hospital. Billy's account also indicates some positive aspects of patient power, for example, organising social events and some participation in decisions in a therapeutic community (see *Box 25.1*). The extent that this is perceived as "real" patient power may depend partly on whether a "consensus" or a "conflict" sociological perspective is adopted, examining, for example, whether such "power" affects areas that are important to patients; helps them to achieve desired goals or influences; or enables control of organisational aims and policies to a marked extent (Byrt 2008b).

Discourse

For Foucault (1991, 2002), one of the most important aspects of power is discourse: "Commonly accepted assumptions that claim to explain reality" (Wilkinson 1999: 21, quoted in Byrt 2008b: 112). Discourse analysis, as part of postmodernist approaches (Brown 2005), partly involves critical

Box 25.1. Billy's commentary: But was it ethically better?

I would like to emphasise that, from my experience, abuses of power in the special (high secure) hospitals were not as high as some people have made out. I never suffered physical abuse, only psychological abuse. I didn't mind cleaning, but would have preferred to do so under my own steam, not be told I had to clean.

However, ethically, they got results. For example, in the early 1980s, there were fewer patients who were overweight, because they were cleaning, kept busy. Patients were less sedentary, diabetes and diseases related to lethargy were less common, and the activity kept patients' weight down. But today, does a softly, softly ethic work? Do patients feel they have to run to nurses? There was no such thing as a one-to-one in the past.

Which is ethically better? The way things were done in the past was brutal, not politically correct. It didn't give a nod to the Human Rights Act, but it worked. There was no nonsense. It's not so much the remit, as its interpretation. In the special hospitals, there were nurses who had worked in the military. I understand that Broadmoor Hospital was built in such a way that it could easily be turned into a barracks.

consideration of why and how individuals in a society or social group "take for granted" that certain values, beliefs and norms are "everyday reality": seen as "true" or "fact", and as self-evident. The questioning of this "reality", and its supporting beliefs and values is seen as absurd by others in the individual's social group because they accord with what is seen as "common sense" and which everyone "knows" to be true (Brown 2005). This may partly explain some of the abuse described by Billy B, e.g. both patients and staff on one ward accepted, "took for granted", that certain types of patient "misbehaviour" would result in a "kicking". As another example, when one of the authors was a student nurse, he was laughed at by nursing staff for addressing an individual with a learning disability as "Mr". This was seen as laughable because many of the staff (and some residents) "knew" that you never addressed someone with a learning disability as "Ms" or "Mr", regardless of her/his preference. The taken for granted, unquestioned discourse, at that time, and in that hospital, was that people with learning disabilities did not have sufficient status to be accorded such titles.

According to Foucault (1991, 1997) and researchers working in a Foucauldian tradition (Mason and Mercer 1998, Fox 1999, Holmes 2006), dominant discourses include beliefs and "knowledge" promulgated by "experts" and other people in elite or otherwise powerful positions, including those with political, economic and professional power (Foucault 1991). Dominant views in a society are influenced by these individuals and by organisations representing their interests (Brown 2005). For example, Foucault

(1971) considers dominant discourses by relatively powerful people and organisations that influenced views about mental illness over several centuries. At different times, these included the church, (mostly lay) proprietors of "madhouses", and increasingly, from the mid-19th century, alienists (later called psychiatrists: Foucault 1971). Brown (2005) points out that present-day societies vary in the extent that there is one or more dominant discourse; and in the extent that competing discourses are enabled, or even encouraged.

Discourse can be considered in relation to Billy B's chapter in various ways. Firstly, until recently, dominant discourses in some forensic mental health services and literature appear to have been predominantly professional and political. In relation to secure hospitals, this is indicated in HM Government inquiries into Ashworth and Rampton Hospitals, which indicate the abusive power over patients of some staff (Department of Health and Social Security 1980, Department of Health 1992a, b). It is comparatively recently that publications about secure services have included the views of patients, although in the UK, (as indicated in *Chapters 18 and 19*), an impetus was given to research in this area by the former National Forensic Mental Health Research and Development Programme (Spiers et al 2005). Organisations such as the Matthew Trust (2010) and WISH (Women in Secure Hospitals) (2010), and legal and independent advocacy services (Garman et al 2005) have also aimed to enable patients in secure services to have an increased voice. The second Ashworth inquiry report, chaired by Fallon, was in response to a patient's concerns, which were largely upheld by the inquiry members (Department of Health 1999). However, a conflict sociologist might argue that, despite this apparently increased "voice", secure hospital patients continue to be relatively powerless, with little choice but to be in the hospital; and with little impact on major decisions affecting their lives (Mason and Mercer 1998, Byrt 2008b, Byrt et al 2008).

The influence of organisational cultures

Discourse in Billy's account can be used to explain, in part, the relatively greater power of staff in the hospitals he describes, and the organisational cultures that supported this (Jacob et al 2009, White et al 2003). The term "organisational culture" refers here to the shared norms, values and beliefs in an institution (Hinshelwood 2001, Marquis and Huston 2009). The Blom-Cooper Ashworth Hospital inquiry report (Department of Health 1992a, b) suggests that, in parts of this high security hospital's organisational culture, there were dominant staff discourses that denigrated patients and perpetuated sexism, racism and homophobia (Potier 1993). Such a culture appears to have continued partly because many staff "took it for granted" that it was a natural part of their working environment. As Billy B comments from his own experience of secure hospitals:

> *Everyone was conditioned. For staff, that was how things were, and patients accepted it.*

Aspects of organisational culture: The secure hospital as total institution

Staff "discourse" can include "taking for granted" institutional cultures which would be considered unacceptable for most other people. "Billy B" and some other service user accounts (Thompson 1972, Laing with McQuarrie 1989) describe organisational cultures of high secure hospitals which are reminiscent of Erving Goffman's (1968) account of "total institutions": organisations in which all aspects of a person's life are subject to surveillance (Foucault 1991, 2002), pervaded by the institution, and dictated by managers and staff and by regimes, routines and rules. Institutional cultures, where the needs of the organisation outweigh those of individuals, have been described in relation to a wide variety of other organisations, including some homes for children and older people (Stanley et al 1999, McKibbin et al 2008). Billy B's account can enable nurses' reflection on the following questions:

> *To what extent do the services' rules, regimes and routines exist:*
> - *For good clinical and safety reasons?*
> - *For the convenience of the organisation/staff?*
> - *Or does no-one know why they exist?*
>
> (Byrt with James 2007: 36)

Similar questions are considered in Kilshaw (1999: 120), who asks: "Can medium secure units avoid becoming total institutions?" Billy B's account indicates that whilst some high secure patients (e.g. in the "gentlemen's club" he describes), had a relatively greater degree of choice and freedom; other people experienced considerable restrictions, e.g. being compelled to scrub floors. Goffman (1968) referred to such processes, which strip people's dignity and identity, as the "mortification of self". However, Goffman (1968) also indicated ways that some people who were subject to total institutions managed to "work the system": that is, avoid surveillance or get away with breaking rules. This is exemplified by Billy's description of patients' midnight feasts and his pretending to the nurse that he had cleaned the toilet ("the water's evaporated off the soap"). In Goffman's observation of a psychiatric hospital:

> *...inmates and staff tacitly cooperated to allow the emergence of bounded physical spaces in which ordinary levels of surveillance and restriction were markedly reduced, spaces where the inmate could openly engage in a range of tabooed activity with some degree of security.*
>
> (Goffman 1968: 205)

Similarly, patients "working the system" is possibly indicated in Billy's account of minor rule-breaking, to which staff turned a "blind eye". Was this because the rules were unrealistic, unnecessary to ensure safety, or impossible to enforce? It is suggested that such questions need to be asked regularly about all rules in secure hospitals (Kilshaw 1999). Should such rule-breaking necessarily be seen as indicative of psychopathology (Goffman 1968, Mason and Mercer 1998)? How many forensic professionals would abide by all the rules if they became secure hospital patients?

Although Foucault (1971, 1991, 2002) indicated the immensely powerful influence of institutions, their "expert" professionals, and surveillance on patients and prisoners. He was:

> *...always at pains to say that resistance is an endemic fact in the world of power relations...There is always something in the social body, and in each person, which evades or wrestles with others' attempt to act on our own ways of acting.*
>
> (Gordon 2002: xx)

Not all total institutions are experienced as unpleasant by their "residents", a point made by Goffman (1968). This is indicated by Billy B's accounts of social environments which were positively valued by high secure hospital patients; and the "gilded cage" private medium secure unit with its wide choice of food and activities. In neither case did patients want to leave. Billy describes a patient who caused staff problems by constantly resisting them, but adds: "Patients who are immune to the institution are very rare. For most of us, the comfort zone erodes our independence, with the provision of things which some patients have never had as children".

Abuse and acceptance of "everyday reality"

Dominant discourses can serve to perpetuate abuse, partly through a process where it becomes seen as "normal", something that "naturally happens" to people who are seen as "other", as less than human, and without the same rights as most people (Horne 2008). Appallingly, abuse of patients has been highlighted in Billy B's and other accounts (Thompson 1972, Laing with McQuarrie 1989, Potier 1993), and in the Blom-Cooper Inquiry into

Ashworth Hospital (Department of Health1992a, b). Billy B describes, in relation to some wards in the past that there was: "A rule by fear: the threat of something happening if you didn't behave"; and states that nursing assistants kicked patients in one hospital.

Penhale states that institutional abuse can occur at three levels:

> *Level 1. Abuse between individuals within the residential setting.*
> *Level 2. Abuse arising due to the regime of the institution.*
> *Level 3. Abuse arising at a system level (broader social structure).*
>
> Penhale (1999: 6)

The Blom-Cooper inquiry into Ashworth Hospital (Department of Health 1992a, b) found evidence of negative discrimination towards patients and other forms of abuse. For example, Potier (1993) outlined the use of many coercive measures at this hospital which denied the basic rights of patients, within safety parameters, to clothing, visits and other things of importance to them.

In relation to dominant discourses, abuse may occur because it is widespread and committed by many people, including those in positions of authority. As Billy B states,

> *Staff...could be complicit with each other. It's amazing how you can accept things that are unethical, and see them as normal behaviour. You accept that the people who are lower down the hierarchical system will get a slap; you accept that the staff will make the decisions about your care.*

Box 25.2 includes an argument that "abuse of power" always occurs in institutions.

Box 25.2. Billy's commentary: It's not possible to have an institution without abuse of power

There is no separation between power and abuse. It is not possible to have an institution with no abuse of power. Abuse can't be eradicated because it's part of human nature, but it can be minimised, policed, targeted. Why are there so many policing bodies currently in secure hospitals?

I don't think you can prevent abuse, because of the different types that exist. Abuse used to be physical, now it's mental: through what nurses write in patients' notes. It's is not possible to eradicate mental abuse because of the nature of the environment. You're asking staff to be powerful, to impose their will, and for patients to be denied things. However, is this because it's the rule, and necessary to ensure safety, or because the nurse has had a rough day?

Conformity to other people's expectations

Billy B's account and other literature suggest that abuse occurs partly because it becomes part of practice which everyone accepts without question. If, as a new staff member, everyone around you is abusive towards patients, it becomes harder to question this, especially if colleagues have more prestige and experience (Rowden 2002). Research on conformity provides some evidence to support this view. For example, studies suggest that student nurses tend to "go along with" what they know to be unsafe or poor nursing practices in order to be accepted by staff. Questioning nursing practice may result in a student nurse feeling uncomfortable and anxious about being given a "bad report" (Sedgwick and Yonge 2008, Levett-Jones and Lathlean 2009). Mason (1997) found that one factor influencing whether nurses secluded patients was the nurses' concern about what colleagues and managers would think of their decision.

In relation to abusive behaviours, the influence of peers and other people in crowds, amongst other factors, has been found to influence the extent that some individuals engage in violent behaviours (Espelage et al 2008, Collins 2009). Milgram (1963) found that subjects could be induced to deliver what they believed to be lethal electric shocks if the researcher giving commands to do so was seen as having authority. Zimbardo et al (1973, 2006) arranged for psychology students to be randomly allocated "prisoner" and "prison guard" roles in a simulated prison. The experiment had to be stopped prematurely because of the extremely negative and cruel ways in which the "guards" treated the prisoners, stereotyped them and perceived them as less than human. Some social psychologists have argued that the results of such experiments indicate the ubiquity of potentially abusive behaviours. In addition, research findings suggest that people who conform may be "rejecting of moral rebels" and resent "those who do the right thing" (Monin et al 2008: 76). However, critics have pointed out that some studies of conformity do not explain why certain individuals fail to conform: for example, through rebelling against the expectations of their social group (Galinsky et al 2008, Dequech 2009). In addition, research has found that individuals vary in their conformity (Imhoff and Erb 2009, Lonnqvist et al 2009). The extent to which laboratory studies on conformity mirror "real life" (Gross 2010) or indicate that subjects are necessarily "evil" (Reeder et al 2008) has also been questioned.

Collins (2009) reflects Billy B's account in pointing out that total institutions are hierarchical, with patients and staff having varying amounts of social status. Billy B refers to rigid divisions between "Us and them", with patients being "told to call staff Sir". Abuse may serve to reinforce the status of the abuser, to show the person perceived to be in an inferior position, who is "boss". Abusive practices may be supported by a discourse that argues that they occur for good reasons: "You have to swear at them because it's all they understand", "It's the only way to ensure safety." To question such beliefs may be seen as "unrealistic", "not based on common sense". Such discourse may be reinforced by attitudes and beliefs about forensic patients, which everybody sees as credible, "knows" to be true. A number of critics have described how forensic patients may become perceived as "other" by both members of the public and some professionals (Mercer et al 1999). "Otherness" refers to specific, labelled individuals being seen as different, deviant and outside "normal" society (Mason and Mercer 1998, Jacob et al 2009). This "othering" may result in forensic patients being perceived as less than human, as not having the same rights and needs as other people (Aiyegbusi 2009). Once individuals are seen only as "evil", they "become 'things' or non-persons as they no longer emit what the 'natural' group considers to be the signifiers of human 'normality'. As a result, this group is thought of as being 'impure' and its members are, therefore, shunned" (Horne 2008: 675). Mercer et al (1999) found evidence for this in their study of forensic nurses' perceptions that some patients were "evil". In contrast, Horne (2008) argued that, ethically, acts should be perceived as "evil", rather than the individuals who perpetrate them.

The power of the pen and the power of the boot

Billy B comments:

> *Nursing evaluations can become a potential abuse of power. One thing that has changed is that the brutality has been replaced by the pen. Instead of a kicking, you get a bad report in your record.*

Foucault (1991) outlined the rise of various professionals who provided types of surveillance, including written observations, with all aspects of prisoners' lives being subject to scrutiny. Goffman (1968) described pathologisation: the assumption that everything the individual said or did was evidence of mental illness. This was found by Rosenhan (1973) who, with other social psychologists, arranged to be admitted covertly to mental health wards. More recently, Davies et al (2008: 99) reported research involving patients in a medium secure unit. These individuals found it particularly difficult "to manage the frustration of living with constant observation and other techniques for their risk assessment and risk management". Davies et al (2008) argue that problems experienced by patients in the medium secure unit affected their expression of aggression, which might have been less likely to occur in a milieu which was "less stressful". The authors refer to methods of assessing and measuring risk that reflected the dominant discourses of mental health professionals, rather than patients' perspectives and experiences. They refer to one individual, who stated, like Billy B, that a staff member tested him by behaving in a certain way to see how he would react.

What can forensic nurses learn from Billy B's account and the related literature?

To what extent can we learn from history (Brown 2005): in this instance, Billy B's own history of his experience in high secure hospitals? It can be argued that the experiences of Billy B and other people can enable those of us who are forensic mental health nurses, or other professionals, to reflect on several areas related to ethical practice.

Firstly, as indicated in *Chapter 11*, there is a need for nurses and other staff to be aware of their own understandable feelings and views concerning patients' offences and behaviours that cause difficulty, e.g. opposition, rejection of interventions and hostility. Opportunities for support and clinical supervision, and relevant education and training need to be provided, with awareness, on the part of managers and clinical supervisors, of the stresses faced by staff, especially nurses, in view of their prolonged contact with patients (Dale et al 1995, Aiyegbusi and Clarke-Moore 2009).

Without high quality supervision and support, there is a danger that staff members' understandably negative feelings remain "unprocessed" (Aiygebusi and Clarke-Moore 2009). Negative attitudes and abuse may be more likely if there is a lack of self-awareness and opportunities for reflection (Stanley et al 1999). The literature suggests that this will affect patient care (Aiygebusi and Clarke-Moore 2009), as reported in Mercer et al's (1999) study, which found that some high secure hospital nurses appeared unable to progress beyond perceptions that patients were "evil". In contrast, Bowers (2002) found that some forensic nurses were able to work effectively with people with "dangerous and severe personality disorder" by adopting reflective strategies. These included acknowledgement of individuals' humanity, focusing on their strengths not just on behaviours, and understanding the underlying reasons for these.

Addressing patients' disempowerment and deprivations

The considerable power imbalances between patients and staff need to be honestly acknowledged, with recognition of the difficulties and deprivations faced by patients (Byrt with James 2007); and the problems of being under surveillance and facing restrictions in a secure hospital (Davies et al 2008).

Patients in secure hospitals are faced, not only with restrictions on freedom and making decisions about their everyday lives, but also with separation from partners, spouses, friends and family, including, for some patients, their children; and with reduced opportunities for emotional and sexual fulfilment (Harner 2004, Aiyegbusi and Byrt 2006). On admission, many patients have uncertainties about the outcome of their court appearances, as well as, for some people, losses in relationships, accommodation and employment (Byrt with James 2007). For patients in high secure hospitals, in particular, these losses are compounded by geographical and social isolation from the people and communities that they know (Mason and Mercer 1998). Enabling patients to maintain contact with their loved ones, families and friends, and with their local communities, may lessen patients' social exclusion and contribute to their recovery (Williams and Dale 2001, Byrt et al 2008). In addition, it is recommended that account needs to be taken of secure hospital patients' perspectives on the problems and deprivations, as well as benefits, from their admission, and of the iatrogenic effects of secure hospitals (Holmes 2006, Davies et al 2008).

Several authors have commented on the need to develop "relational security": to reduce unnecessary power differentials between nurses and patients (Dale and Gardner 2001, Aiygebusi and Clarke-Moore 2009, Department of Health 2010b). This involves attempts to forge therapeutic alliances, despite the difficulties (Kirby and Cross 2002, Aiygebusi and Clarke-Moore 2009); and to find "common ground": areas that patient and nurse agree that they can work on (Lowe 1992, McDougall 2000). Active listening and attempts to empathise with patients' experiences may also help to increase patient empowerment (Aiygebusi and Clarke-Moore 2009), although a conflict theorist (e.g. Szasz 2000) would argue that this was not "real" empowerment, since few forensic patients are able to make choices to leave hospital, or about their relationships and other important areas of their lives (Byrt 2008b). In addition, some critics have questioned the extent that forensic nurses can successfully combine the psychotherapeutic and physical security aspects of their role (Schafer 2002, Holmes 2006). (Security aspects of nursing in acute mental health settings are considered by Cowman and Bowers 2009.) Is it possible for a forensic nurse to be involved in in-depth counselling with patients one moment, and searching their bedrooms the next? This may or may not affect the therapeutic relationship and communication, but the ethical implications appear to have been little considered by the Nursing and Midwifery Council (Byrt 2005) or in mental health nursing textbooks (e.g. Barker 2009, Norman and Ryrie 2009). Does the discourse in such textbooks realistically reflect what mental health nurses actually do, especially in relation to aspects of physical security and surveillance, which involve much of forensic nurses' work in the UK? This

Box 25.3. Billy's commentary: Nurses being human

I would like nurses to demonstrate that they have human reactions: for example, admit it if they're in a bad mood. But are staff free to say they were wrong, admit, for example, that they were authoritarian? (An example where a nurse admitted this, and apologised to a patient is given in Ford et al, 2010: 88f).

Another example of ethical care is the dividing line between staff being human and willing to talk about themselves if this furthers their relationship with the patient (Stuart 2009), or being robotic and refusing any sort of therapeutic disclosure. If nurses are like that, how can patients be expected to disclose?

question is related to one that has often been debated in relation to many areas of nursing (Thompson et al 2006): How can forensic nurses most effectively have regard for "respect for persons" (Kant 1969: deeply valuing the individual and her/his autonomy) and maintain a duty of care to ensure the safety of the patient and other people, whilst avoiding the misuse of power (Burrow 1998) (see *Chapter 2*)?

Billy B describes social environments on wards with rigid divisions between staff and patients (see *Box 25.3*), as well as apparently more beneficial environments, such as therapeutic communities and the "gentleman's club" in one hospital. It can be argued that a priority in managing change in secure hospitals is to assess and improve the quality of, not only physical security, but also the social and physical environment (Dale and Lynch 1996, Byrt 2007). A priority, described in relation to effecting change at Ashworth Hospital, following the Blom-Cooper Inquiry (Department of Health 1992a, b) was to eliminate authoritarianism and abuse of power (Dale et al 1995), similar to the situation described by Billy B. Research suggests that high levels of authoritarianism and aggression on mental health wards are associated with worsening of symptoms in people with schizophrenia and with patient dissatisfaction (Timko and Moos 2004, Wilson et al 2008). A relevant assessment is the Essen Climate Evaluation Scale (EssenCES): "a short questionnaire for assessing the social climate of forensic wards" (Schalast et al 2008: 49). This has been used to measure aspects of therapeutic staff–patient relationships; and the extent that social environments are therapeutic and safe (Schalast et al 2008).

Can abuse be totally eliminated in secure hospitals?

Billy argues that this is impossible (*Box 25.2*). We suggest that a distinction can be drawn between actions, attitudes and speech which are *intentionally* abusive; and those which, whilst (from staff perspectives) are intended to be for the benefit of patients, and necessary to ensure safety, are *perceived by patients* as abusive. For example, a patient's leave may be suspended by staff because there is evidence that she/he is likely to harm self or others whilst away from the hospital. Professionals may not (and always should not) intend to abuse the patient, but in the authors' experience, the patient might well perceive the suspension of leave as abusive. Another example relates to seclusion. Research findings suggest that most patients report detrimental effects from seclusion which they could perceive as abusive (Sailas and Fenton 2006, Bergk et al 2010, Mayers et al 2010). However, there is also evidence that patients and staff could feel abused if they are assaulted (Howard and Hegarty 2003, Abderhalden et al 2006); and it is sometimes concluded that seclusion is the only way to prevent violence towards others (see *Chapters 16 and 17*). Forensic nurses and other forensic mental health professionals often appear to have to implement measures to ensure safety which patients experience as coercive, regardless of staff intentions (Holmes 2006, Bergk 2010). However, it has been argued that education to increase nurses' therapeutic skills may result in a reduction of the use of coercive measures (Dale et al 1995, Abderhalden et al 2006).

Managing change

It can be concluded that improvements in patient care, including the elimination of intentionally abusive practice, can occur only through effective leadership and management, which have been identified as crucial to facilitating change (Dale et al 1995, Jones and Jenkins 2007, Marquis and Huston 2009). Dale et al (1995) argue that there needs to be clear leadership and management on the part of senior nurse managers, but that staff at all levels and patients also need to be involved in owning, and putting forward, ideas for change. In addition, understanding the difference between formal and informal organisation appears to be essential to successfully bringing about change (See *Box 25.4*). A strong informal organisation may sabotage efforts to implement change.

An early researched example, related to formal and informal organisation, concerned a large, institutionalised psychiatric hospital in North America. Many senior nurses and doctors tried to institute changes, but these did not succeed in the long term because of the successful efforts of nursing aides (similar to healthcare assistants) to sabotage the changes. These staff members were the main "culture carriers" in the hospital. The researchers concluded that the changes were unsuccessful because the aides were not involved at all by the senior staff who imposed the innovations. The aides were expected to co-operate with the changes, without being consulted or otherwise involved. In addition, they had low status in the hospital, their contributions to patient care were not recognised, and they received little

Box 25.4. Formal and informal organisation

In considering the needs and goals of organisations (e.g. wards, community services), and in effecting change, it is important to differentiate between formal and informal organisation:

"The nature of the formal organisation is normally dictated by the senior managers and may include such elements as the working environment, shift patterns and staff numbers" (Dowding and Barr 2002: 118). Formal organisation includes the formal roles of staff (director of nursing, ward manager, staff nurse, healthcare assistant) and the procedures and policies of the unit. The formal organisation of health services is often represented in official written statements (e.g. trust annual reports, organisational charts, policy files). Formal organisation is the "public face of the organisation", with managerial statements representing the "official version", rather than "what really happens" (Dowding and Barr 2002).

"The informal organisation, on the other hand, exists within the formal structure in order to support people's social and psychological needs" (Dowding and Barr 2002: 118f). The informal organisation includes staff relationships which are outwith individuals' official roles: e.g. groups of staff who pass on information over coffee breaks. Such aspects of the informal organisation generally involve individuals' needs or goals, which may accord with, or sharply differ from those of the formal organisation.

Formal and informal organisational goals

In bringing about change, it is necessary to be clear about the following:

- What are the goals of:
  - The formal organisation (e.g. the NHS trust managing a service)?
  - The informal organisation?
  - The intended change?
- Formal structure and processes to meet the needs of the organisation to meet formal goals.
- Informal structure and processes to meet needs of the informal organisation, e.g. staff's ability to cope with the job or to obtain support or various satisfactions.
- Change may be facilitated if managers recognise the informal organisation and nurses' needs related to this (Dale et al 1995).
- In bringing about change, it is necessary to consider that the need for the formal organisation to change may clash with the needs of the informal organisation. In the latter, individuals may wish to maintain the status quo: e.g. because this is more personally rewarding or less threatening.

(Marquis and Huston 2009)

education relevant to their work. The researchers concluded that these factors contributed to the lack of effective or permanent change (Cumming and Cumming 1962).

In this example, the informal organisation of aides had, in the long term, greater effects on patient care than the formal organisation: the hospital managers' decisions, and written statements about, changes in the care of patients. In contrast, Dale et al (1995) outline attempts to involve all staff, as well as patients, in changes at Ashworth Hospital. This account and other literature suggests that, in order to change abusive and other poor practice, it is essential to support all staff, involve them in changes, and provide essential clinical supervision, education and training (Dale et al 1995, Marquis and Huston 2009, Miller et al 2009, Tuck 2009).

In addition, the literature suggests that, in order to effect changes, it is necessary to understand the needs and goals of grassroots staff who are part of a secure hospital's informal organisation. Recognising the motivations of staff appears to be crucial (Tuck 2009). Abusive practices may arise partly to make nurses' work more "bearable". For example, stigmatising patients as "evil" and "othering" them as less than human, may be a way of defending against unbearable feelings about the offences that patients have committed, and the emotional demands that very needy patients place on the forensic nurse (Aiyegbusi and Clarke-Moore 2009). Menzies (1960) referred to such mechanisms as individual and social "defences against anxiety". Examination of such motives is not about excusing abusive practices, but is concerned with understanding and preventing them through, for example, managerial support, clinical supervision, education and training (Walker 2007, Watson and Kettles 2007).

Clear articulation of oganisational goals and values and clinical supervision

A clear articulation of organisational goals and values, shared by all participants, is stressed by various authors as essential to implementing change (Dale et al 1995, Jones and Jenkins 2007). Some authors argue that non-judgemental attitudes are essential in preventing abusive practice, including not labelling or perceiving individual patients only in terms of their offence, but seeing them as whole people (Dale et al 1995, Williams and Dale 2001). This view contrasts with Billy B's comment that, from his past experience:

> *Patients are stigmatised and traumatised by staff. The opportunity to stigmatise people is there. OK, they're trained to shut out stigmatising thoughts, but they're only human.*

Billy B adds that: "Staff are influenced by how they've been brought up", referring to the socialisation into stigmatising attitudes towards individuals with mental health problems that occurs in wider society from an early age (Morris 2006). This can result in forensic patients internalising these attitudes: "Patients may self-stigmatise: feel unworthy, feel labelled 'bad', 'ill'." Bartlett (2004) refers to the "double stigmatisation" that forensic patients experience in relation to their experience as offenders and as people with mental health problems.

Effective clinical supervision is seen as crucial in enabling professionals to be self-aware, to consider any negative attitudes and perceptions they may hold, and to reflect on the effectiveness of their interventions (Jennings 2001, Walker 2007, Mackie 2009). This appears to be essential in eliminating the types of abuse described by Billy B and referred to by Dale et al (1995).

Reflective practice, based on clinical supervision, is also relevant to abuses of power, such as "testing of patients" described by Billy B; and to a critical consideration of written records about patients. "The pen is mightier than the sword" (Bulwer-Lytton 1839, quoted in *The Phrase Finder* 2010); and care is needed, as Billy B suggests, to avoid writing statements that are judgemental, and express the professionals' opinion or their negative mood, rather than being based on evidence and discussion with the patient, and where possible, writing records and care plans with her/him. This contrasts with Billy B's experience: "Some staff feel that everything that patients say or do must be recorded. They may feel they must take their training literally, and see psychopathy in every word and action."

Also of importance, is avoiding documenting trivial information which has no bearing on the individual's health, welfare or risk (Davies et al 2008). Clinical supervision and other means to reflective practice should also enable honest self-awareness, acknowledgement of mistakes, and "non-defensive practice" (Mackie 2009), in contrast to Billy B's experience:

> *We're told: "You must learn by this", but I've never known a nurse thank me if the errors of their ways are pointed out by advocacy. They see it as effrontery, they don't accept it. They wonder why patients are complaining. It's OK for nurses to challenge patients' behaviour, but not vice versa.*

The roles of lawyers, advocates and commissioners

Finally, Billy B comments on the increased involvement of legal and other advocates as one of the main reasons for a lessening of physical abuse in high secure hospitals:

More people are watching, and there is nowhere to take people for a kicking. Also, there are now more legal people: different bodies like the Mental Health Act Commission (now part of the Care Quality Commission 2010), and visiting advocacy groups, so the opportunity for unethical behaviour has been reduced.

The role of legal and other advocates, including those of voluntary organisations (Matthew Trust 2010, Together 2010, WISH 2010) and frequent visits by the Care Quality Commission (2010) appear to be crucial to enabling forensic patients to have an increased voice (Garman et al 2005, Kenny 2005):

Until there is a commitment to total user involvement and advocacy... users will continue to suffer through lack of knowledge of their rights and responsibilities, and the inability to effectively express their needs.
(Lees and Withington 2001: 120)

The extent that abusive practices can be avoided in secure hospitals relates, in part, to questions of discourse, considered at the beginning of this chapter. In preventing abuse, it is suggested that managers of secure services and professionals need to consider the question: To what extent does our service enable the voice of patients, and the victims/survivors of offences and individuals and organisations representing their rights, needs and interests? How much power do these people have, compared with individuals and organisations with dominant discourses, including politicians, Government departments and the media?

References

Abderhalden C, Hahn S, Bonner YDB, Galeazzi GM (2006) Users' perceptions and views on violence and coercion in mental health. In: Richter D, Whittington R (eds) *Violence in Mental Health Settings. Causes Consequences Management*. Springer, New York

Aiyegbusi A (2009) The dynamics of difference. In: Aiyegbusi A, Clarke-Moore J (eds) *Therapeutic Relationships with Offenders. An Introduction to the Psychodynamics of Forensic Mental Health Nursing*. Jessica Kingsley, London

Aiyegbusi A, Byrt R (2006) Gender and sexuality. In: National Forensic Nurses' Research and Development Group: Woods P, Kettles AM, Byrt R, Addo M, Coffey M, Collins M, Doyle M, Garman G, Watson C (eds) *Aspects of Forensic Mental Health Nursing: Interventions with People with 'Personality Disorder'* Quay Books MA Healthcare Ltd, London

Aiyegbusi A, Clarke-Moore J (eds) (2009) *Therapeutic Relationships with Offenders. An Introduction to the Psychodynamics of Forensic Mental Health Nursing*. Jessica Kingsley, London

Anonymous (2000) The experience of being a black patient. In: Kaye C, Lingiah T (eds) *Race Culture and Ethnicity in Secure Psychiatric Practice: Working with Difference*. Jessica Kingsley, London

Barker P (ed) (2009) *Psychiatric and Mental Health Nursing: The Craft of Caring* (2nd edn). Arnold, London

Barker P, Stevenson C (eds) (2000) *The Construction of Power and Authority in Psychiatry*. Butterworth Heinemann, Oxford

Bartlett A (2004) Fashions in psychiatric care: Implications for sense of self. In: Crisp AH (ed) *Every Family in the Land: Understanding Prejudice and Discrimination Against People with Mental Illness*. Royal Society of Medicine Press, London

Bergk J, Flamme E, Steinert T (2010) Coercion Experience Scale (CES) Validation of a questionnaire on coercive measures. *BMC Psychiatry* 10(5): 1–10

Bowers L (2002) *Dangerous and Severe Personality Disorder: Response and Role of the Psychiatric Team*. Routledge, London

Brown CG (2005) *Postmodernism for Historians*. Pearson Longman, Harlow

Bulwer-Lytton E (1839) Richlieu or the conspiracy. In: The Phrase Finder (2010) Available from: www.phrases.org.uk/meanings/the-pen-is-mightier-than-the-sword.html [Last accessed 16 May 2010]

Burrow S (1998) Therapy versus security: Reconciling healing and damnation. In: Mason T, Mercer D (eds) *Critical Perspectives in Forensic Care: Inside Out*. Macmillan, Basingstoke

Byrt R (2005) Forensic mental health nurses' involvement in physical security: Points for consideration. Unpublished paper sent on behalf of the National Forensic Nurses' Research and Development Group as a response to the Review on Mental Health Nursing

Byrt R (2007) Towards therapeutic environments: Alternatives and solutions. In: National Forensic Nurses' Research and Development Group: Kettles AM, Woods P, Byrt R, Addo M A, Coffey M, Doyle M (eds) *Forensic Mental Health Nursing: Forensic Aspects of Acute Care*. Quay Books MA Healthcare Ltd, London

Byrt R (2008a) Power and participation in forensic services: An introduction. In: National Forensic Nurses' Research and Development Group: Kettles AM Woods P, Byrt R (eds) *Forensic Mental Health Nursing: Capabilities Roles Responsibilities*. Quay Books MA Healthcare Ltd, London

Byrt R (2008b) Negative control or life saving? Perspectives on power. In: National Forensic Nurses' Research and Development Group: Kettles AM Woods P, Byrt R (eds) (2008) *Forensic Mental Health Nursing: Capabilities Roles Responsibilities*. Quay Books MA Healthcare Ltd, London

Byrt R, Hart L, James-Sow L (2008) Patient empowerment and participation: Barriers and the way forward. In: National Forensic Nurses' Research and Development Group: Kettles AM Woods P, Byrt R (eds) *Forensic Mental Health Nursing: Capabilities Roles Responsibilities*. Quay Books MA Healthcare Ltd, London

Byrt R, James L (2007) Towards therapeutic environments: Challenges and problems. In: National Forensic Nurses' Research and Development Group: Kettles AM, Woods P, Byrt R, Addo M A, Coffey M, Doyle M (eds) *Aspects of Forensic Mental Health Nursing in Acute Mental Health Settings*. Quay Books MA Healthcare, London

Care Quality Commission (2010) Available from: www.cqc.org.uk [Last accessed 16 May 2010]

Collins R (2009) *Violence: A Microsociological Theory*. Princeton University Press, Princeton NJ

Cowman S, Bowers L (2009) Safety and security in acute admission wards in Ireland and London: A comparative study. *Journal of Clinical Nursing* 18(9): 1346–53

Cumming J, Cumming E (1962) *Ego and Milieu. Theory and Practice*. Atherton Press, New York

Dale C, Gardner J (2001) Security in forensic environments: Strategic and operational issues. In: Dale C, Thompson T, Woods P (eds) *Forensic Mental Health: Issues in Practice*. Bailliere Tindall/Royal College of Nursing, Edinburgh

Dale C, Lynch J (1996) Blueprint for healthcare. *Nursing Management* 3(6): 22–4

Dale C, Rae M, Tarbuck P (1995) Changing the nursing culture in a special hospital. *Nursing Times* 91(30): 33–5

Davies J, Godin P, Heyman B, Reynolds L, Shaw M (2008) Ecological validity and risk management in forensic mental health services. In: Petersen A, Wilkinson I (eds) (2008) *Health Risk and Vulnerability*. Routledge Taylor and Francis Group, Hove

Department of Health (1992a) *Report of the Committee of Inquiry into Complaints about Ashworth Hospital. Vol. 1*. Cm 2028 – 1. HMSO: London. (Chair: L. Blom-Cooper) HMSO, London

Department of Health. (1992b) *Report of the Committee of Inquiry into Complaints at Ashworth Hospital. Vol. 2. Case Studies*. Cm 2028 – II iHMSO: London. (Chair: L. Blom-Cooper) HMSO, London

Department of Health. (1999) *Committee of Inquiry into the Personality Disorder Unit Ashworth Special Hospital. Vol. 1*. Cm 4194 – II.. HMSO: London. (Chair: P. Fallon) The Stationery Office London

Department of Health (2010a) *Clinical Governance and Adult Safeguarding. An Integrated Process*. February 2010. Prepared by A. Morgan. Department of Health, London

Department of Health (2010b) *Your Guide to Relational Security. See Think Act*. Department of Health, London

Department of Health and Social Security (1980) *Report of the Review of Rampton Hospital (Boynton Report)* Cmnd 8073. HMSO, London

Dequech D (2009) Institutions, social norms and decision – theoretic norms. *Journal of Economic Behavior and Organization* 72: 70–8

Dowding L, Barr J (2002) *Managing Change in Health Care*. Prentice Hall, London

Espelage DL, Wasserman S, Fleisher M (2008) Social networks and violent behavior. In: Flannery DT, Vazsonyi AT, Waldman ID (eds) *The Cambridge Handbook of Violent Behavior and Aggression*. Cambridge University Press, New York

Foucault M (1971) *Madness and Civilisation: A History of Insanity in the Age of Reason*. Tavistock Social Science Paperback, London

Foucault M (1991) *Discipline and Punish. The Birth of the Prison*. Translated from the French by Alan Sheridan. Penguin Books, Harmondsworth

Foucault M (2002) *Power. Essential Works of Foucault 1954–1984. (Volume 3)* Translated by R. Hurley and Others. Penguin Books, London

Ford K, Byrt R, Dooher J (2010) *Preventing and Reducing Aggression and Violence in Health and Social Care: A Holistic Approach*. M & K Publishing, Keswick

Fox KJ (1999) Changing violent minds: Discursive correction and resistance in the cognitive treatment of violent offenders in prison. *Social Problems* 46(1): 88–103

Galinsky AD, Magee JC, Gruenfeld DH Whitson JA, Liljenquist KA (2008) Power reduces the press of the situation: Implications for creativity, conformity and dissonance. *Journal of Personality and Social Psychology* 95(6): 1450–66

Garman G, Kelly R, Waldon S (2005) Setting up a successful patients' council. *Mental Health Practice*. 6(97): 20–2

George S (1998) More than a pound of flesh: A patient's perspective. In: Mason T, Mercer D (eds) *Critical Perspectives in Forensic Care: Inside Out*. Macmillan, Basingstoke

Goffman E (1968) *Asylums. Essays on the Social Situation of Mental Patients and Other Inmates*. Penguin Books, Harmondsworth

Gordon C (2002) Introduction. In: Foucault M (2002) *Power. Essential Works of Foucault 1954–1984. (Volume 3)*. Translated by R. Hurley and Others. Penguin Books, London

Gross R (2010) *Psychology. The Science of Mind and Behaviour* (6th edn). Hodder Arnold Hachette, UK

Harner HM (2004) Relationships between incarcerated women: Moving beyond stereotypes. *Journal of Psychosocial Nursing and Mental Health Services* 42(1): 38–46

"Harry" (1999) The sharp end of Broadmoor: A look at developments in nursing at Broadmoor Hospital from a patient's perspective. In: P Tarbuck; B Topping-Morris, P Burnard (eds) *Forensic Mental Health Nursing. Strategy and Implementation*. Whurr Publications, London

Hinshelwood RD (2001) *Thinking About Institutions: Milieux and Madness*. Jessica Kingsley, London

Holmes D (2006) Governing the captives: Forensic psychiatric nursing in corrections. *Perspectives in Psychiatric Care* 41(1): 3–13

Horne M (2008) Evil acts not evil people: Their characteristics and contexts. *Journal of Analytic Psychology* 53: 669–90

Howard R, Hegarty JR (2003) Violent incidents and staff stress. *British Journal of Developmental Disabilities* 96(1): 3–21

Imhoff R, Erb H-P. (2009) What motivates nonconformity? Uniqueness seeking blocks majority influence. *Personality and Social Psychology Bulletin* 35(3): 309–20

Jacob JD, Gagnon M, Holmes D (2009) Nursing so-called monsters: On the implication of abjection and fear in forensic psychiatric nursing. *Journal of Forensic Nursing* 5: 153–61

Jennings L (2001) Clinical supervision. In: Dale C, Thompson T, Woods P (eds) *Forensic Mental Health: Issues in Practice*. Bailliere Tindall/Royal College of Nursing, Edinburgh.

Jones R, Jenkins F (eds) (2007) *Key Topics in Healthcare Management. Understanding the Big Picture*. Radcliffe Publishing, Oxford

Kant I (1969) The Moral Law: Kant's Groundwork of the Metaphysics of Morals. London. Hutchinson. (Translated by Paton HJ) Cited in: Thompson IE, Melia KM, Boyd KM, Horsburgh D (eds) (2006) (5th Ed) *Nursing Ethics*. Churchill Livingstone/Elsevier, Edinburgh

Kenny PJ (2005) The place of a legal representative or advocate working for their client. In: Wix S, Humphreys M (eds) *Multidisciplinary Working in Forensic Mental Health Care*. Elsevier, Edinburgh.

Kilshaw J (1999) Can medium secure units avoid becoming total institutions? In P Tarbuck; B Topping-Morris, P Burnard (eds) *Forensic Mental Health Nursing. Strategy and Implementation*. Whurr Publications, London

Kirby SD, Cross D (2002) Socially constructed narrative interventions. A foundation for therapeutic alliances. In: Kettles AM, Woods P, Collins M (eds) *Therapeutic Interventions for Mental Health Nurses*. Jessica Kingsley, London

Laing J with McQuarrie D (1989) *Fifty Years in the System*. Mainstream, Edinburgh

Lees N, Withington J (2001) Involving service users. In: Dale C, Thompson T, Woods P (eds) *Forensic Mental Health: Issues in Practice*. Bailliere Tindall/Royal College of Nursing, Edinburgh.

Levet-Jones T, Lathlean J (2009) "Don't rock the boat": Nursing students' experiences of conformity and compliance. *Nurse Education Today* 29: 342–9

Lonnqvist J-E., Walkowitz G, Wichardt P, Lindeman M, Verkaslo M (2009) The moderating effect of conformism values on the relations between other personal values, social norms, moral obligation and single altruistic behaviours. *British Journal of Social Psychology* 48: 525–46

Lowe T (1992) Characteristics of effective nursing interventions in the management of challenging behaviour. *Journal of Advanced Nursing* 17: 1226–32

McDougall T (2000) Violent incidents in a forensic adolescent unit: A retrospective analysis. *Nursing Times Research* 5(2): 87–98

McKibbin J,Walton A, Mason L (2008) *Leadership and Management in Health and Social Care for NVQ/SQV, Level 4*. Heinemann, Harlow

Mackie S (2009) Reflecting on murderousness: Reflective practice in secure forensic settings. In: Aiyegbusi A , Clarke-Moore J (eds) *Therapeutic Relationships with Offenders. An Introduction to the Psychodynamics of Forensic Mental Health Nursing*. Jessica Kingsley, London

Marquis BL, Huston CJ (2009) *Leadership Roles and Management Functions in Nursing. Theory and Application* (6th edn) Wolters Klower Health Lippincott Williams and Wilkins, Philadelphia

Mason T (1997) An ethnomethodological analysis of the use of seclusion. *Journal of Advanced Nursing* 26: 780–9

Mason T, Mercer D (eds) (1998) *Critical Perspectives in Forensic Care: Inside Out*. Macmillan, Basingstoke

Masterson A, Maslin-Prothero S (1999) Power, politics and nursing. In: Mastersonson A, Maslin-Prothero S (eds) *Nursing and Politics. Power Through Practice*. Churchill Livingstone, Edinburgh.

Matthew Trust (2010) Available from: www.matthewtrust.org/index.htm [Last accessed 16 May 2010]

Mayers P, Keet N, Winkler G, Flisher AJ (2010) Mental health service users' perceptions and experiences of seclusion and restraint. *International Journal of Social Psychiatry* 56(1): 60–73

Menzies I (1960) A case study in the functioning of social systems as a defence against anxiety: A report on a study of the nursing service of a general hospital. *Human Relations* 13: 95–121

Mercer D, Mason T, Richman J (1999) Good and evil in the crusade of care. *Journal of Psychosocial Nursing and Mental Health Services* 37(9): 13–17

Milgram S (1963) Behavioral study of obedience. *Journal of Abnormal Psychology* 67: 391–8. Cited in: Gross R (2010) *Psychology. The Science of Mind and Behaviour* (6th edn). Hodder Arnold Hachette, UK

Miller G, Paterson B, McKenna K (2009) Changing the culture of care. In: Hughes R (ed) *Reducing Restraints in Health and Social Care*. Quay Books MA Healthcare Ltd, London

Monin B, Sawyer PJ, Marquez MJ (2008) The rejection of moral rebels: Resenting those who do the right thing. *Journal of Personality and Social Psychology* 95 (1): 76–93

Morris G (2006) *Mental Health Issues and the Media: An Introduction for Mental Health Professionals*. Routledge Taylor and Francis Group, London

Norman I, Ryrie I (eds) (2009) *The Art and Science of Mental Health Nursing. A Textbook of Principles and Practice*. McGraw Hill Open University Press, Maidenhead

Nursing and Midwifery Council (2002) *Client–Practitioner Relationships and the Prevention of Abuse*. Nursing and Midwifery Council, London

Nursing and Midwifery Council (2009) *Clear Sexual Boundaries*. Nursing and Midwifery Council, London.

Onyskiw JE (2005) A concept analysis of abuse. In: Cutcliffe JR, McKenna H (eds) *The Essential Concepts of Nursing. Building Blocks for Practice*. Elsevier. Churchill Livingstone, Edinburgh

Parry-Crooke G (2000) *Good girls: Surviving the Secure System. A Consultation with Women in High and Medium Secure Settings*. WISH/University of North London, London

Penhale B (1999) Introduction. In: Stanley N, Manthorpe J, Penhale B (eds) *Institutional Abuse. Perspectives Across the Life Course*. Routledge, London

Potier MA (1993) Giving evidence: Women's lives in Ashworth maximum secure psychiatric hospital. *Feminism and Psychology* 3: 335–47

Reeder GD, Monroe AE, Pryor JB (2008) Impressions of Milgram's obedient teachers: Situational cues inform influences about motives and traits. *Journal of Personality and Social Psychology* 98(1): 1–17

Rosenhan DL (1973) On being sane in insane places. *Science* 179: 250–8

Rowden R (2002) Empowerment in forensic mental health. In: Dooher J, Byrt R (eds) *Empowerment and Participation: Power Influence and Control in Contemporary Health Care*. Quay Books, Dinton Salisbury.

Sailas E, Fenton M (2006) *Seclusion and Restraint for People with Serious Mental Illness*. The Cochrane Library 2006 (1) (CD001163)

Schafer PE (2002) Nursing interventions and future directions with patients who constantly break rules and test boundaries. In: Kettles AM, Woods P, Collins M (eds) *Therapeutic Interventions for Mental Health Nurses*. Jessica Kingsley, London

Schalast N, Redies M, Collins M, Stacy J, Howells K (2008) EssenCES, a short questionnaire for assessing the social climate of forensic psychiatric wards. *Criminal Behaviour and Mental Health* 18(1): 49–58

Sedgwick M, Yonge O (2008) "We're it", "we're a team", "we're family" means a sense of belonging. *Rural and Remote Health 8. Electronic Version*. Cited in: Levett-Jones T, Lathlean J (2009) "Don't Rock the Boat": Nursing Students' Experiences of Conformity and Compliance. *Nurse Education Today* 29: 342–9

Spiers S, Harney K, Chilvers C (2005) Service user involvement in forensic mental health:

Can it work? *Journal of Forensic Psychiatry and Psychology* 16(2): 211–20

Stanley N, Manthorpe J, Penhale B (eds) (1999) *Institutional Abuse. Perspectives Across the Life Course*. Routledge, London.

Stuart GW (2009) Therapeutic nurse–patient relationship. In Stuart GW (ed) *Principles and Practice of Psychiatric Nursing* (9th edn). Mosby Elsevier, St. Louis

Szasz T (2000) The case against psychiatric power. In: Barker P, Stevenson C (eds) *The Construction of Power and Authority in Psychiatry*. Butterworth Heinemann, Oxford

Thompson IE, Melia KM, Boyd KM and Horsburgh D (eds) (2006) *Nursing Ethics* (5th edn). Churchill Livingstone/Elsevier, Edinburgh

Thompson P (1972) *Bound for Broadmoor*. Hodder and Stoughton, London

Timko C, Moos RH (2004) Measuring the therapeutic environment. In: Campling P, Davies S, Farquharson G (eds) *From Toxic Institutions to Therapeutic Environments: Residential Settings in Mental Health Services*. Gaskell, London

Together. (2010) Available from: www.together.uk.org/ [Last accessed 16 May 2010]

Tuck G (2009) Forensic systems and organizational dynamics. In: Aiyegbusi A, Clarke-Moore J (eds) *Therapeutic Relationships with Offenders. An Introduction to the Psychodynamics of Forensic Mental Health Nursing*. Jessica Kingsley, London

Walker H (2007) Issues in multi-professional working. In: National Forensic Nurses' Research and Development Group: Kettles AM, Woods P, Byrt R, Addo M A, Coffey M, Doyle M (eds) *Aspects of Forensic Mental Health Nursing in Acute Mental Health Settings*. Quay Books MA Healthcare, London

Watson C, Kettles AM (2007) Forensic educational aspects of acute mental health care: Policy, characteristics, skills and knowledge. In: National Forensic Nurses' Research and Development Group: Kettles AM, Woods P, Byrt R, Addo M A, Coffey M, Doyle M (eds) *Aspects of Forensic Mental Health Nursing in Acute Mental Health Settings*. Quay Books MA Healthcare, London

Westwood S (2002) *Power and the Social*. Routledge, London

White C, Holland D, Marsland D, Oakes P (2003) The identification of environments and cultures that promote the abuse of people with intellectual disabilities: A review of the literature. *Journal of Applied Research in Intellectual Disabilities* 16(1): 1–9

Wilkinson G (1999) Theories of power. In: Wilkinson G, Miers M (eds) *Power and Nursing Practice*. Macmillan, Basingstoke

Williams P, Dale C (2001) The application of values in working with patients in forensic mental health settings. In: Dale C, Thompson T, Woods P (eds) *Forensic Mental Health: Issues in Practice*. Bailliere Tindall/Royal College of Nursing, Edinburgh

Wilson PA et al (2008) Scale development of a measure to assess community-based and clinical intervention group environments. *Journal of Community Psychology* 36(93): 271–88

WISH (2010) Available from: 222.womenatwish.org.uk/ [Last accessed 16 May 2010]

Zimbardo PG (1973) On the ethics of intervention in human psychological research with special reference to the "Stanford Prison Experiment". *Cognition* 2(2): 243–55. Cited in: Gross R (2010) *Psychology. The Science of Mind and Behaviour* (6th edn). Hodder Arnold Hachette, UK

Zimbardo PG (2006) On rethinking the psychology of tyranny: The BBC Prison Study. *British Journal of Social Psychology* 45(1): 47–53

Index

P

R

S